The natural way to a better pregnancy

*To the big, round, fecund fertility goddess
and all women everywhere
who have embodied her incarnation*

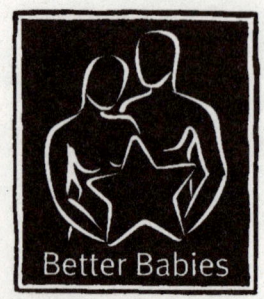

the *natural* way to a better pregnancy

Francesca Naish and Janette Roberts

DOUBLEDAY
SYDNEY • AUCKLAND • TORONTO • NEW YORK • LONDON

THE NATURAL WAY TO A BETTER PREGNANCY
A DOUBLEDAY BOOK

First published in Australia and New Zealand
in 1999 by Doubleday

Copyright © Francesca Naish and Janette Roberts, 1999

All rights reserved. No part of this publication may be reproduced, stored in a retrieval system, transmitted in any form or by any means, electronic, mechanical, photocopying, recording or otherwise, without the prior written permission of the publisher.

National Library of Australia
Cataloguing-in-Publication Entry

Naish, Francesca.
　The natural way to a better pregnancy.
　Bibliography.
　Includes index.
　ISBN 0 86824 795 2.

　1. Pregnancy. 2. Prenatal care. 3. Pregnant women –
　Health and hygiene. I. Roberts, Janette. II. Title.

　618.2

Bantam books are published by
Transworld Publishers,
a division of Random House Australia Pty Ltd
20 Alfred Street, Milsons Point, NSW 2061

Random House New Zealand Limited
18 Poland Road, Glenfield, Auckland

Transworld Publishers (UK) Limited
61–63 Uxbridge Road, Ealing, London W5 5SA

Random House Inc
1540 Broadway, New York, New York 10036

Edited by Amanda O'Connell
Cover design and text design by Liz Nicholson, design BITE
Cover photograph by Louise Lister
Illustrations by Deborah Clarke
Index by Keyword Editorial Services
Typeset in 10/14 Candida by Midland Typesetters Pty Ltd
Printed by Griffin Press, Netley, South Australia

10 9 8 7 6 5 4 3 2 1

The information provided in this book is intended for general information and guidance only, and should not be used as a substitute for consulting a qualified health practitioner. Neither the authors nor the publisher can accept any responsibility for your health or any side-effects of treatments described in this book.

Contents

About the authors vii

Acknowledgements ix

Note to readers xiii

Foreword xv

Chapter 1	Your better pregnancy	1
Chapter 2	How you and your baby grow	12
Chapter 3	Eating well	26
Chapter 4	Nutritional supplementation	55
Chapter 5	A healthy lifestyle	68
Chapter 6	A clean environment	81
Chapter 7	Detoxification	97
Chapter 8	Allergies and infections	107
Chapter 9	Exercise	124
Chapter 10	Reducing stress and thinking positively	144
Chapter 11	Antenatal testing	172
Chapter 12	Choosing your carer	192
Chapter 13	Natural treatments and remedies	204

Sources and recommended reading 256

Contacts and resources 265

Appendices

1	Reproductive health: diet summary	276
2	Nutritional content of organic versus non-organic foods	281
3	Nutrients lost when wheat is refined	282
4	Nutritional deficiencies and symptoms	283
5	Diet and lifestyle questionnaire	285
6	Herbs to avoid during pregnancy	291
7	Essential oils to avoid during pregnancy	299
8	Acupressure points to avoid during pregnancy	301
9	Tips for travellers	303
10	Drinking water	305
11	Preconception health care	309
12	How to prevent miscarriage	323

Glossary 328

Index 333

About the authors

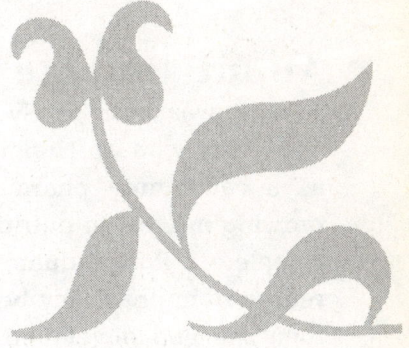

About Francesca

Francesca Naish was born in England in 1946. She studied mathematics at Sussex University, but after arrival in Australia, when in her late twenties, established a Natural Birth Control practice in Paddington, Sydney. This grew into The Village Healing and Growth Centre, one of the first holistic health-care practices in Australia. Since 1994 she has trained health professionals in the use of her unique Natural Fertility Management techniques, and has recently established agencies in New Zealand, Malaysia, the United States and England. In 1995, after 20 years in clinical practice, she established The Jocelyn Centre in Woollahra, Sydney. This is the first clinic in Australia to specialise in natural methods for fertility management, reproductive health and preconception health care.

Francesca is a qualified naturopath, herbalist and hypnotherapist. She writes extensively for the press, appears regularly on radio and television and is sought after as a public speaker and lecturer. She also pioneered the teaching in Australia of natural vision improvement.

She has written three previous books: *The Lunar Cycle* (1989), *Natural Fertility* (1991) and *The Natural Way to Better Babies: Preconception Health Care for Prospective Parents* (co-authored with Janette Roberts) in 1996. Francesca has two sons and lives in the Sydney suburb of Bondi with her family.

About Janette

Janette was born in Sydney in 1947 and graduated from Sydney University with an Honours Degree in Pharmacy in 1968. Her career as a community pharmacist spanned almost twenty years, but a growing interest in nutritional and environmental medicine led her to complete a Postgraduate Diploma in Clinical Nutrition in 1983. She retired from pharmacy before the birth of her first son in 1985, but by then she had developed a specific interest in preconception health care, which she has promoted in Australia on behalf of the British Foresight Association since 1987. Her first book, *The Natural Way to Better Babies: Preconception Health Care for Prospective Parents* (co-authored with Francesca Naish), was published in 1996.

Janette makes frequent appearances on radio and television, and presents public lectures to prospective parents and workshops and seminars to health professionals around Australia and New Zealand. In 1998 she and two partners established one of the first Vitality and Longevity Centres in Australia. It is situated in the Sydney suburb of Balmain where Janette lives with her two sons.

Acknowledgements

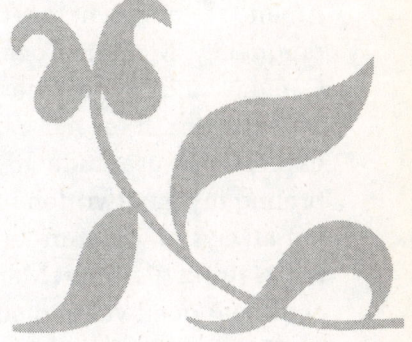

Francesca's acknowledgements

Any book written on such a universally relevant subject as pregnancy is bound to have been influenced by the experiences and expertise of countless women and men—so here is where I pay tribute to generations of midwives and wise women, to those doctors whose prenatal and birthing practices have been woman-centred in their approach, and to all those who have written on this topic. I can only hope to give a small contribution to the mass of published, broadcast and personally transmitted information and lore that surrounds this almost mystical experience of pregnancy.

'There is nothing new under the sun' and in many ways this book is just a reminder. At a time when so much that appears new (i.e. technology and drugs) threatens to eclipse the knowledge of centuries, it is perhaps relevant to re-examine traditional approaches and adapt them to the demands of modern lifestyles and conditions. So many people have written on this topic, that I can't begin to acknowledge all their contributions, though some particularly useful books are noted in Sources and Recommended Reading.

I would like to thank especially: Jane Bennett and Cheryl Dingle for the section on yoga; Vicki Turner for her insightful contributions as her own long-awaited pregnancy progressed; Kerry Bone and Amanda Haberecht for their research into which herbs to avoid in pregnancy; Melanie Koeman for the 'water purifiers' appendix; Miriam Camara and Sally Charles for advice on acupressure points and Melinda Smith for her expertise in aromatherapy. I would also like to express my gratitude to Karina Quinlan, for her patience in interpreting my handwritten first drafts, where inspiration and legibility did not always go hand-in-hand, and to all the staff at The Jocelyn Centre for Natural Fertility Management and Holistic Medicine, for their continual goodwill and support.

Thanks are due to Lynne McTaggart, editor of the excellent book and newsletter *What Doctors Don't Tell You*, for permission to include the information on travel vaccines. You can find further details of these publications in Sources and Recommended Reading. Thanks too to the *International Herald Tribune* for permission to reproduce 'Prenatal Nightmare—Medicine's Oracle of Delphi'. You will also find, in Contacts and Resources, where to obtain the Australian Bush Flower Essences. My thanks to Ian White for the information on which essences may be helpful during pregnancy. Further thanks go to Liz Courtney and Tonia Port, our book agents, for their skills and support, and the important role they played in turning a book and a concept into a series, and to Shona Martyn and Fiona Henderson of Transworld Publishers for their enthusiasm and commitment to the ongoing series of *Better Babies* books. Thanks also to our editors, Amanda O'Connell and Belinda Yuille, our designer, our illustrator, our proofreader and our indexer, who have all made valuable contributions.

This is also where I publicly express my gratitude to my co-author Janette, without whom writing a book would be considerably more of a chore and less of a joy. If it wasn't for her extensive knowledge, her enthusiasm for and dedication to populating the world with 'better' babies, our books would be far less informative and the world a poorer place.

Two important acknowledgements remain—firstly to my children, partner and carers for their roles in my own memorable experiences of pregnancy. Secondly, to all pregnant women everywhere and through all time, who have felt the extraordinary inner glow that comes with new life within, and have had the privilege of taking part in one of life's eternal mysteries.

Janette's acknowledgements

I spent the first 35 years of my life childless, with a passionate commitment to staying that way. I can still only marvel at the change that occurred—a change which not only saw the blossoming of my dormant maternal instinct, but which encompassed an amorous embrace of totally natural child-bearing and raising methods. It was also a change which has taken my life in increasingly exciting and stimulating directions.

This book is just one of those directions, and the people who must take some credit for it, and its stable-mates, are numerous. The list must begin with my mother Margaret who certainly had a 'better pregnancy' at a time when it was, in many ways, much easier to do so, although the diet recommended by her naturopath, and which she faithfully followed, in 1947, was considered completely radical.

The Foresight Association and Dr Stephen Davies, of the UK, and Dr Robert Buist from Sydney, NSW, sparked my interest in preconception health care. Having faith in the full preconception health care program gave me the further confidence to follow a completely natural course through both my pregnancies and births. My midwife Sue Sagewood affirmed everything I believed in and supported me in avoiding the screening and diagnostic procedures which are now a routine part of an 'elderly primagravida's' pregnancy.

It has been, to a large degree, my very positive experiences and those of a few others, and the less than positive experiences of many more women who have shared their stories, which prompted this book and its subsequent titles. Publicists Liz Courtney and Tonia Port deserve very special thanks because they have ensured that my words will actually reach an audience, and Shona Martyn and Fiona Henderson of Transworld Publishers have been equally enthusiastic about the project.

The writing of this book was done under very different circumstances from *The Natural Way to Better Babies*. This time a pressing deadline, the concurrent need to submit an edited version of *Better Babies* to its US publisher, and a schedule of preconception health care lectures and seminars, had me wishing that school pick-up was at 7.30pm rather than 2.30pm and also, sometimes, longing for a 'regular' job. However, my children, to their credit, have survived having their mother glued to a computer screen. At least they now know how I feel when they are glued to the television.

My exercise schedule, so much a regular part of my life for so many years, was slotted in at 6am, and I am grateful to Ivan Waters of BOO Personal Training for rekindling the enthusiasm which I lost along with those early morning starts. John de Voy's chiropractic adjustments and Nola Ainsworth's massages ironed out the kinks I acquired from sitting too long at the keyboard, and I thank them both.

Martha Lourey, while involved in studying for her Master's degree, still found the time and enthusiasm to provide valuable advice. Her vast experience of all aspects of exercise and her special interest in, and knowledge of, exercise during pregnancy proved invaluable. Morris Karam, of Balmain Life Fitness, also put aside his busy schedule, as he did for *Better Babies*, to add his comments to the exercise chapter. Cheryl Dingle of Castlemaine Iyengar Yoga Studio went, once again, beyond the call of duty to provide the information and the models for the section on yoga during pregnancy.

Without my co-author Francesca, and her valuable and extensive clinical skills, this book would be just a shadow. Our writing partnership is a dream, and even when I have to incorporate her endless handwritten annotations, I am in awe of her ability to write a first draft in longhand without an amendment or a deletion.

To Bill Moore, go my thanks for all sorts of things. His implementation of all those personal diet and lifestyle changes in which I firmly believe, is a belief in me. His unequivocal support for my life's purpose, and his prompting and goading, have given me the confidence to take my message to the world, and his shared enthusiasm for our new joint project, the Balmain Wellness Centre, will change the public perception of health care as we enter the new millennium. It's just a shame he hasn't got more time to spare because he's a damn good proofreader too.

Fortunately, my dear friend Barry Smith-Roberts, who has supported me in ways too numerous to mention, brought his expertise to that role as well, and I am truly grateful for his generosity.

Note to readers

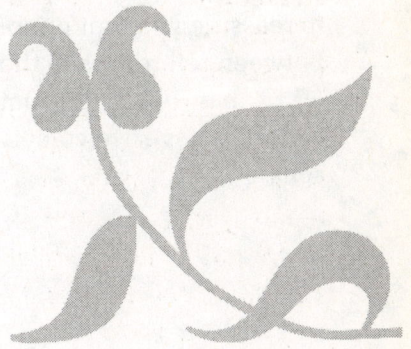

In this book we deal with both self-help and practitioner-guided treatments. If you are in any doubt about what you should do on your own or what requires professional help, always seek help. But be sure that the medical advice you receive is from a practitioner who has a commitment to using as natural and non-interventionist approach as possible.

The herbs and supplements that we recommend will be available from a number of different sources including holistic and natural health practitioners, health food stores and pharmacies. Supermarkets also carry an increasing range of supplements and remedies, but wherever you purchase your products, make sure that they fulfil the dosages that we recommend.

In the case of nutritional supplements we have given clear guidelines regarding dosages for general use. Herbal and other natural remedies come in a variety of forms, and it is therefore not possible to give similarly clear-cut guidelines for dosage. Whether the product is a tablet, capsule, loose herb, fluid extract or powder, if it is sold through a retail outlet it will have clear directions for use on the container and you should follow those. If you are in any doubt or if you have specific concerns it is always advisable to consult a natural health practitioner. You can take a copy of our book to your practitioner for reference.

Frequently, we have referred to your baby as 'he'. We would like to reassure you that our only reason for doing so is to distinguish easily between references to the mother ('she') and the baby. Though neither of us has been fortunate enough to have a daughter we would certainly have welcomed such an addition to our brood of delightful sons.

Foreword

We believe that your pregnancy should be a truly wonderful time, but we know that your pregnancy will only be truly wonderful if it is a 'better' one. Pregnancy is not an illness—it is a perfectly normal physiological event, another cycle in your sexual and reproductive life, and we certainly don't believe it's necessary for you to suffer a long list of complaints and discomforts in order to have a child.

Many of the conditions which are considered par for the course when you're pregnant can be prevented or can be readily treated by natural means. We know that the achievement of a 'better' pregnancy isn't as difficult as you might think and we also know that a healthy, stress-free, full-term pregnancy is an important factor in having physically, mentally and emotionally healthy children. Along with an uncomplicated birth and breastfeeding relationship, it's a wonderful way for your whole family to begin its life together. We firmly believe that all of these things are essential for the optimum health of families today, and essential for the health of future generations of families.

This book looks at all the factors which contribute to a better pregnancy. They include a nutritious diet, a healthy lifestyle, a clean environment, regular exercise and mental and emotional wellbeing, and we suggest natural and practical steps to help you achieve them all. We sincerely hope that after reading this book you will be inspired to strive for a better pregnancy (and the continuum which can and should easily follow) and in doing so give your whole family a much 'better beginning'.

This excellent start to your child's and your family's life can be made even better if both prospective parents attend to their health before conception. If you haven't yet conceived, then you will have an ideal opportunity to put our recommendations into effect before your pregnancy begins, when it is easier to implement the full program.

Your better pregnancy

chapter 1

There is little doubt that, even though having a baby unites almost all women in an experience which is exceedingly commonplace, pregnancy still remains alluring and seductive, an exciting, mysterious and endlessly fascinating state. Pregnancy is a very special time indeed.

ENJOY IT

Today, you are unlikely to experience more than one or two pregnancies in your lifetime, so it is important that each one brings you great joy and happiness. Your pregnancy is a time to be savoured and cherished, it is a time to be remembered with fondness and affection. It is a time when you should feel more alive, more special, more nurtured than at any other time in your life. You should be really and truly 'pregnant'—not just pregnant with new life, but pregnant with the anticipation of what the new life will mean. You should be filled with the simple wonder of a baby growing in your belly, excited by the thought of bringing that baby to birth, looking forward to every aspect of nurturing your baby, anticipating with eagerness your new life as a mother and your life together as a family.

DON'T ENDURE IT

When you are pregnant you should feel physically, mentally and emotionally on top of the world. Therefore we think it unfortunate that so much of what you hear, so much of what you read and so much of what you and those close to you experience leaves you with the impression that morning sickness, stretch marks, constipation, haemorrhoids, varicose veins, heartburn, dizzy or fainting spells, increased skin pigmentation, bleeding gums, falling hair, cramps and oedema are a normal part of pregnancy or simply the price that you pay for having a baby.

For these are just some of the conditions which are termed 'minor discomforts'. They might perhaps seem minor to the medical expert who is writing about them, they might even seem minor when you are reading about them, but if you're actually suffering from them, they can make your pregnancy more of an endurance test than a time of great joy, excitement and anticipation.

Apart from these 'minor discomforts' there are of course the more serious complications such as hyperemesis (excessive vomiting), placenta praevia, toxaemia and prematurity which can make your pregnancy a very distressing time indeed.

But we firmly believe you can avoid many minor discomforts, not to mention more serious complaints. Pregnancy definitely can, and should, be more than just an endurance test which will result in the birth of a child.

BE CONFIDENT

You should be absolutely certain of the physical and mental health of your baby, not worried about possible poor outcomes, not dependent on a battery of screening and diagnostic tests to reassure you. You should be safe and secure in the knowledge that you are doing everything possible to create an optimally healthy environment in which your child can develop and grow. We believe that you can easily achieve all of these things and that when you do, not only is your pregnancy a whole lot 'better', but the whole family gets a 'better beginning'.

Of course, the earlier you start the better, but the most important thing you can do is to focus on all the very positive things that you are doing now. Maybe your pregnancy caught you unawares, or your baby was planned but you're uncertain how good your preconception preparation was. Don't dwell on what might have been forgotten. Positive thoughts and emotions produce a certain type of chemical in the brain and that beneficial chemical will be transmitted to your growing baby. Affirm 'better' pregnancy and 'better' baby to yourself every day. Thinking positively produces positive results. Remember, it's never too late to begin. At all stages of your pregnancy there is an enormous amount you can do to ensure that you have a 'better' baby, who will then have a 'better' chance of growing into a healthy well-adjusted child and adult.

OLDER OR YOUNGER MUM?

Experts reckon that the prime time, in physical terms, for a woman to conceive and bear children is from her late teens to early twenties, and yet more and more couples are delaying their child-bearing for 20 years or more. What does this delay mean? At age 20, your chances of having a Down syndrome child are 1 in 2000, but at age 43 your chances are 1 in 50. If we take all chromosomal abnormalities into consideration, at age 25 your chances of having a baby with an abnormality are 1 in 527, but at age 45, your chances are 1 in 23.2.

Just as you now make a considered decision to delay having a baby, you can make a similarly conscious decision to ensure that your baby is as healthy as possible.

If you have already conceived, and are an older mum, then it is very important that you follow our healthy guidelines during your pregnancy and 'put the clock back' as much as you can. We'd also like to reassure you that Down syndrome babies are being effectively treated with nutritional medicine, and some genuine breakthroughs are being made.

What if you're at the opposite end of the spectrum and you're going to be a teenage mum? Although a lack of physical maturity can result in some increased difficulties, you should be in peak condition, and relatively fit compared to older mothers. With this advantage, and even if your pregnancy was unplanned, with attention to all our recommendations for pregnancy health care, it is possible for very young couples, just as it is for older parents, to reduce the risks to themselves and to their baby. You can significantly improve your chances of preventing the problems associated with teenage pregnancy, like the increased perinatal death rate, increased rate of postpartum haemorrhage and more. Just remember—look after yourself and your baby.

AN OPTIMALLY HEALTHY LIFESTYLE

To put it very simply, an optimally healthy lifestyle aims to ensure that there is an adequate supply of all those nutritional factors which you and your growing baby need and an absence of all those factors which might compromise your reproductive or general health, or which are harmful to foetal development. A healthy lifestyle gives you the best chance of an easy labour and a successful breastfeeding experience as well.

In the following pages we're going to show you how to achieve and maintain that level of optimum health. We'll tell you all the positive things you can do and we'll tell you what to avoid as well. We'll also tell you how to implement all of our recommendations. We know that we make a lot of recommendations, but the great majority of them are really only common sense, and we know that putting them into place can make a huge difference to your pregnancy and your baby's health.

Obviously there are numerous issues that you will be able to deal with on your own without expert help and we're going to cover those in detail. We'll give you lots of helpful hints which will make those issues easier to address. There are, though, some areas where you'll need help from a trained practitioner. We'll cover those in detail too, but a good way to approach them is to go to your practitioner armed with our book.

NATURAL TREATMENTS

Self-help and naturopathic remedies may be used to relieve many of the 'symptoms' of pregnancy and are often more appropriate than orthodox medical treatments. Natural remedies work by bringing systems back into balance, rather than by merely disguising symptoms, and we have holistic, natural suggestions to cover most conditions. The use of natural remedies also encourages you to tune into your body's signals, to trust your body's ability to grow a healthy baby, to become intuitive and to believe in your own inner wisdom. This is all wonderful preparation for birthing, breastfeeding and mothering generally, when you must rely to a very large degree on your intuition and be able to believe in the very real value of your 'maternal instinct'.

TRUST YOUR INSTINCTS

The medical model of child-bearing and raising often negates intuitive feelings, denies the power and wisdom of maternal instinct and ignores the spiritual aspects of becoming a family. We want to discuss the importance of trusting your intuition, of relying on those very strong maternal feelings and of regaining some sort of spiritual understanding of what you do when you create life and become a parent. We want to emphasise how profoundly transformative the whole process of conceiving, being pregnant with, giving birth to, and nurturing a baby can be.

We also want to draw your attention to the inappropriate or excessive use of medical technology. Largely due to our twentieth-century love affair with science and technology, we have tampered with, or medicalised, many aspects of conception, pregnancy, birth and breastfeeding. In doing so we have really lost sight of the fact that, while awe-inspiring in its complexity, the whole reproductive cycle is a normal, natural process, not an illness requiring constant medical surveillance or intervention, however well-intentioned that surveillance or intervention may be.

We firmly believe that you must allow all the marvellous, normal, natural functions to proceed without interference if you are to have optimal reproductive outcomes and families with optimal physical, mental and emotional health. We believe that families have been disadvantaged in their embrace of the medical paradigm which presently overwhelmingly governs their reproductive lives. We hope our book can go some little way to recovering what has been lost. We hope we may be able to show families how they can redress the balance and regain something of the robust health, the optimism and the wonder which should be an integral part of becoming a family!

WHICH PREGNANCY FOR YOU?

To illustrate our point better, we would like to follow two women through their pregnancies. The first story involves a woman who has planned and prepared for her pregnancy for some time and who cares well for herself and her baby during the following nine months. The second account involves a woman whose history is a little different.

Consciously pregnant

In a softly lit room, an oil burner fills the air with a subtle perfume. In this room a couple are preparing to conceive their child. After many months of actively avoiding harmful lifestyle factors and environmental pollutants, and of nurturing themselves with nutritious, uncontaminated food and positive affirmations, they know that they are both in the state of optimal physical and mental health which is necessary if their baby is to enjoy the same robust good health.

Today, they know, from observing the woman's cervical mucus, that she is fertile and they have abstained from sex over the last few days to increase the man's sperm count. They have also carefully prepared the room in which they will make love and they are both excited at the prospect of 'conceiving consciously' and of being able to welcome their child's existence from its very earliest moments. They are confident that this act of love will lead to the conception of their baby.

The charting of cervical mucus and temperature is now a routine part of this woman's life, and when her at-rest body temperature is still elevated 20 days later this couple knows that their long-awaited child is a reality, even though it is, at this stage, no larger than an apple pip. The woman has already noticed some subtle changes in her body, but the delight that she and her partner experience in having the conception confirmed beyond any doubt is overwhelming, and they both know that the months of preconception health care were well worthwhile.

This elated expectant mother suffers a little morning sickness during the first few weeks, but she finds relief by eating small nutritious snacks at frequent intervals. She drinks ginger tea as well. She also feels more tired than usual, so she gets as much rest as she can during the day and goes to bed early. Despite not feeling quite her usual self, she still makes a special effort to continue her routine of eating well and exercising moderately and she is also careful to avoid as much chemical and electromagnetic pollution as possible.

By the time her first antenatal visit is due, she has already decided that she would prefer to be in the care of a midwife, so she seeks out a birthing centre where she will see the same group of midwives for all of her antenatal visits. The midwives, whom she comes to know during the pregnancy, will attend the birth as well. The sort of care she has chosen is non-invasive and non-technological. Her midwives use manual palpation to assess the position and size of her baby and the only other tests she has routinely are those for blood pressure, ferritin and zinc levels, and at each antenatal visit her urine is tested for sugar and protein.

She decides against ultrasound scans and also against chorionic villus sampling (CVS) and amniocentesis. She has absolutely no doubt that her baby is healthy and growing well. She is quietly confident that everything she is doing to avoid harmful environmental and lifestyle factors, while eating well, supplementing her diet appropriately, exercising moderately and keeping stress levels down, is providing her child with an optimally healthy environment in which to develop.

Her pregnancy progresses with only minor discomforts. She and her midwife always discuss treatment options. These vary, but include osteopathic adjustments, acupressure, herbal and homoeopathic remedies and nutritional support. She experiences the expected discomfort of extra pressure on her bladder, less space in her stomach and an altered sleep pattern. But she doesn't actually mind the latter—she is sure this is nature's way of preparing her for nursing her baby through the night. Throughout the nine months she listens attentively to what her body is telling her.

She changes her exercise routine from one which involves high impact activity to something much less jarring, takes time to focus her attention on her growing baby, gets lots of rest, eats nutritious meals (smaller but more frequent than in the past) and simply revels in the delights of being pregnant. Her partner helps her with some stretching exercises and together they share the wonder of observing their baby's increasingly strong movements which send ripples across her growing belly.

She finds all of her senses heightened and knows that she looks as she feels—radiant and very special. As the months pass she looks forward to giving birth and nurturing her baby. She is sure that the processes of labour, birth and breastfeeding will be uncomplicated and she will cope with them as easily as she has with the conception and pregnancy. She affirms these facts to herself every day.

Too good to be true? It certainly isn't! We're pleased to tell you that it happened to Janette, despite being aged 37 and 42 when she was pregnant with her two sons. We've taken no poetic licence either.

'Falling' pregnant

A couple try to conceive for three years before they decide to seek help at a clinic for assisted reproduction. They are accepted into the program, but are given no counselling about self-help measures which could improve their fertility quite significantly. They continue in their stressful lifestyle and unhealthy habits, hoping for a technological miracle. However the ill-effects of prescribed drugs and the stress of the program's procedures exact a heavy toll, both physically and emotionally, and after four failed IVF attempts the couple decides that their marriage is unlikely to survive if they continue with the program.

But within two years, and very much to their surprise, the woman conceives. Her pregnancy is considered a possibility only after she has consulted her doctor because of constant nausea and vomiting and desperate tiredness. Her periods have always been irregular and she cannot remember the date of her last one. The positive blood test is immediately backed up by an ultrasound scan, and although the 'diagnosis' delights both prospective parents, physically this woman still feels wretched, and her nausea and vomiting continue for some time.

Finally she seems to regain her interest in food and decides that it is time to think about eating well and cutting down her caffeine and alcohol consumption. Her obstetrician has suggested she limit both and also prescribes supplements of folic acid and iron. However the iron (which is inorganic) makes the woman constipated and she develops haemorrhoids, and small varicose veins in her legs. She also notices stretch marks appearing on her breasts and belly. But despite these and other minor discomforts all seems to be progressing well, and she is reassured by the regular scans which are part of her routine antenatal visits.

This woman and her husband have a video film taken of their baby during one of these scans and are surprised to see the way their child tries to move away from the sound waves as the test is in progress. She remembers clearly the baby's increased activity at the time; she even remarked on it to the technician. However her doctor has assured her that the test is 'as safe as watching television'. To allay any further anxiety, he orders an alpha fetoprotein (AFP) test at 16 weeks. He tells her that a high result on this test could indicate the presence of a neural tube defect such as spina bifida. A low level could indicate a Down syndrome baby.

He does not tell her that the uncertainty about her 'dates' may also have contributed to the positive test results which are returned. She and her husband now spend an extremely worrying and anxious few weeks while they wait for the results of the subsequent amniocentesis which will confirm or deny their worst fears. However these results indicate that all is well and they realise they have worried unnecessarily. They try to get back to thinking positively about the eventual outcome of the pregnancy.

By the end of the second trimester this woman has gained 15 kilograms and feels and looks extremely ungainly. Her doctor warns her that she must try to limit her weight gain so she makes some attempts to cut her food intake and she starts to do a little exercise, but neither seems to have much effect on her upward weight spiral. Towards the end of the third trimester, her blood pressure becomes a matter of concern and she is ordered to bed to rest. She is told that toxaemia of pregnancy can be life-threatening to both her and her child, so she takes her bed-rest very seriously. Her doctor has also indicated that an elective caesarean section is the most likely outcome, since he does not believe in putting either of his patients at risk. The final weeks of her pregnancy drag by. Even though she is sure she is in good hands she is not much comforted by the thought of a caesarean since she has been hoping for a natural birth. Now she is worried and also a little depressed and just wants to get things over and done with.

The choice is yours

Two stories of two women expecting their first baby: there's probably no doubt in your mind which woman you would prefer to be. But does the second story sound more familiar than the first? Perhaps it reminds you of someone you know or maybe it even brings back memories of your own experience. We've certainly seen enough to know that this is what a pregnancy is like for far too many women. But don't despair, by the time you've finished reading our book you'll know that it can be different and that the 'better' pregnancy isn't just a figment of our imagination. You'll also know that it's not so very difficult to make the difference!

So what do you need to do to give yourself the very best possible chance of having a story which more closely resembles the first than the second? What do you need to do to give you and your baby (and the whole family for that matter) the very best possible start?

IT'S YOUR RESPONSIBILITY

The achievement of a physically, mentally and emotionally healthy pregnancy which results in the birth of a healthy baby is not just a happy accident. You must be prepared to make an effort! You have to accept some responsibility if all the marvellously complex and interdependent processes of the full reproductive cycle are to proceed smoothly. But when you take that responsibility, not only will you feel much more positive about the eventual outcome, the eventual outcome will itself be much more positive.

Your partner's contribution

Parenting is a joint effort and the sooner your partner becomes involved, the better for the whole family. You need your partner's support and one of the best ways he can give that is to keep you company in your efforts to give your baby a really healthy environment in which to grow. The more support he can give you, the more involved he's going to feel in the pregnancy and the more bonded he's going to feel to his baby.

He can help you prepare lots of really healthy meals; he can take supplements when you take yours; he should give up coffee and cigarettes and alcohol (it will be much easier for you if he does); he can get started on an exercise program with you. Always remember, this baby is very much the product of you both!

AFFIRM YOUR ATTITUDE

Remember, you can make an enormous difference to your own general health during your pregnancy. Make it a better pregnancy.

Remember, there are lots of good reasons for using natural alternatives and for avoiding the high-tech approach to your pregnancy. Make it a natural pregnancy.

Remember, everything positive that you do will contribute to a much more positive outcome. Make it a better outcome.

Remember, the responsibility for the healthy development of your baby rests largely with you. Make it a better baby.

Affirm all of these facts to yourself every day.

chapter 2
How you and your baby grow

A 'better' pregnancy is one which is free of many of the 'symptoms' which are often considered par for the course. A better pregnancy is free of vomiting and varicose veins, and of hair loss and haemorrhoids. These conditions (and a host of others that are equally distressing) don't have to go hand in hand with being pregnant. But no matter how much better your pregnancy, there are some symptoms which are absolutely unavoidable and these are linked to the extraordinary growth which occurs within you and the changes which your body undergoes. In the following paragraphs we'll look briefly at some of the normal physical, mental and emotional changes which happen to you during those momentous nine months.

HOW *YOU* CHANGE AND DEVELOP

Your pregnancy will last for nine lunar months, or about 266 days from the date of conception. So the actual duration of pregnancy relates to the lunar calendar (which has of course been connected with women and fertility from time immemorial). More commonly, your due date is calculated as 40 weeks following the first day of your last menstrual period, or as nine calendar months (first, second and third trimesters). Calendar months are of course an entirely arbitrary, man-made construct. Just as women have menstrual cycles of slightly different lengths, just as children grow at different rates, just as we are all physically different, babies grow in utero at varying rates too. In reality, a pregnancy of anywhere between 38 and 42 weeks is still well within normal range. Therefore, when you are given the expected date of your baby's birth, we suggest you don't set too much store by it. Treat it as a rough approximation only, and rest assured that your baby will be born when good and ready. However, if you are aware of your fertility and conceive consciously, you should have a very good idea of your due date (which may differ from the one your doctor calculates).

First signs of pregnancy

If you've been charting your temperature as part of your fertility awareness, the first sign that you have conceived will be a temperature that has remained elevated for 20 days. This may be accompanied by increased urination, tender nipples, and a dragging sensation not unlike menstrual pain.

Reduced energy in the early weeks

During the first 12 weeks (first trimester) your baby is growing at an extremely rapid rate and massive hormonal changes are also taking place in your body. More significant changes and more growth occur during this period than during any other of the whole pregnancy. If you focus on the work your body is doing and the extraordinarily rapid development of the embryo, you won't be surprised by the fact that you've got less energy than normal.

This is a great opportunity to get into the habit of taking some 'time-out'. If you're working throughout your pregnancy, make time to put your feet up for 30 minutes after work and if you're at home with small children, 'Playschool', or a teenager who lives nearby, can be effective short-term babysitters.

You'll probably experience several weeks of unaccustomed

lethargy, but don't be frustrated by this. Just listen to what your body is telling you. Slow down, rest whenever you can, get plenty of sleep. This is a great opportunity to get into the habit of an afternoon siesta. These are habits for which you have a valid excuse and which you can keep up for years. For as long as your baby nurses through the night, your sanity and sometimes your survival can depend on taking that 'time-out'.

Breast and nipple changes

Your breasts will become larger and your nipples will change in the early weeks of your pregnancy. The areola, which is the circle of darker skin surrounding the nipple, will darken further. The areola is also bumpy with tiny raised glands (Montgomery's tubercles) which will become larger as well and this may be one of the first signs that you've conceived. Your nipples will also become quite tender, especially if this is your first baby. This could be a good time to start exposing them very briefly to the sun, which is probably the only process which might be at all useful in preparing them for breastfeeding.

Not surprisingly (at least we don't think it's surprising) adequate nutritional status (particularly zinc and vitamins C and E) is the best prevention for cracked nipples. Nursing babies also do a wonderful job of toughening up nipples and rest assured that very small or inverted nipples will all rise to the occasion. As your pregnancy progresses you will probably be able to squeeze some colostrum from your nipples. Colostrum is the rich yellow substance which precedes the breast milk and there's no need to rub it off as it dries.

Nipple 'treatment'?

We definitely don't recommend any of the horrific treatment which has been recommended in the past as 'nipple preparation'. Nipples are made of extremely sensitive erectile tissue, in case you hadn't noticed. In that they're a little like the penis, so we can only wonder at suggestions to scrub nipples with a nailbrush or rub them with surgical spirit or alcohol. These must definitely be the suggestions of misogynists—we doubt these individuals would subject their similarly sensitive organs to such treatment.

It's certainly worth remembering that breastfeeding, despite what you might have been led to believe, is a completely natural, uncomplicated function. It's no more remarkable than your digestion really, it's just that your breasts are a lot more attractive (and visible) than your intestines. But all sizes of breasts and all shapes of nipples, belonging to all sorts of women, have managed successfully to breast-feed all manner of babies through millennia (otherwise none of us would be here). Remember that these women managed to do this without the benefit of creams, lotions, potions and certainly without nailbrushes!

Your bladder needs emptying often

The bane of the pregnant woman—the need to urinate frequently—will make itself felt in the very early weeks. By the end of the pregnancy, and with the 8-12 glasses of water we're going to recommend (you'll come to the reasons why shortly) sloshing around inside you, you'll be heartily fed up with the whole thing. Unfortunately there's no remedy for this; you'll just have to grin and bear it. Physiological changes—such as the expanding uterus which puts pressure on your bladder—are the cause. We don't recommend you stint on the water treatment either as drinking less will just undermine the health of your kidneys rather than solving your problem. You may prefer not to drink too much late at night, however.

Morning/evening/anytime sickness

Some very slight nausea may be a feature of the early weeks and this may be unavoidable due to the massive hormonal changes which are taking place. You might feel a bit seedy at any time during the day or night, and you might wonder how this condition ever became known as 'morning sickness'.

Eating can help to overcome this feeling (truly!), but it's sometimes difficult to know exactly what sort of meal you fancy. It's very easy when you feel like this to reach for refined or sugary snacks, but you're better off avoiding these, as well as tea and coffee. Small frequent meals, or simply a succession of nutritious snacks, in which you include lots of complex carbohydrates (fruit, vegetables and grains; almonds are also good) will give you a lot of relief because they'll help to keep your blood sugar levels stable, and by the end of the first trimester this seedy feeling should completely pass.

If you're constantly feeling really nauseated, or if you're actually vomiting, then this will obviously affect your eating habits at the very time when regular nutritious meals are vitally important. So you definitely shouldn't consider excessive nausea or vomiting to be normal (despite the fact that many pregnant women seem to suffer from these conditions). There are lots of natural remedies which can give you relief (see Chapter 13 for more information), and we promise you won't have your head over the hand basin for the whole nine months. As we said at the beginning of the book you should enjoy your pregnancy—not just endure it!

Sleep may not come easily

Your sleep patterns will change and these changes appear to be due to a number of factors. It seems certain, however, that even from the very earliest days, Nature is preparing you for the coming months or years (yes, it can sometimes be years, but remember the benefit of the afternoon nap!) when your baby will be nursing through the night. As the size of your belly increases, it may be hard to find a comfortable sleeping position, and all of your best efforts to induce slumber may find you lying very wide awake.

After sleeping soundly for six or eight hours for most of your life, sleepless periods can come as an unpleasant surprise. Instead of worrying about them, however, you can use the time constructively. Practise your relaxation techniques (we describe some in Chapter 10). Play some quiet ambient music. Do some deep breathing or stretching exercises (see Chapter 9). Practise some visualisations or affirmations (see Chapter 10). Anything which is soothing, peaceful, beautiful or inspirational is much better food for midnight meditations than a random clutter of thoughts about nursery colour schemes or baby accessories.

Even reading will sometimes allow you to fall asleep again without too much trouble. Just make sure that your reading material is appropriate; no murder mysteries please. There are also lots of natural remedies you can try if your insomnia is a real problem. (For more information see Chapter 13.)

Braxton-Hicks contractions: a dress rehearsal for your uterus

As your pregnancy progresses you'll start to experience practice (Braxton-Hicks) contractions. These are painless but you'll feel the muscles of your uterus contract and your belly will feel hard and tight. This is nothing to be alarmed about, it's simply your uterus having a trial run. These contractions will increase in intensity and frequency during the last month, but their efficiency will be enhanced if levels of nutrients such as calcium and magnesium are in plentiful supply.

A sense of joy and wellbeing

The latter part of your pregnancy should be a time of excitement and fulfilment. You should be able to focus on the miracle of the new life growing within you, free of the discomforts which are a major concern for many women. The tiredness and nausea which you may have experienced in the early weeks should have disappeared now. For the first time you can feel the wonderful fluttering of tiny limbs. Your skin glows and as the months pass you should be filled with a great sense of joy and wellbeing as you eagerly await the birth of your child. The fact that you are caring for yourself and your baby in every possible way is already sending that baby a number of very important messages. These are loving, caring and nurturing messages which it seems almost certain your child can understand long before you can hold him in your arms.

One door closes, another opens

The latter stage of your pregnancy is the time to bring to a close those things that you no longer have any use for. You might need to put your career on hold or leave your job. But rather than see this as a loss, think of it simply as the ending of one cycle and the beginning of another. Human life is not a linear progression from birth to death—this is a purely Western perception. In reality, life is a succession of cycles—beginnings and endings, new beginnings and more endings. One door closes and another one opens.

However, it's really important that you acknowledge the ending of one cycle. You need to give some recognition to this permanent and final end. Inevitably some sort of mourning must take place, and when you have done this you can be really free to welcome the new cycle. You'll probably know instinctively what sort of ritual will help you to mark the passing of your life without children. Janette remembers putting her white pharmacist's uniforms into the washing machine for the very last time. She knew she wasn't going to miss the job of washing, whitening and ironing them. Believe it or not, nature actually helps you to mark your passage from woman to mother too.

As the time to give birth draws closer, you'll find yourself, whether you like it or not, cleaning windows and cupboards, shifting furniture around and generally getting ready for your baby's arrival. It's that famous 'nesting instinct', and it's not a myth or a figment of someone's imagination. Nature's amazing—she knows it's going to be a very long time before you clean out those cupboards again. As for the windows, well . . .

Nature also makes sure that by the time your pregnancy draws to a close you're looking forward to getting rid of that baby from your belly. It's hard to believe when for so long all you wanted was to 'be pregnant', when your pregnancy has been so much 'better', and when you've enjoyed the whole nine months so thoroughly. But finally, the day will come when all you want is to go into labour and stop the endless phone calls from your mother asking, 'Anything happening yet?' When all of that happens you'll know that your baby's arrival isn't very far away!

HOW YOUR BABY DEVELOPS

When you consider in a little detail how your child develops from the time of conception to the moment of birth, then it becomes obvious just how important it is that his development takes place in an optimally healthy environment. What follows is not a day-by-day description of embryonic and foetal development, for that has been written about and even photographed in extraordinary detail elsewhere. The following paragraphs are just a very broad overview of what happens following conception and during your baby's growth and development.

It's a miracle
In simplifying and abbreviating the story of the growth and development of your baby, we don't mean to make light of the whole process.

For truly, it's nothing short of a miracle that, for the most part, embryonic and foetal development proceed according to plan. The complexity of the whole process of creation of a human being is truly awe-inspiring.

Your baby begins as a single cell, the product of the union of egg and sperm, which contains the full complement of genetic material which will lead to the development of a unique individual with a blend of characteristics from both parents. But there is actually more to embryonic and foetal development than just this blending and mixing of genetic material. There is more to the mental and physical attributes of your baby than the right proportions of DNA from his mother and father.

The presence of an adequate supply of all essential nutrients and an absence of harmful factors are the other determinants of development. You might have a mix of DNA which codes for well-proportioned limbs, attractive facial features and superior brain size, but if there's an absence of any of the vitamins, minerals or essential amino or fatty acids, or if there's an excess of toxic products, this baby will be unable to realise its full genetic potential. Conversely, a plentiful supply of essential nutrients can sometimes mean that a gene which is linked to deleterious characteristics will not be expressed.

Embryonic development begins

But back to our story ... The single cell which is the beginning of your baby now splits into two, and the two cells split into four, and the four into eight and so on, until the cluster of cells resembles a blackberry. As this cluster continues to divide it makes its descent of the Fallopian tube.

The Fallopian journey

This journey is facilitated by the action of the cilia. These are small hair-like projections which line the Fallopian tube and they waft the fertilised egg gently downwards. The tube itself also helps the downward progress with a pulsating movement (which is dependent on hormonal activity). Not surprisingly the health of the cilia and the efficiency of the movement of the Fallopian tube are closely linked to your general health. The journey takes about a week to complete and along the way the developing cell cluster is nurtured and fed by secretions from the tube. The healthier you are, the healthier these secretions will be.

Implantation occurs

With the Fallopian journey complete, the cell cluster implants in the endometrium which is the blood-rich lining of the uterus. This lining has thickened under the influence of progesterone which is the hormone secreted following ovulation. Again, the health of the endometrium has its basis in good nutrition and overall general health. The cluster of cells sends out roots into the blood and nutrient-rich endometrium and those roots start to draw up food to nurture the cells. The roots spread out into the uterine lining and as this early establishment of a foetal–maternal blood supply occurs, you will frequently experience the sort of pain that signals you are about to menstruate. But this month your period never arrives.

A tadpole, a seahorse or a baby?

The cellular growth now continues at a very rapid rate and pretty soon that cluster of cells is composed of two distinct layers. The outside layer is already doing its job of nourishing your baby and will become the placenta. Your baby develops from the inner cells. *Fourteen days* after conception those inner cells are made up of three distinct types. The ectoderm, or outer layer, will become your baby's nervous system, hair, skin and nails. The mesoderm, or middle layer, will form connective tissue, urinary tract, bones and muscles, and the endoderm, or inner layer will form the lining of the intestinal tract, liver and other organs.

About *21 days* after conception your baby has a distinct big round top which is the head and a thin curved tail. Then the body begins to grow from the back and eventually joins at the front, a little like a cardigan being buttoned up. During the *fourth week*, the spinal cord and the brain begin to take shape and the protective back bones also form. Your baby doesn't look distinctly human yet, but has features which are common to many embryos.

The face and throat are starting to grow and rudimentary eyes, ears, nose and mouth are present. The formation of organs such as the stomach, intestines, liver and kidneys has also begun and the embryo has blood vessels, blood and a heart. The skin covering its body is as thin as rice paper and about *25 days* after fertilisation the heart begins to beat under the skin. The body is still bent almost double so that its head nearly touches its tail. Ten days later the embryo is about 12 mm long and little buds which will become its arms and legs have formed.

Arms, legs and face continue to develop, with fingers and toes appearing and limbs growing longer. Your baby has some early reflexes and also has prints on his feet and palms. His organs are now under the control of the brain and by the end of the *seventh week* he is able to respond to touch. If you could touch your baby's hands or eyelids he would close them. Although his arms are growing longer they still aren't long enough to touch each other, although he can touch his face. By the *tenth week* nails are forming, and hair appears on his head, upper eyelids and eyebrows. You can now tell whether your baby is a boy or a girl and the kidneys start to secrete small amounts of urine.

By *12 weeks* your baby is about 7.5 cm long, weighs about 30 g, and is able to open and close his mouth. He can also swallow and make some facial expressions. He can move and bend his arms and legs as well, but his eyes are now closed while they undergo further development.

Nutrients necessary for rapid cell division

From fertilisation to the end of the first 12 weeks, your baby is called an embryo, and the rapid development proceeds according to a very strict timetable. During that time, the embryonic mass increases by a factor of 2.5 million, cells differentiate into specialised tissue and all the organs form. However this cell differentiation and organ formation waits for no-one. For example, at day 28 or 29 the neural tube closes. You may already know that if there is insufficient folic acid present at this time, then the neural tube will fail to close properly and a baby with spina bifida will result. However, *all* nutrients, not just folic acid, are required to create a healthy baby and if there is a deficiency in any nutrient, the development of the embryo will go forward regardless. So during this critical period any nutritional lack (or toxic excess) can have a profound and permanent effect on your baby's physical and mental development.

From embryo to foetus

Now that you've reached the end of the first trimester (12 weeks) the embryo changes its name and becomes a foetus. Your baby's now about as long as your little finger, but it's still a little too early for you to feel any of those movements that he's starting to make. Although you can't feel anything, your baby can make swimming motions with his arms and legs and he can turn somersaults in his warm watery environment.

At *14 weeks* your baby completely fills up your uterus. Lanugo, which is a downy fuzz, starts to cover his whole body. Now your baby has prints on his fingers and his bones are beginning to harden. This process begins at the middle of each long bone and works towards the ends, although the hardening won't be complete until your child is a young adult in his twenties! About this time you may start to feel your baby's first movements. These are actually quite hard to distinguish, especially if you are pregnant for the first time. Initially you might mistake them for a 'windy' tummy, but finally you will be able to differentiate those tiny subtle flutterings, like the stirring of gossamer wings.

At *five months* your baby is about 25 cm long and weighs almost 500 g. Hair is starting to grow on his head and his skin no longer looks like rice paper. He begins to store a little fat and some vernix appears. This is the thick, white, creamy substance which protects his skin from becoming waterlogged. He now makes some primitive breathing movements, and may develop hiccups as he sucks in some of the amniotic fluid. You will certainly know if he's hiccupping!

At *six months* your baby is about 30 cm long and weighs 750 g. His eyes are open again and if he is born at this stage he will try to breathe and will have a slim chance of survival.

At *seven months* he has grown to 40 cm and weighs 1.5–1.75 kilograms. From now on he will gain about 250 g each week and is practising sucking movements in preparation for breastfeeding. He can put his fingers into his mouth and may already have a habit of sucking his thumb.

As your baby grows bigger he is no longer able to float and turn so easily. He now curls up tightly in the foetal position with his knees under his chin, arms crossed over his chest and head bent forward. He is getting fatter and less wrinkled and you can easily feel his movements as he pushes off against the springy muscle of your uterus. You and your partner can clearly see the movements as they send ripples across your belly.

At *nine months* your baby is about 50 cm long and weighs 3–3.5 kilograms. He is plump and smooth, usually with not much vernix left on his skin and is now all ready to be born.

Foetal growth and brain development continue
From 12 weeks to full term at approximately 40 weeks, the mass of your baby increases by a factor of 230. Compare this to the rapid increase in the very early weeks when the foetal mass increases by a factor of well over 2 million. Any adverse nutritional influences which you might experience during the latter period of your pregnancy can only affect the growth of your baby, although the foetal brain continues to develop rapidly throughout the entire 40 weeks (and for three years after birth as well), so obviously nutritional status continues to be critically important.

Foetal awareness increases gradually

It is now known that the process of birth is not the trigger for your baby's consciousness. The switch is not suddenly turned on at nine months to give full illumination, but may be likened more to a dimmer switch, with awareness gradually increasing throughout the time in utero.

Hearing your voice
At six months your baby can hear your voice and also responds unmistakably to loud sounds. At the Paris V University in France, Dr Marie-Claire Busnel, Head of Research in the Department of Genetics, Neurogenesis and Behaviour, is investigating foetal hearing. Her findings suggest that unborn babies can distinguish between two syllables and between male and female voices. Further research at the University of North Carolina found foetuses were even able to recognise a story read aloud by their mothers every day for six weeks. Findings such as these have prompted some bizarre attempts to accelerate the rate at which a baby learns. Loudspeakers strapped to the mother's abdomen relaying music, the alphabet and foreign languages have been devised. These devices have not been shown to have any benefits, but may actually be harmful, since over-stimulation of some of your baby's developing senses may inhibit the development of others.

Reacting to stress
While there is no doubt that your unborn baby has capabilities and a level of awareness with which it was not previously credited, that awareness almost certainly develops best in a normal, healthy, loving,

stress-free environment. Dr Vivette Glover, a research scientist in London's Queen Charlotte Hospital writes, 'Exposure to stress in utero has long-term implications for brain development.' She has shown that babies who have a foetal blood transfusion through their abdomen (as opposed to through the placental cord where there is no nerve supply) show high rises in stress hormones.

Stress for the foetus may also be generated by many of the screening and diagnostic procedures which are used routinely. The *Foresight Newsletter* (Autumn 1997) reports that San Diego psychologist Dr David Chamberlain, president of the Association for Pre and Perinatal Psychology and Health, is continually amazed by foetal behaviour. 'When you do ultrasounds you can see twins relating to each other and during amniocentesis the foetus often guides the needle away. It's an astonishing thing to observe,' he says. He believes there can now be no question that foetuses learn and remember during their time in the womb. This new understanding, that the foetus has an awareness of noise, stress, anxiety, sorrow and pain, makes it even more imperative that your baby's life in utero is free of as many physical and emotional stressors as possible. While isolated stressful or unhappy events are unlikely to have long-lasting effects, there is now no doubt that constant exposure to physical or mental stress in utero will adversely affect your baby's development. This knowledge simply reinforces the need for a better pregnancy which contains an abundance of all the helpful factors.

First steps
At seven months your baby opens his eyes and the world takes on a warm red glow. His fingernails look like tiny seashells. Those tentative stepping movements he makes by pressing a foot against your uterus now help him turn upside down in readiness for his journey down the birth canal. During the last weeks before the birth your baby starts to get plump and you feel very large and very full of baby indeed!

BIRTH APPROACHES

During the last weeks copper levels rise and zinc packs into the placenta. These high copper levels are thought to trigger the phenomenon of birth. Somewhere between 38 and 42 weeks after your last menstrual period you will start to experience some pain which is not unlike the period pain you might have experienced back then. The mucus plug which has sealed the neck of the cervix will come away, or there might be a gush of amniotic fluid or perhaps just a slow trickle. When these signs appear you will know that at last your labour is beginning and that your pregnancy is very nearly at its end.

chapter 3

Eating well

We don't believe we're overstating the case when we say that the most important area you need to attend to during your pregnancy is your diet. Your diet is important because all those marvellously complex and interdependent processes, which constitute the full reproductive cycle, don't just happen in a vacuum. The basic building blocks necessary for your baby's growth and for the many changes going on in your body won't materialise out of thin air.

NUTRIENTS ARE ESSENTIAL

What you eat (and digest and absorb—we'll talk more of that in a little while) is the source of all the nutrients which must be present in plentiful supply if you are to have a better pregnancy and a better baby. The health of your uterus and placenta, the development of the embryo exactly according to plan, and every other aspect of your reproductive health, including the production of a plentiful supply of high quality breast milk, are dependent on an adequate supply of vitamins, trace minerals and essential amino and fatty acids.

Increased needs during pregnancy

A diet which is good enough to sustain you in adult life may fail to support you adequately during reproduction. When you're pregnant your need for a particular nutrient may increase several-fold. Requirements for nutrients such as folic acid, the whole vitamin B-complex, vitamin C, zinc, calcium and magnesium increase by 30–100 per cent during pregnancy, yet your food requirements only increase by a modest 15–20 per cent. These figures should dispel the popular misconception that pregnancy means eating for two. To be more accurate, what you really need during your pregnancy are *nutrients for two*.

Insufficient nutrients

We now know a great deal about what happens when there are not sufficient nutrients for two. Many hundreds of studies have been carried out since the early part of this century.

Dr Weston Price, an American dentist, and Francis Pottenger, a contemporary, were two of those very early researchers. Their studies, conducted in the 1930s, showed that native peoples who ate their traditional unrefined diet had robust physical and mental health. It didn't matter whether the diet was one rich in dairy products—unpasteurised milk, butter, cream and cheese—as favoured in Swiss villages; fish with oats made into porridge or oatcakes as eaten along the Scottish coast; game animals together with grains, tubers, vegetables and fruit as consumed by hunter–gatherers in Canada, America, Australia and Africa; or seafood eaten by the Polynesians and Maoris. The foods that allowed people of every race to be healthy were whole natural foods—meat with its fat, organ meats, wholemilk products, fish, insects, whole grains, tubers, vegetables and fruit. Many traditional communities also enhanced the vitamin content of grains and tubers and made minerals more available by soaking, fermenting, sprouting and sour leavening. Of further interest was the fact that the diets of healthy native groups contained at least 10 times more vitamin A and D than the American diet of Weston Price's day.

Not surprisingly, when a community switched to a refined Western diet with the emphasis on foods containing sugar, white flour and chemically altered vegetable oils, there was marked physical and mental deterioration, as well as a decrease in the efficiency of the birthing process.

Unfortunately, diets of whole natural uncontaminated food are eaten in very few communities today, and the discrepancies in trace mineral and vitamin contents are even more marked than they were in the time of Weston Price.

Nutrient lack causes 'conditions' of pregnancy

Weston Price's studies, which are documented in his book *Nutrition and Physical Degeneration: A Comparison of Primitive and Modern Diets and Their Effects*, were carried out more than 60 years ago, and since then many other researchers have clearly shown that infertility, miscarriage, premature and stillbirth, prolonged labour, reduced birthweight, inability to breastfeed, and poor health in the newborn can be directly attributed to deficiencies of vitamins, trace minerals and essential amino and fatty acids. It has also been shown that inadequate amounts of these nutritional factors can lead to stretch marks, varicose veins, breakthrough bleeding, gestational diabetes, toxaemia and many other 'conditions' of pregnancy.

Genes influenced by nutrition

Compromised nutrition is at the very foundation of compromised reproductive health. But, as well, many congenital defects, which were once considered to be due solely to genetic factors, can be manipulated at will by inducing a deficiency in one or more of the essential nutrients. Furthermore, the effects of a defective gene may be suppressed in the presence of an optimal supply of a particular nutrient.

Nutrient lack in utero affects health in adulthood

Recent studies carried out in the UK show that early nutritional experiences have an effect in adult life. Compromised nutrition in utero has a powerful influence on the development of chronic degenerative disease. Poor foetal growth is a strong predictor for hypertension, diabetes and mortality from cardiovascular and chronic obstructive airways disease in adulthood. Professor Barker of the University of Southampton (and author of *Mothers, Babies and Disease in Later Life*), says:

> 'Undernutrition in foetal life has a permanent, detrimental effect on the baby's metabolism, hormonal response, immune function

and organ development and increases susceptibility to disease in later life, including cardiovascular disease, diabetes and respiratory illness.'

Your partner's nutrition

An adequate supply of all essential nutrients is important for prospective fathers too. They aren't exempt from the need to eat well just because their sperm have done their work. Fathers need to support their partners wholeheartedly in their efforts to have a better pregnancy. There's nothing more demoralising or likely to foster resentment than your partner continuing with a junk food diet while you pursue the healthiest possible option. Any mother-to-be will be much more motivated to eat well if her partner actively supports her efforts and her healthy food choices.

Eating well now is also good training for all the years to come when as parents you'll be setting an example for your children to follow. Studies have demonstrated that children adopt the eating patterns of their father, so that's a pretty heavy responsibility for the guys to get used to!

BEST SOURCES OF ESSENTIAL NUTRIENTS

To ensure your changing body and your growing baby receive an adequate supply of all the basic building blocks it's important that your food has the highest possible nutritional value. For this reason we recommend that you eat fruit and vegetables which have been organically grown, and animal produce which has been raised in a free-range manner and fed on organically grown fodder. Weston Price, Pottenger, and many others have clearly shown that optimal health (which translates into a better pregnancy) is achieved only by eating healthy food which is grown on healthy soil!

Organic produce

The basis of organic or sustainable farming (as it is also known) is truly healthy soil. Organic farming uses a variety of techniques to achieve this healthy soil. The processes vary, but they may begin with green manuring in which a clover crop is allowed to grow for several months. This puts organic matter as well as nitrogen back into the soil. Composting, which follows, takes a further three months, and ensures that the soil contains an adequate supply of nutrients before the crops are planted.

Before planting, seedlings may be hand selected so that the weaker ones are discarded. In general only seasonal crops are grown. These are rotated, with the same crop going back into the same soil only after two or three season's rest. Companion planting as a method of deterring (or attracting) pests is also practised. Complete pest eradication is not considered desirable, since there is then no food for natural predators. If necessary there may be very limited use of low toxicity natural sprays. Weeding is frequently done by hand.

The fruit and vegies from sustainable farms may be smaller than conventionally grown produce and sometimes they will display blemishes which would be unacceptable in non-organic food. However, organic produce tastes great, undoubtedly because it has a much higher trace mineral content. Some of these differences in nutritional value were determined in a study carried out at Rutgers University in the United States. The vegetables examined were spinach, lettuce, cabbage, tomatoes and snap beans. The organically grown spinach contained twice as much calcium, four times as much magnesium and 117 times as much manganese. The other organically grown vegetables were similarly rich in trace elements and the tomatoes were found to have 1900 times more iron than the negligible amount found in tomatoes grown by non-sustainable methods.

A further 12-year study found that desirable substances such as cobalt, boron and magnesium were significantly higher, and undesirable substances (such as nitrates) were lower in organic produce.

Charts detailing the results of these studies are reproduced in Appendix 2.

Whole unrefined foods

Fortunately for you, nature is very clever. When you eat whole, unrefined foods you also receive the full complement of vitamins and minerals which are necessary for your body to metabolise those foods completely. For example, all of the B-complex vitamins and minerals such as zinc, chromium and magnesium, which are needed for the breakdown of complex carbohydrates, exist alongside those complex carbohydrates.

When whole foods are refined, partitioned or otherwise broken down, however, a large percentage of the naturally occurring nutrients are removed. For example, grains such as whole wheat and brown rice are an important source of B-complex vitamins and trace minerals, but when you eat white flour or white rice you get only a tiny fraction of the original concentration of these nutrients, because most of them have been removed in the refining process.

The B-complex vitamins have many important functions during reproduction, but only 23 per cent of the vitamin B1, which is present in whole wheat, is retained in white flour after milling. Only 20 per cent of vitamin B2 is retained, only 19 per cent of vitamin B3, only 50 per cent of vitamin B5, only 29 per cent of vitamin B6 and only 33 per cent of folic acid. Check the chart in Appendix 3 which shows the percentage of all vitamins and minerals which are removed during the milling of whole wheat.

Zinc is an essential trace element with similarly important functions during pregnancy, but most zinc is lost from food during refining processes (78 per cent of zinc is removed when we refine flour, 98 per cent is lost in the production of refined sugar). The story with chromium and magnesium is similar.

Whole foods mean energy

As well as their various roles in reproduction, the B-complex vitamins readily found in whole foods are needed for energy production. Complex carbohydrates are broken down by your body, in the presence of these vitamins and some minerals, to form glucose. Glucose is then further broken down to yield carbon dioxide, water and energy. This energy is not just a by-product of the breakdown of complex carbohydrates, it's what keeps your body's machinery running. As well, your baby depends entirely on this energy for his growth. Clearly any deficiency in B-complex vitamins (or minerals such as zinc and chromium) will mean that this production of energy is compromised. This can leave you feeling tired, run-down or even depressed, and can compromise foetal development.

Whole foods deliver zinc

Zinc is also needed for the breakdown of complex carbohydrates, but has some other very important functions as well. It is a part of over 200 enzyme systems in the body and is involved in every aspect of reproduction. In fact many researchers feel that it is the most important trace element for the pregnant woman.

Zinc is necessary for proper fertility in both the male and female. Zinc is one of the nutrients necessary for proper formation of elastin chains in connective tissue, so it is needed to maintain the integrity of your growing belly and breasts. It is also necessary to ensure that your uterus will contract efficiently during labour and that your perineum will stretch fully to allow your baby to be born easily. Zinc is needed to ensure appropriate foetal growth. Adequate zinc levels can prevent premature births, toxaemia and postnatal depression. Zinc is intimately involved in the correct formation and function of the foetus's brain and immune system. Zinc is necessary for proper taste sensation. Adequate zinc levels can prevent many congenital abnormalities, and can also ensure that your baby is easy to settle and does not cry excessively. You can see what we mean when we say that zinc is important.

You'll only give yourself the best possible chance of getting enough of this extremely important mineral, and enough of the B-complex vitamins as well, when you eat whole unrefined food. But there are other reasons for eating a whole food diet as well.

Get the co-factors too

There are co-factors occurring in foods such as whole grains which aid the digestion, absorption and metabolism of the food. We are at last beginning to recognise what holistic practitioners have maintained for many years; that whole food has something else—a life force, an energy, 'chi', or whatever you want to call it—which makes it better able to sustain life than the partitioned product which is devoid of such energy. Many researchers have shown conclusively that optimal health (and remember the word optimal does not merely denote the absence of disease) can only be achieved by eating whole food grown on healthy soil!

POOR SOURCES OF ESSENTIAL NUTRIENTS

You might think that if fruit and vegetables thrive, this must surely indicate the health of the soil in which they are grown and the health of the produce itself. Unfortunately, this is not always the case.

Inorganic produce

A great deal of the soil in Australia is low in essential trace elements, particularly magnesium and selenium because of the great age of the continent.

Then for the most part, Australian primary producers use non-sustainable or non-organic farming methods which aggravate the problem of soil already low in many essential trace elements. Non-sustainable farming techniques involve continual use of the land, with no period of lying fallow, crops of a single variety which are generally not rotated, and the use of fertilisers of the inorganic type which contain only nitrogen, phosphorus and potassium.

This means that the levels of many micronutrients such as calcium, chromium, cobalt, iron, magnesium, manganese, molybdenum and zinc continue to fall with use of the land. Since these micronutrients are never replenished, crops have increasingly low levels of trace elements to draw upon. These crops will be more susceptible to disease and will require more frequent applications of fertiliser.

Inorganic fertilisers certainly boost the plant's growth, but they don't give it time to absorb the nutrients remaining in the soil. These nutrient-deficient, disease-susceptible crops must be sprayed repeatedly with pesticides. Further nutritional deficits arise from the use of these compounds, particularly those of the organophosphate type. Organophosphates destroy choline-containing enzymes, which prevents the uptake of manganese by the plant. Manganese is involved in bone growth and development and also in the formation of certain enzymes which affect the glandular secretions underlying maternal instinct.

To sum up, fruit and vegetables grown using non-sustainable or non-organic farming techniques have trace mineral contents many times lower than produce grown using sustainable methods. They may be large, but their size may be due simply to high concentration of water. Non-organically grown produce is also usually rather tasteless. Not surprisingly, animals and birds which have been intensively farmed or battery bred will display corresponding differences in nutritional value from those which have been fed organically and grazed in a free-range manner. Also, since many contaminants, such as pesticides, are stored in fat, non-organic animal produce will contain higher levels of harmful substances as well as lower levels of beneficial nutrients.

Refined/partitioned foods

We've just discussed how all the B-vitamins and some minerals are necessary for the metabolic breakdown of complex carbohydrates. These vitamins and minerals are needed for the metabolic breakdown of refined carbohydrates too. In other words they're needed for the metabolism of all the products which contain white flour, white rice and refined sugar. But you'll remember that, unlike complex carbohydrates, refined carbohydrates have been separated from the nutrients which are necessary for their metabolism.

Clearly, if 100 per cent of the vitamin or mineral is necessary for the complete metabolic breakdown of a product like white bread, and if only about 30 per cent of that nutrient is actually present, the deficit must be made up from somewhere. In the case of the metabolism of refined carbohydrates, the body's stores will be raided, and when they are depleted, deficiencies will develop. These can lead, in extreme cases, to conditions such as pellagra and beri-beri. Less severe cases will lead to a state of sub-optimal general health, sub-optimal health during pregnancy and sub-optimal foetal development.

Is refined but fortified an alternative?

Breakfast cereal and bread manufacturers obviously have some doubts about the value of partitioning food and throwing away the nutrient-dense portion; hence their desire to put some vitamins and minerals back! They try to improve on the original product by fortifying cereals with nutrients in amounts beyond the initial concentrations, or with nutrients which were not even there in the first place. For example, many cereals are fortified with vitamins A and C which they have never contained, and calcium and iron are frequently boosted way beyond naturally occurring levels. It is far better for you to eat the whole grain as nature intended and receive nutrients in their naturally occurring and balanced state.

Empty calories

Put simply, highly refined products are nothing more than empty calories, and frequent consumption of white flour and sugar-containing products will lead to a number of nutrient deficiencies. The B-complex vitamins and minerals such as magnesium, manganese, zinc and chromium are particularly affected. These sub-clinical deficiencies will mean you have a much reduced chance of a better pregnancy and better baby. Ironically, a reduced level of these nutrients will create a craving for more sugary foods and a vicious cycle is established.

Sugar

Unlike the refining of whole wheat, which leaves a small percentage of nutrients in white flour, the refining of sugar cane to white sugar leaves no nutrients at all and provides nothing to sustain a better pregnancy. Unfortunately sugar is not always called 'sugar'. Sugar comes in many guises and there are many names by which it is known. Manufacturers often include several different types of sugar in one product (see box). You need a degree in biochemistry to recognise that all of these are forms of sugar. Clearly, all of these substances should be avoided if you're trying to attain adequate nutritional status.

All types of sugar increase your body's needs for minerals such as zinc and chromium and all the B-complex vitamins. Vitamin B6, which is the nutrient necessary for the formation of progesterone, the hormone which maintains your pregnancy, is particularly affected. Folic acid, which is vitally important during the early stages of pregnancy, when the neural tube is closing,

---

SUGAR'S MANY NAMES

Glucose
Dextrose
Sucrose
Fructose
Maltose
Galactose
Mannose
Syrup
Lactose
Modified carbohydrate
Xylitol
Sorbitol
Mannitol
Invert sugar
Brown sugar
Raw sugar
Molasses
Malt extract
Malt
Corn starch
Honey

is also part of the B-complex range and is adversely affected too.

Sugar consumption interferes with calcium absorption and therefore with bone formation. Sugar also increases the formation of serotonin. When this chemical transmitter is present in excess there is a tendency to aggressive behaviour, and of course this chemical messenger is not confined to your bloodstream, but will enter the foetal circulation as well.

WHAT TO EAT FOR OPTIMAL HEALTH

Hopefully we've made it clear that your needs for all nutrients during pregnancy are much higher than at other times. We hope you're now aware that a diet of organically grown whole food is the most nutritious diet. We hope you can see why this is the only diet which can provide all the nutrients your body needs to manufacture pregnancy hormones, maintain the health of your uterus and placenta, keep the collagen sound as your breasts and belly grow, and ensure that your baby's development proceeds according to its blueprint. We hope you realise that eating really well will give you the best chance of a healthy full-term pregnancy and a healthy baby.

But knowing these things isn't enough. You need to be able to put that knowledge into practice. Therefore we're going to give you some much more specific information, often by means of point form guidelines, about exactly what to eat and what to avoid. If you follow all of these guidelines you'll be well on the way to ensuring that you have adequate nutritional status and that both you and your developing baby will have an ample supply of nutrients from which to draw. (A summary of our recommendations is set out in the Reproductive Health Diet found in Appendix 1.)

Fruit and vegetables

Fresh vegetables and fruit which have been organically grown can provide a wide range of essential nutrients and they are alkali-promoting foods as well. If your system is too acidic (that is, not sufficiently alkaline), toxic metals are more likely to be absorbed and radiation becomes more of a hazard. Vegetables, with some fruit, should make up a very high proportion of your diet.

- ✔ At least 40 per cent of your total food intake (not just of your main meal) should be made up of vegetables.
- ✔ Eat a combination of raw and cooked vegetables.
- ✔ Juices are a good way to increase your consumption of raw vegies. Try carrot, celery or beetroot. You can add any others (including dark green leafy ones).
- ✔ Whether you eat or drink your vegetables, you should always aim to eat as wide a variety as possible, focusing particularly on the dark green leafy varieties and any which are red or orange in colour, which are high in beta-carotene (a precursor of vitamin A) and the essential bioflavonoids, which potentiate the action of vitamin C and have an important role to play in keeping the vascular system elastic as your blood volume expands. Avocadoes are also high in many essential nutrients.
- ✔ When eating salads, it is important to think beyond the traditional lettuce and tomato combination. When choosing a lettuce for a salad, select one with dark leaves since it will contain a higher concentration of minerals. Add chopped fresh herbs such as parsley, watercress or basil, and non-leguminous sprouts (but avoid alfalfa during pregnancy).
- ✔ While root vegetables such as carrots are best broken down by grating, juicing, lightly steaming or stir-frying, nearly all other vegetables are easily prepared by chopping or shredding. Always eat them immediately once they've been chopped to minimise nutrient loss.
- ✔ Steaming and stir-frying are the preferred methods of cooking your vegetables. Always cook for the minimum possible time since too much heat destroys nutrients. Cooked vegies should still be crunchy, not a limp soggy mess.
- ✔ Eat no more than two or three pieces of fruit daily. While fruit is an important food, you need to remember that it is also quite high in sugar. Even fruit sugar in excess can contribute to nutrient loss, and this applies particularly to fruit that is juiced.

- ✘ Even juices with no added sugar are still very high in fructose (fruit sugar) and studies have shown that as little as two glasses of unsweetened orange juice can reduce immune function by up to 50 per cent for three hours after ingestion.
- ✘ Dried fruits should be avoided too since these products are very

high in sugar and may contain chemical additives.
- ✗ Green potatoes should be avoided since they contain a toxin which is especially harmful to the developing foetus. Don't try to peel off the green part; throw the whole potato away, even if it is only very slightly tinged with green.

Grains

You should eat whole grains and avoid white flour, white rice and products containing sugar.

- ✓ Eat brown rice and pasta made from the whole grain. Many whole grain pastas are now available, and while the whole wheat varieties may seem a little heavy at first, those made from other grains such as corn are lighter in texture.
- ✓ Many interesting breads are now available from your health food store or organic supplier. These are usually made from organically grown whole grain flour which has been stone ground, but do make sure they are free of additives.
- ✓ Try other grains. Rolled oats, whole wheat, buckwheat, brown rice, quinoa, barley, corn and cracked wheat can be used to make all sorts of dishes.

- ✗ Avoid all refined grains such as white bread, rice and pasta. Green pasta is often only white pasta with colouring added.
- ✗ Avoid all foods containing white flour and sugar, such as cakes, biscuits, pastries and soft drinks.
- ✗ Avoid other forms of sugar (see box, page 35), including honey, Nutrasweet and even concentrated fruit sugar.

Protein

There is some debate about the amount of protein that pregnant women should consume. The World Health Organisation (WHO) recommendations, which suggest 36 g per day during pregnancy (rising to 43 g daily during lactation) are in sharp contrast to the US National Research Council (NRC) which recommends 70 g daily during pregnancy. The WHO levels are a reflection of the much more meagre diets consumed by two-thirds of the world's population while the NRC recommendations are designed for Western consumers. You certainly don't need more than 70 g daily. On pages 44–46 we talk more about the appropriate balance of protein, carbohydrate and fat.

In fact, too much protein can lead to a rise in the production of urea which has a diuretic effect and will increase the excretion of minerals such as calcium. Increasing amounts of protein in Western diets correspond with an increasing incidence of osteoporosis. It is interesting to note that communities of Eskimo (Inuit) eating their traditional diet of whale, seal and fish, have undoubtedly the highest rate of protein consumption in the world (and well above average calcium consumption as well). They also have the highest incidence of osteoporosis. The Inuit consume between 250–400 g protein, along with about 2000 mg calcium every day.

Animal protein

Primary protein is protein from an animal source and it contains all the essential amino acids. Fish, chicken, red meat, eggs and dairy produce are all types of primary protein.

- ✔ Fish is the most appropriate type of primary protein because it's low in saturated fats, which you want to avoid. It should be eaten at least two or three times a week. If it's deep-dwelling, cold-water fish then it is particularly high in essential fatty acids and is also less likely to be contaminated by pollution. Such choices include mackerel, mullet, salmon, taylor, trevally and sardines.
- ✔ Canned and frozen fish may be eaten occasionally, but you will only receive the full nutritional value of fish if it is freshly caught, freshly bought and freshly prepared.
- ✔ Oysters are particularly high in zinc, but the level of contaminants is often high as well, so we don't recommend you eat oysters too often. This caution applies to prawns and other bottom-dwelling coastal seafood too.
- ✔ Red meat and chicken should be organically fed and raised in a free-range manner. It's important to realise that some birds and animals may be free-range, but their fodder may not be organically grown.
- ✔ Goat's milk, cheese and yoghurt are preferable to products made from cow's milk. Even though unpasteurised dairy produce is nutritionally superior to pasteurised produce (remember Weston Price's studies), unpasteurised products are best avoided during

pregnancy, since they can be a source of the organism which causes listeriosis. Listeriosis is a flu-like disease which can cause miscarriage and stillbirth. Yoghurt made from cow's milk can be eaten without problems by most people (even those sensitive to cow's milk and cheese) but it should be fresh and natural (no sugar) and contain acidophilus and bifidus lactobacilli.

- ✘ Avoid large fish high in the food chain such as tuna, swordfish and shark since they can be contaminated with mercury.
- ✘ Avoid battery-bred and raised animal produce which may have been fed antibiotics and hormones.
- ✘ Avoid organ meats (such as liver and kidneys) from non-organically fed animals. These organs are the detoxification routes for the animal and are likely to contain high levels of pesticides and heavy metals.
- ✘ Avoid mince since it is usually made from organ meats. If necessary select some *lean* meat and ask your butcher to mince it for you. Alternatively, use mince made from organic meat.
- ✘ Avoid sausages and delicatessen meats which contain organ meats as well as chemicals such as nitrites. (You can ask your butcher to make sausages using a lean cut of organically raised meat.)
- ✘ Avoid dairy products made from cow's milk. Wherever you can, substitute soya, goat's or sheep's milk produce (but make sure it's been pasteurised, to avoid any risk of listeriosis). Remember that low-fat products are still made from cow's milk and are often quite highly processed. Cow's milk is a very common allergen and can cause congestion in the mucous membranes. This can compromise the digestion and absorption of nutrients, and can also adversely affect the health of the reproductive system.

Plant protein

Secondary proteins are proteins of plant origin, and, unlike primary proteins, they do not contain the full complement of essential amino acids. For this reason, if you favour a vegetarian diet, the appropriate combination of vegetable protein should be eaten each day. This involves combining any two from the following groups:

- Nuts
- Grains/seeds

* Legumes/pulses

Such combinations will ensure you obtain the full complement of amino acids.

✔ You could combine brown rice with cashews, pumpkin seeds with hazelnuts, corn with lentils and so on. Of course, traditional diets, based on combinations such as rice and beans, or nuts and seeds, addressed the issue of plant protein combining long before we knew anything about amino acids.
✔ When buying nuts, make sure they are fresh (specialist shops may be more informed about the age of their stock). Eat them soon after purchase. They should taste sweet, not bitter. Store all nuts in a cool place and away from light. (In the fridge is a good spot.)
✔ Grains include corn, rice, wheat, barley, rye, quinoa, oats.
✔ Legumes (pulses) include lentils, split peas, dried beans of all types, chickpeas and soya beans. Soy products such as tofu and tempeh, and legumes are all excellent forms of plant protein and can also assist your body's own efforts to detoxify.

✘ Nuts which are not fresh, or which have not been stored appropriately, can do more harm than good. This is because the oils which they contain go rancid very quickly. This leads to the production of free radicals—compounds which can cause damage to DNA, proteins and the membranes that make up cell walls.
✘ If you can, ensure that your soya beans are not genetically engineered. At this stage we really have no idea of the long-term effects of eating food which has been altered in this way, so it is definitely best to avoid eating genetically engineered food.

Fats and oils

You must have some oils and fats in your diet because they are a source of the oil-soluble vitamins (vitamins A, D and E) which are important both for your health and for your baby's development. Vitamin A is essential for healthy eyes, hair, skin and teeth and good bone structure. Vitamin D is also necessary for growth of bones and teeth and it aids the absorption of calcium as well. Vitamin E is important as an anti-oxidant (which means it protects against free radical damage) and a deficiency can lead to prolonged difficult labour and compromised foetal development. Oils and fats are also a source of the essential fatty acids which are necessary for the production of hormone-like substances which regulate many body processes. They are necessary for the growth of the placenta and for your baby's brain and eye development, especially in the last 12 weeks of pregnancy. You must eat the right types of oils (and avoid saturated animal fats and polyunsaturated vegetable oils) to obtain the correct balance of essential fatty acids. It is important that your fats and oils are from organically grown and fed sources wherever possible, as fat is the primary reservoir of pollutants and toxins. This applies to animal foods, oil bearing vegetables (such as avocado) and nuts.

- ✔ Use olive oil for stir-frying. This is a mono-unsaturated oil and unlike polyunsaturated oils will not become saturated on heating. Saturated fats and oils must be avoided since they block the metabolism of the essential fatty acids which are so important for your baby's brain and eye development. Make sure the olive oil is cold-pressed and (preferably) organically grown. Canola and sesame oils are possible alternatives.
- ✔ Use lots of organically grown cold-pressed olive (or flaxseed, pumpkin, walnut, safflower or sunflower) oil on salads. If never heated, these are high in essential fatty acids. Add chopped fresh herbs, garlic or lemon juice to add flavour.
- ✔ Butter, although it falls into the category of saturated animal fats, is still preferable to margarine, and can help to get rid of mercury from the body.
- ✔ If you want an alternative to butter, try spreading your bread with tahini, hummus, mashed banana, avocado or soya mayonnaise. You can also try dunking your bread in cold-pressed olive oil (make sure it's organically grown).
- ✔ Choose lean cuts of red meat, trim off all the fat, skin the chicken.

- ✘ Avoid margarine, which may contain harmful chemical additives as well as up to 30 per cent of 'trans' fatty acids which block the metabolism of essential fatty acids.
- ✘ Avoid fried foods and animal fats. These contain saturated fats which also interfere with the correct balance of essential fatty acids.
- ✘ Avoid delicatessen or processed meats such as salami and

sausages. These are high in saturated fat as well as harmful chemicals.

Additives

Salt
Too much salt adversely affects mineral or electrolyte balance and causes fluid retention. Fluid retention (oedema) is a common problem in the latter part of pregnancy and may indicate toxaemia which is a very serious condition. Recent studies indicate that too little salt can also be a problem and that salt should be added 'to taste'. In other words, don't use it indiscriminately in your cooking or on your food, avoid heavily salted, pre-prepared foods and use your body's in-built discretion to add small amounts of sea, rock or Celtic salt (*not* table salt) to individual foods, if required. It's important, however, that your taste is not depraved by deficient zinc levels, or by previous excessive salt consumption.

Chemicals
Almost all foods which are found in packets, cans or bottles have some sort of chemical added to help retain texture and taste and to improve shelf life. These chemicals may include preservatives, colourings, artificial sweeteners and flavourings, emulsifiers and 'extenders'. Apart from the fact that some may be the cause of intolerance or sensitivity reactions, such as skin conditions or respiratory distress, your body uses up many essential nutrients to detoxify these substances. You must remember too that what constitutes a relatively small dose of a chemical additive for an adult is actually a very large dose for the developing foetus.

- ✔ Sea, rock or Celtic salts may be used in moderation since they contain important trace minerals. Avoid ordinary table salt.
- ✔ Add flavour with garlic, black pepper, ginger, parsley, basil, chives etc.

- ✘ Be aware that most pre-prepared foods contain a high level of salt.

✘ Almost everything in a can, bottle or packet will contain added chemicals.
✘ Breads made from 'baker's flour' are of particular concern since breadmaking flour (even the wholemeal variety) contains dozens of additives. These include chemicals to make the flour easy to handle and chemicals to enhance the keeping qualities of the loaf. Few packaged breads are free of preservatives, although there are some whole grain exceptions.

The correct balance

The dietary recommendations we've just outlined will give many of you enough to do. But some of you might be prepared to go one extra step. Just as important as what you should be eating (and what you should be avoiding) is the appropriate balance of all those good foods. Balancing carbohydrate, protein and fat in the right proportions not only means a better pregnancy, with plenty of energy, mental clarity and appropriate weight gain, it means a healthier baby too.

We all tend to eat too many carbohydrates. Since the mid 1980s we have all been exhorted to eat more complex carbohydrates such as whole grains, fruit and vegetables and reduce our intake of protein and fat. But increasing obesity and fatigue levels closely parallel this increased consumption of grains, starches and sugars.

That doesn't mean that complex carbohydrates have to go—in fact we've talked at length about the reasons for eating whole unrefined grains and lots of vegetables with some fruit. But you must balance the carbohydrates with sufficient quality protein and fat. Balance is the key word. When you achieve the appropriate balance you also balance two key hormones: insulin and glucagon.

You can think of insulin as the 'saving' hormone—it tells your body to save fat. Glucagon, on the other hand, is the 'spending' hormone—it takes energy from the fat cells to be used as fuel. When these two hormones are well balanced, your weight gain during pregnancy will be right for you and your blood sugar levels won't fluctuate. Stable blood sugar levels mean you will be less likely to suffer from morning sickness, fatigue and emotional instability and they also mean your baby will receive a constant supply of glucose for his energy needs.

How do you get your body into that state of balance between insulin and glucagon?

1. Work out your daily protein requirements—at one meal you need an amount of protein that is the same size as (and no thicker than) the palm of your hand. Now increase that amount by one-third (for your pregnancy), by a further quarter for light activity, by one-third for moderate activity (30 minutes of exercise on three days per week) and by a half for strenuous activity (60 minutes of exercise on five days per week). You already know the most appropriate proteins to select.

2. Now the next step is to add your carbohydrates. Here you have to consider that there are two types of carbohydrates: risk-reducing (low glycaemic) or risk-promoting (high glycaemic). Which category a food falls into depends on the amount of carbohydrate present in the food and the amount of fibre it contains. Foods that are low in carbohydrate and high in fibre or water are risk-reducing and it is those foods which you should select wherever possible. These include asparagus, bok choy, broccoli, brussel sprouts, cabbage, capsicum, cauliflower, chickpeas, cucumber, eggplant, kidney beans, lentils, lettuce, mushrooms, onion, spinach and tomatoes. Low-risk fruits include apples, apricots, berries, grapes, melons, oranges, peaches, pineapple and strawberries. The moderate-risk foods (which can still be eaten, but in smaller amounts) include baked beans, corn, carrots, peas, potatoes, squash, sweet potato, bananas, dates, figs, mango, papaya, fruit juices and all the assorted pasta, breads and grains.

3. Because of the differences in animal and vegetable protein and because there are risk-reducing and risk-promoting carbohydrates, it is possible to achieve the correct balance in a number of different ways. Here are some examples of how to fill an average-sized dinner plate:
    - Let's say your *animal protein* takes up one-third of your plate, then you select *low-risk carbohydrates* to take up two-thirds of the plate (e.g. beef and vegetables, in a 1 : 2 ratio)
    - If your *animal protein* takes up one-third of your plate, then you select *moderate-risk carbohydrates* to take up one-third of the plate, leaving one-third of the plate empty (e.g. chicken and pasta, in a 1 : 1 ratio)

- If your *vegetable protein* takes up half of your plate, then you select *low-risk carbohydrates* to take up half of the plate (e.g. tofu and vegetables/lentils, in a 1 : 1 ratio)
- If your *vegetable protein* takes up half of your plate, then you select *moderate-risk carbohydrates* to take up one-third of the plate (e.g tofu and rice)

4. Next you add healthy fats to each meal—these reduce your blood sugar and insulin response to a meal and are a very important part of achieving the balance between insulin and glucagon. Here is a list of the healthy fats:
   - For dressings and sauces (do not heat)—olive, flax, pumpkin, walnut, canola, safflower and sunflower oils (all cold-pressed)
   - In cooking—olive, sesame, canola oils
   - Seeds—flax, pumpkin, sesame, sunflower
   - Nuts—walnuts, hazelnuts, almonds
   - Avocado
   - Eggless or soya mayonnaise

5. Drink plenty of water—but drink it in between meals so that it doesn't interfere with your digestion. We give more details about water consumption in just a moment.

You can add snacks in between meals—work out the appropriate proportions the same way, but halve your protein allowance. You shouldn't go more than four hours without a meal or a snack. This method of eating is known as 'the zone insulin system' or 'the zone diet' and you'll certainly have a better pregnancy if you always *stay in the zone*.

Water

Water is essential for life. About 75 per cent of your body is made of water. Without adequate water intake to replace what your body uses as it breathes, sweats and excretes, your cells and tissues will not be adequately hydrated and waste products won't be properly eliminated. You'll find lots more information about the importance of water purification and consumption in Chapter 7 and Appendix 10.

✔ Drink plenty of fresh, purified water. We recommend 8–12 glasses daily. Bottled (still; spring) water is another option, but it is not as reliably free of contaminants (as this depends on where it is collected) and will be more expensive in the long run than buying a good quality purifier.

✔ A slice of lemon (or lime) in your glass of water will make it taste more interesting and make it more easily absorbed by your body.

✔ Herb and green teas can be very helpful, but should not take the place of purified water. The water for your tea should also be purified, as boiling does not remove toxins, only bacteria. Toxins will be concentrated by boiling. Herb teas should not be used if the herb appears in the list of contra-indicated herbs in Appendix 6, though the amount of any harmful constituent absorbed from a tea will be negligible.

✔ Green (unfermented) tea is particularly high in anti-oxidants (which protect against free radical damage). Black tea also contains anti-oxidants, though the advantage may be lost when milk is added, and caffeine content may be high as well.

✘ Avoid drinking with meals, as this will dilute the digestive juices in your stomach.

✘ Avoid mineral (sparkling) water, which may be high in sodium (salt) and should only be used occasionally.

✘ Avoid soft drinks and coffee and teas which contain caffeine. We'll talk more about the reasons for avoiding caffeine in Chapter 5. Unfortunately decaffeinated tea and coffee are not a good alternative, as undesirable chemicals are used in the caffeine removal process. Although some coffees are decaffeinated using a water process, these are still better avoided, as caffeine is not the only harmful constituent in coffee. Some teas which are naturally low in caffeine may, however, be drunk in moderation (no more than 2 cups daily) and cereal or dandelion based coffee substitutes are fine as long as they don't contain sugar.

PREPARING FOOD FOR OPTIMAL HEALTH

Now that you know which foods are best for you, here are some hints on how to prepare them to ensure you obtain maximum nutritional benefit.

- ✔ Vegetables should be scrubbed, not peeled. Lots of the nutrients are found in (or just under) the skins (e.g. potatoes).
- ✔ Cut vegetables just before cooking or eating them since exposure to the air destroys nutrients (especially vitamin C).
- ✔ Steaming and stir-frying are the preferred methods of cooking. Vegetables should still be crisp and brightly coloured. Cooking for the minimum period of time is another way to minimise nutrient loss.
- ✔ Dry bake vegetables such as pumpkin, kumera and potato.
- ✔ If you feel that you aren't getting an adequate supply of vegetables with your meals, top up with vegetable juices.

All of the above methods of preparing and cooking foods are designed to minimise nutrient loss. The methods we suggest you avoid are those which destroy nutrients. These methods include the following:

- ✘ Roasting, frying or boiling foods (these methods use too much fat or heat).
- ✘ Microwaving, although convenient, destroys protein structures and the enzymes that you need to aid absorption of nutrients. Even defrosting frozen food in a microwave oven will have this effect, so avoid microwaving altogether.

MAKING DIETARY CHANGES

You might now realise that a complete overhaul of your eating habits is in order. Maybe it's just a minor overhaul that's required. But we know that both major and minor changes to eating habits can be difficult to make because there's sometimes complete confusion about where to begin. Hopefully the suggestions which follow will dispel the confusion and will help you put the necessary changes into place.

Buy organically grown produce

A switch to eating organically grown produce can be made quite easily. Where once organic produce was only found in tired heaps at the local village markets, there are now many retail outlets which supply this type of produce, and in most capital cities there are home delivery services as well. You'll find the word 'organic' or 'biodynamic' appearing on more and more labels, although remember there will be nutrient losses when food has been put in a packet, can or bottle. Fresh is definitely best and your organic supplier should be able to tell you what 'grade' the farm has been given if you are in any doubt about the source of the organic produce. While you may find that organic produce is slightly more expensive than regular fruit, vegetables and meat, we feel that the long-term benefits and savings far outweigh the short-term extra expense. Organic animal produce may be less readily available than organic fruit and vegetables, but since many contaminants are stored in fat, it's well worth seeking out a supplier.

Set goals

- Set some realistic goals and when making changes to eating habits, don't try to make them all at once.

- But do remember that you haven't got forever to implement these changes. Your changing body and your growing baby need those nutrients right now.

- Get rid of all those sugary, salty, refined foods and drinks straightaway.

- Replace white bread with brown; white rice with brown rice.

- Eat an orange, apple (or any other fruit) and drink some water, instead of drinking juice.

- This week you could start your day with a nutritious breakfast and mid-morning snack, then next week include a healthy lunch and afternoon tea. Before you know it you're eating and snacking well all through the day.

Dealing with cravings

- One sugar hit leads to another. Heavy consumption of products containing sugar can lead to fluctuating blood sugar levels and when your body is in the too low phase (hypoglycaemic) you will crave more sugar to get it back into the normal (or the elevated) phase. These unstable blood sugar levels are a significant contributing factor in morning sickness.

- Do remember that human beings have a natural affinity for sweet foods. The theory is that there was an evolutionary advantage to those who selected the piece of fruit. (Do you feel better now that you've got an excuse?) So if you simply can't get through your day without a sweet fix, a date or two is preferable to a chocolate bar. If sweet cravings are really bad, consider supplementing with some extra magnesium (especially if the cravings are for chocolate), and GTF (Glucose Tolerance Factor) chromium to help control those blood sugar levels. Zinc deficiency also affects taste sensation, leading to cravings, so you may need more zinc too. There's a simple test for this which we'll explain in the next chapter (on supplements). The problem is that refined carbohydrates (white flour, bread and rice, alcohol and all forms of sugar), reduce these nutrients, leading to further cravings. This is because carbohydrates require these nutrients (and the B-complex vitamins) for their metabolism, but have lost them during the refining process, so take them from your body instead. This vicious cycle is another reason why going 'cold turkey' on sugary foods is necessary.

- Be aware that soft drinks may contain up to seven teaspoonful of sugar, and be careful too of excessive consumption of fruit juices which will contain a lot of 'natural' sugar. It's better to eat a whole apple or orange and have a drink of water instead.

- Pregnant women have a reputation for weird food cravings which, so the belief goes, should be indulged. Endless cartoons depict the male of the species heading off at some ungodly hour to locate whatever it is that his partner fancies. Cravings for charcoal, chalk and other oddities have been reported. However, we believe weird food cravings are a sign of nutrient deficiencies and shouldn't be indulged but rather should be a warning sign that your nutrition is in need of serious attention.

Shopping trips

- Shop at the organic produce store. Chances are that most of your food choices will be of the right sort.

- If you need to shop at the supermarket, go when you're well fed. You're much less likely to be tempted by inappropriate snacks.

- Avoid shopping with children (this may be a luxury you'll only enjoy if this is your first pregnancy). Otherwise, we wish you well as you negotiate the aisles full of inappropriate food choices, all of which your children will know intimately from their (occasional, we hope) television viewing.

- Avoid shopping with your partner, unless he's a dedicated health-food expert (on second thoughts, don't leave him at home, just educate him and let him do it all for you).

- Work out menus for the week ahead and shop for the menu.

- Read labels. By this we mean the list of ingredients, not the advertising. Be aware of all the various guises of sugar (remember all the words ending in 'ose', honey, corn, starch, malt, molasses, syrup etc.). Some processed cereals may contain almost 50 per cent refined sugar, and are therefore almost completely devoid of essential nutrients.

- You might consider the cost of whole, fresh, high-quality produce prohibitive. But when you compare this to refined, processed and packaged foods, you should also factor doctors' visits and pharmaceuticals into the cost of the latter, both during your pregnancy and your family's life. And don't forget the cost to the environment! Then the cost of whole, fresh, uncontaminated food becomes bargain basement stuff.

Eating out

- Eat food you have prepared at home more often. Restrict eating out and getting takeaways to special occasions only.

- Eat a good breakfast before you leave home, then you'll have less need of snacks and takeaways. If a bowl of muesli or a cooked breakfast is too heavy for you, have some fresh fruit with natural yoghurt and add a handful of nuts and seeds.

- Carry healthy snacks with you at all times. Almonds, which can stabilise blood sugar levels, are convenient and good for alleviating that seedy feeling of early pregnancy.

- Take a packed lunch from home. Prepare a big bowl of salad vegies the night before (leaving them whole). Add some whole grain bread with red salmon or goat's cheese. Try an avocado with a dressing of olive oil and chopped herbs.

- When you do eat out and you've no choice but the white rice option, just relax and forget about it, but don't make it an excuse to slip back into unhealthy habits. Remember, it's what you eat 90 per cent of the time that counts!

Eating at home

- Make sure you have a variety of delicious, healthy foods to munch on when hungry. This avoids trips to the corner shop where you will usually only find inappropriate snacks.

- The added time taken to chew a meal which is high in complex carbohydrates such as brown rice means that you'll actually have to set aside some time to finish a meal. This is not only much healthier for your digestive system but it's actually very good training for family life.

- Have good whole grain bread and nut spreads from the health food store available at all times. (Remember to keep nut products in the fridge.)

- Keep carrots, celery, cherry tomatoes and button mushrooms handy. If your emphasis is always on fresh vegies, salads and fruit, you should always have something nutritious to snack on.

- Keep a selection of nuts and seeds in the fridge too.

Food preparation

- Find a good recipe book with the emphasis on whole unrefined foods and minimal preparation. (We are planning a Better Babies cookbook, but meanwhile we have suggested some titles in Recommended Reading.)

- Make your own soups. Use all the vegies in your fridge and throw in some lentils, split peas or barley with some herbs and spices. Do as much of this preparation as you can in the food processor to avoid excessive cooking.

- Bake your own bread from organically grown, stoneground flour.

- Cook some brown rice and put it in the fridge. Then it's ready to mix with sweet things such as stewed fruit, or savoury foods such as salmon and tomatoes, spiced up with a little tamari.

- Make the food look attractive—nothing looks better or more inviting than fresh, carefully prepared food.

- Change your methods of cooking. Replace roasting and deep-frying with steaming and stir-frying.

- Grow your own vegies, keep your own chooks. Just make sure your garden isn't full of lead and pesticides. Chooks are even better than a compost heap or a worm farm—they produce eggs as well as fertiliser!

Stay motivated

- Answer the food-related questions in Appendix 5, and see how you rate.

- Refer frequently to this chapter.

- Pin your diet summary on your kitchen wall (see Appendix 1).

- Say an affirmation. For example, 'Better food, better pregnancy, better baby' or 'I need nutrients for two'.

- And remember—don't despair, forget the guilt, one or two transgressions won't really do you any harm—it's what you eat 90 per cent of the time that counts.

Start your exercise program

You might wonder what exercise has to do with changing your eating habits, but you'll soon discover that the endorphins which are produced when you exercise regularly are wonderful things. Not only are they mood enhancers, but they are also appetite suppressants so they can help you to make the necessary improvement to your diet.

WEIGHT GAIN DURING PREGNANCY

Before we leave this very important topic of diet we just want to say a word about weight gain during pregnancy. If you attend faithfully to all of our nutritional and lifestyle guidelines during pregnancy, your weight gain will be adequate, but may be considerably less than what obstetricians and gynaecologists presently consider normal. However, they rarely see truly well-nourished women eating a whole food, unrefined diet. The weight gains of women eating a refined Western diet are often very substantial, due to over-consumption of refined carbohydrates and fat. Some of this weight gain may also be due to oedema (fluid retention), a condition which is also based in faulty nutrition. We are certainly not advocating that you attempt to limit your weight gain (10–13 kilos is about average). We are simply saying that if you faithfully follow the diet we recommend, you will gain the appropriate amount of weight for you and your baby.

Once you've attended to your diet and started on your exercise program (see Chapter 9 for details) you should be feeling quite positive and enthusiastic about some of the other changes which you need to make, and believe it or not, once you're in this positive frame of mind, these changes seem to fall quite naturally into place. In the following chapters we'll talk more about what these other changes are.

Nutritional supplementation

chapter 4

You might think that nutritional supplements are superfluous if you're faithfully following all the guidelines we've just laid down for eating well. Lots of people do and we hear comments like this one all the time.

'I like to get all my vitamins and minerals from my diet.'

In response we usually reply, 'We'd like you to be able to get all your nutrients from your diet too.'

However, you frequently don't (or can't) and we recommend you take a comprehensive and balanced combination of supplementary vitamins, trace minerals and essential fatty acids as an insurance policy, at the very least. It's important that you take this combination of supplements during the whole time that you're breastfeeding as well as during your pregnancy. In fact there are so many studies to show the benefits of supplementation with regard to every aspect of your health through every period of your life, we wonder why you'd ever stop.

A HEALTHY DIET IS NOT ENOUGH

Unfortunately, a great deal of confusion and uncertainty surrounds the use of nutritional supplements, particularly during pregnancy. It seems that the full impact of thousands of scientific studies which fill dozens of peer-reviewed journals in the USA, UK, Europe and Australia hasn't yet filtered down to all health professionals and some of them are still in the dark ages of believing that, 'Anyone who eats a reasonably varied diet will have an adequate supply of vitamins and minerals and taking supplements only creates expensive urine.' This was how her lecturer introduced the subject of nutrition to Janette when she studied pharmacy (and that wasn't quite in the dark ages either; only a little over 30 years ago).

What this vast body of nutritional research shows is that in between optimal health (which means a better pregnancy) and a frank deficiency state such as scurvy, there exists a large grey area of sub-clinical deficiencies of many kinds. Unlike 'frank' or undisguised deficiency states, sub-clinical deficiencies are disguised. However, these sub-clinical deficiencies are responsible for many of the problem conditions of pregnancy and are also implicated in more serious reproductive failures such as infertility, miscarriage and premature birth. But many health professionals, particularly those who are caring for women during their reproductive years, are not well informed about recent nutritional studies. Their training has frequently devoted no more than a few hours to this enormously complex and important subject. Because their knowledge is inadequate or outdated, these professionals still often caution women against routine supplementation during pregnancy, or inappropriately prescribe one or two isolated nutrients.

WHY SUPPLEMENT THROUGH PREGNANCY?

Nutritional needs may double during pregnancy

Probably the most compelling reason for supplementing during pregnancy is those increased nutritional needs of which we've already spoken. During your pregnancy your nutritional needs may double—remember we said you need *'nutrients for two'*. But remember we also said you're definitely not *eating for two*. Your food intake should only increase by about one-fifth.

Nutritional needs vary in individuals

Every individual is biochemically different and it may be impossible for some of you to receive an adequate nutrient intake from diet alone (no matter how nutritious it is). This biochemical individuality appears to explain to some extent the heightened folic acid (folate) requirements which are observed in some individuals. It seems that about 10 per cent of the white population has a genetic variability in an enzyme involved in folate metabolism. When this enzyme is impaired, folate requirements increase and when these are not met during early pregnancy, the risk of a baby with a neural tube defect increases. As more research is done, it is certain that other enzyme defects which are linked to various other essential nutrients will be revealed.

Nutrient content of food is variable

Remember too that the nutrient content of the food you've been eating most of your life is variable for a number of reasons. Australian soil is very old and non-sustainable farming methods have further depleted it of essential nutrients. For example, the uptake of zinc from soil is seriously disrupted by non-organic agricultural methods. Animals are grazed on fodder which has been grown on these impoverished soils and they may be fed antibiotics and hormones. They are dipped or drenched in a variety of chemicals. As we've already pointed out, there is serious doubt about the health and nutritional value of the produce grown and raised by non-sustainable farming methods. Even if you switch to organic whole foods right now, there'll still be deficits to make up from a lifetime of eating non-organic produce.

Pollution takes a toll on nutrients

You live in a very polluted environment. You can do a great deal to reduce your personal chemical exposure in the home, the garden and at work and we're going to discuss that in Chapter 6, but exposure to pollution is unavoidable, and your body requires many essential nutrients to detoxify the heavy metals, chemicals and additives found in food, the water supply and in the air. For example, zinc, which is vital for you and your baby, is used by your body to excrete toxic metals such as cadmium and lead, and food colourings of the tartrazine group also increase the excretion of zinc. Other nutrients are used to protect the body from the effects of radiation.

Lifestyle factors deplete nutrient levels

Before reading this book you may have smoked and drunk alcohol, tea, coffee and Coca-Cola, all of which draw heavily on your stores of zinc. You may have lived a lifestyle which was stressful. Stress increases requirements for zinc and all the B-complex vitamins. You may have used oral contraceptives which have a profoundly adverse effect on zinc and folate status as well as that of most other nutrients. Zinc status is also disrupted by copper IUDs, and by the use of inorganic iron supplements. Gastrointestinal malabsorption, caused by allergies or other conditions, may have been a problem for some of you. All of these factors, and others such as growth (even muscle growth during exercise) and illness, significantly increase your requirements of essential nutrients.

WHICH SUPPLEMENTS SHOULD I TAKE?

We recommend the following general daily dosages of supplements during pregnancy. Of course you should always consult a professional if you have any serious health concerns.

SUPPLEMENT	DAILY DOSAGE
Vitamin A	10,000 IU *or* 6 mg beta-carotene (choose mixed carotenes if available)
B-complex vitamins	B1, B2, B3, B5: 50 mg B6: 50 mg, or 100 mg if nauseated (can be higher: if necessary up to 250 mg to prevent nausea)

B12: 400 mcg
Choline, Inositol, PABA: 25 mg
Biotin: 200 mcg
Folic acid: 500 mcg (increase this to 1000 mcg if you have suffered a previous miscarriage, if there is a history of neural tube defects in your family, or if you are over 40 years of age)

Vitamin C	1–2 g (take the higher dose if you are exposed to toxicity or in contact with, or suffering from, infection)
Bioflavonoids	500–1000 mg (helpful for preventing miscarriage and breakthrough bleeding)
Vitamin D	200 IU
Vitamin E	500 IU (increasing to 800 IU during last trimester)
Calcium	800 mg (increasing to 1200 mg during middle trimester when your baby's bones are forming, or if symptoms such as leg cramps indicate an increased need)
Magnesium	400 mg (half the dose of calcium)
Potassium	15 mg or as cell salt (potassium chloride, 3 tablets)
Iron	Supplement only if need is proven; dosage depends on serum ferritin levels (stored iron) If levels < 30 mcg per litre, take 30 mg If levels < 45 mcg per litre, take 20 mg If levels < 60 mcg per litre, take 10 mg This test for ferritin levels should be repeated at the end of each trimester, and we give further details in Chapter 11.
Manganese	10 mg

Zinc	20–60 mg, taken last thing at night on an empty stomach (dose level to depend on results of zinc taste test, which ideally should be performed at two monthly intervals during your pregnancy; see page 172–174 for details)
Chromium	100–200 mcg (upper limit applies to those with sugar cravings or with proven need)
Selenium	100–200 mcg (upper limit for those exposed to high levels of heavy metal or chemical pollution). Selenium is best taken away from vitamin C, but can be taken with zinc.
Iodine	75 mcg (or take 150 mg of kelp instead)
Acidophilus/Bifidus	Half to one teaspoonful, one to three times daily (upper limits for those who suffer from thrush)
Evening primrose oil	500–1000 mg two to three times daily
MaxEPA (or deep sea fish oils)	500–1000 mg two to three times daily
Garlic	2000–5000 mg (higher levels for those exposed to toxins)
Silica	20 mg
Copper	1–2 mg (but only if zinc levels are adequate)
Hydrochloric acid and digestive enzymes	For those with digestive problems. There are numerous proprietary preparations which contain an appropriate combination of active ingredients. Ask your health practitioner, pharmacist or health food shop for guidance, and take as directed on the label.
Co-enzyme Q10	10 mg daily

The importance of zinc

When your zinc status is inadequate your taste sensation is impaired. This impairment means that the subtle flavours of fruit and vegetables are lost, and you will tend to favour very sweet or very salty foods which will invariably be unhealthy food choices. To restore the flavour of the healthy food choices you need to improve your zinc status. As your zinc status improves, your ability to taste subtle flavours improves, and you can start to change your eating habits without too much distress.

Testing for zinc deficiency

This is a test that we recommend you repeat every two months during your pregnancy. It's extremely simple, and merely involves taking 5 ml of a solution of zinc sulphate into your mouth. (You can buy this solution or have it made up at your local pharmacy.)

We call this the zinc taste test.

If you experience a strong, unpleasant taste promptly, your zinc status is adequate, but you still need to maintain it with supplementation (at the lower end of our recommended dose range). This supplementation can be taken in tablet form.

If you experience something which is more like a dry furry sensation, your zinc status is marginal. If you experience no taste at all, you are zinc deficient. In both instances you must supplement using a liquid product. (You can use the same product you used for the taste test or a more concentrated form which contains the necessary co-factors and which is available as a proprietary product.) Full instructions and dosage guidelines for the test are given in Chapter 11.

White spots on your fingernails are another sign of zinc deficiency! You'll probably notice that lots of people have them. Your observations bear out the fact that zinc deficiency is widespread amongst the general population. In fact it's now considered to be the most widespread deficiency in the Western world. In Australia a CSIRO study published in *Nurtritional Research* in 1991 showed that the diets of 67 per cent of Australian men and 85 per cent of women were below the recommended daily allowance in zinc. However, whichever marker you're using, and whether you're zinc deficient or not, you'll still need to take some form of zinc supplement.

Incidentally, markers like white spots on the fingernails and no taste sensation, while they may appear a little unscientific to some people, are actually quite useful benchmarks. (In fact, if the zinc taste test shows that you are zinc deficient, you can assume that your nutritional status is generally below par.) These and other physical markers, which indicate a variety of nutrient deficiencies, can be more instructive than blood levels, since the body's homoeostatic mechanisms will always endeavour to keep blood levels constant. (Refer to Appendix 4.)

Zinc supplementation

If your zinc status is quite compromised then the liquid preparation is the best way to improve it quickly, simply because if you are zinc deficient your zinc absorption from a tablet preparation is impaired—it's a vicious cycle isn't it? You must continue to supplement with the liquid preparation until you experience a definite taste sensation with the taste test. Then you can revert to supplementing with tablets, which you should also be using if your zinc status is already adequate. This will ensure that levels of this very important nutrient are maintained throughout your pregnancy.

These tablets should contain zinc chelate, in combination with zinc's co-factors magnesium, manganese, vitamin A and vitamin B6. Zinc should always be taken away from food and other supplements (though it can be taken with selenium). Last thing at night, on an empty stomach, is a good time.

HINTS ON TAKING YOUR SUPPLEMENTS

You might wonder how on earth you'll find time to take all these supplements—or find the space to store them. Rest assured, there are a number of multivitamin and mineral formulae available which contain approximately the dosages of nutrients we've recommended above. You could start by visiting a health food shop or pharmacy. Remember to take your supplements daily and bear in mind the following do's and don'ts.

Avoid isolated nutrients and mega-doses

If you demonstrate an increased need for a particular nutrient (e.g. white spots on your fingernails indicating a zinc deficiency), you should avoid supplementation with a single nutrient in isolation, or a nutrient taken in mega-doses. This is because one nutrient taken in excess over a period of time can lead to a deficiency in another.

Take folic acid with other B vitamins

The Medical Research Corneil Study, published in *The Lancet* in 1991, represented the work of eight years in 33 international centres. It showed that folic acid taken before and around the time of conception can prevent neural tube defects, but it is particularly important that you take your folic acid supplement in tandem with other B-complex vitamins. Folic acid supplements are now routinely given to women who are thinking about having a family. But folic acid is one of the B-complex group of vitamins. These vitamins never exist on their own in nature. They occur together and they work together and in some instances they can substitute for one another.

This means that supplements of single B vitamins should not be given. If you take one of this group of nutrients alone, or in mega-doses, over an extended period, you can induce a deficiency in one of the other members of the group. So if folic acid is given alone over months or years (especially in the high doses which are often prescribed), a deficiency in one of the other B vitamins will be induced. Folic acid also interferes with zinc absorption, so not surprisingly, since both zinc and the B vitamins are involved in many aspects of reproduction, such a deficiency could lead, ironically, to a baby with a condition just as disabling as the one you have been trying to avoid.

Avoid inorganic iron or isolated calcium supplements

Similarly, inorganic iron supplements which are frequently prescribed for anaemia compete with zinc for uptake and metabolism. Since zinc is probably the most important trace element for the pregnant woman, iron supplementation (if it is proven necessary) should contain an organic compound (such as iron chelate) and should only be given in combination with a full range of essential trace elements, fatty acids and vitamins. Too much calcium (which is often routinely prescribed during pregnancy) can also reduce the uptake of zinc (which is rarely prescribed along with the calcium, although zinc is probably more important). Calcium can only be utilized properly in the presence of an adequate (and proportional) supply of magnesium and vitamin D.

Avoid mega-doses of Vitamin C

Vitamin C is a powerful anti-oxidant which protects against the toxicity of heavy metals, pesticides and other environmental pollutants, and also against the activity of mutagens which affect the chromosomes in sperm and ova. Vitamin C is necessary for hormone production, for the metabolism of essential fatty acids and must be present for the proper absorption of iron. It is important for the maintenance of you body's immune function and for the production of collagen. It promotes the integrity of skin, tissue and bone, and protects them from invasion by foreign organisms. Lack of vitamin C during pregnancy has been linked to an increased risk of miscarriage, spontaneous rupture of the membranes, and brain tumours in the offspring.

It's obviously important that you get adequate doses of vitamin C daily. We recommended between 1–2 g of vitamin C daily during your pregnancy, but suggest you take much larger doses only if they've been prescribed by your health practitioner. Mega-doses of vitamin C may put stresses on your kidneys, which are vulnerable during pregnancy.

Take Vitamin A in moderation

Vitamin A is important for the integrity of all the mucous membranes—the linings of the mouth, vagina and intestines are kept healthy in the presence of vitamin A, so this is an important nutrient for both the mother and the foetus. A deficiency of this nutrient can lead to breakdown of these membranes and invasion of the surfaces by infectious organisms such as thrush. Vitamin A is also essential for healthy eyes, skin, hair and teeth and for good bone structure. The formation of both red and white blood cells depends on vitamin A, as does the formation of all the hormones involved in reproduction and lactation. If vitamin A is deficient, there may be appetite loss and poor digestion, which will lead to further nutrient deficiencies.

Vitamin A deficiency in the foetus can result in eye defects of all sorts, including the complete absence of eyes. Hydrocephalus, heart defects, defects of the genito-urinary system, hernia of the diaphragm, deformed penis and undescended testicles are other conditions which have been linked to vitamin A deficiency.

However, it is now widely recognised that too much vitamin A during pregnancy can be teratogenic. In other words, vitamin A in high doses can lead to birth defects. The Orthoplex Report, October 1993, states that a review of the literature reveals a total of 18 affected pregnancies where the mother took 25 000 IU–500 000 IU daily. More recent research by Rothman et al. at Boston University shows vitamin A may pose a danger when women take more than 10 000 IU per day.

While there is no doubt that reports exist of teratogenicity, it is important that you do not avoid modest amounts of vitamin A, because there are probably more incidences of congenital abnormalities due to a deficiency than there are incidences of teratogenic effects from an excess. Studies around the world have supplemented pregnant women with 6000 IU of vitamin A per day, and have demonstrated a lowering of the incidence of birth defects. Weston Price actually referred to the fat soluble vitamins as 'catalysts' or 'activators' upon which the assimilation of all the other nutrients depended. We consider 10 000 IU daily to be perfectly safe, but recommend that you do not exceed this dose. To be extra confident, you may prefer to take the equivalent dose of beta-carotene (6 mg) which is entirely non-toxic and which your body will convert to vitamin A as required. The latest research indicates that 'mixed carotenes', which occur in natural sources, may be the preferred approach to supplementation.

Don't forget essential fatty acids

Multivitamin and mineral supplements don't usually contain essential fatty acids so you need to include these very important nutrients in a separate supplement.

Take your supplements at mealtimes

Supplements should be taken regularly every day if they're going to have the maximum benefit. If you take them immediately before, during or straight after a meal they'll be better absorbed. The only exception is your zinc supplement which should be taken alone, not with food or other supplements (except selenium). Selenium should also be taken separately from food or supplements containing vitamin C (e.g. fruit and vegetables). Luckily, selenium and zinc can be taken together, so keep them by your bed to remind you to take them last thing at night (or first thing in the morning).

Get organized

Having to count out the required number of tablets each morning is time-consuming, and you can make life easier for yourself if you do your dispensing once a week—line up seven containers (old tablet vials are ideal, as are film canisters, but even plastic bags will do), and put a day's supply of tablets into each container. Then you can take the container with you through the day and take a few tablets with each meal. This will avoid any feeling of indigestion, which is not only uncomfortable, but will reduce nutrient absorption.

Digestive enzymes aid absorption

If you have digestive problems you can add a supplement of hydrochloric acid with pancreatic enzymes to aid absorption of all nutrients from food or supplements. You can also use 'bitter herbs', such as dandelion leaves or chicory, which act as a digestive tonic and can be added to your green salads.

What if tablets and capsules are hard to swallow?

You might find that supplements in tablet or capsule form are difficult to swallow. This sometimes happens when you're pregnant, particularly if you're suffering from nausea. Janette found that the half dozen supplements which she tossed down at one gulp every morning before her pregnancy needed to be taken one at a time once she was pregnant (and often later in the day) if they were to go down and stay down, and many of Francesca's patients find they need an alternative approach.

Micelles, which are soluble forms of vitamins and minerals, can be helpful in this case. Alternatively, powdered supplements can be taken. Since these may not contain the oil-soluble vitamins such as A and E, nor the essential fatty acids, these must still be taken separately. Essential fatty acids can be taken as an oil, which can be added to drinks, or simply swallowed.

START YOUR SUPPLEMENTATION PROGRAM WITHOUT DELAY

In the preceding pages we've briefly outlined the reasons we recommend supplementation during pregnancy. We've tried to make the reasons more cogent by using zinc and folic acid as examples of nutrients which are adversely affected by biochemical, dietary, lifestyle and environmental factors. However, zinc and folate are not unique. As we've tried to make clear, *all* of the nutrients have important roles to play during your pregnancy. However, all nutrients are lost or destroyed in ways which are similar to zinc and the B-complex vitamins. Therefore, if you consider that almost everything we eat, all of our lifestyle habits and everything in our environment are implicated in causing some sort of nutrient loss, you'll want to start on your supplementation program without delay.

An immediate start on your comprehensive supplementation program can help you improve your eating habits as well as your general nutritional status. The regular use of nutritional supplements can help to eliminate cravings for sweets and chocolate (chromium and magnesium are particularly useful) and can also regulate the mood swings and erratic behaviour which often lead to smoking, drinking and consumption of drinks containing caffeine. Not only will your diet improve, but you'll find your healthier lifestyle easier to adjust to.

But do remember that nutritional supplements cannot take the place of a whole food diet, a healthy lifestyle and a clean environment. A comprehensive, well-balanced vitamin, mineral and essential fatty acid supplementation program is only an insurance policy, not a substitute.

chapter 5

A healthy lifestyle

There is no doubt that various lifestyle factors such as the regular consumption of the social drugs, nicotine, alcohol and caffeine, and the use of either prescribed or recreational drugs, adversely affect general health. You shouldn't be too surprised that these habits adversely affect your reproductive health as well, and you certainly shouldn't be surprised that they affect the health of your developing baby.

Yet cautions against the use of these socially acceptable substances during pregnancy are often only very modest. Of course nicotine, alcohol and caffeine are not only widely consumed, but are often consumed by the very doctors and midwives who should be giving cautions about their use. This is undoubtedly the reason that cautions against any form of drug use during pregnancy are not much more forceful.

A BETTER PREGNANCY IS DRUG-FREE

Our recommendation is that all drugs, social or otherwise, should be completely avoided while you're pregnant. Cigarettes, alcohol, caffeine and other drugs not only adversely affect various organ systems, they also compromise the nutritional status which you're trying hard to improve. So there's no doubt they will seriously compromise your health during pregnancy and will also affect your ability to give birth easily and breastfeed successfully. Obviously if your general health is compromised, your baby's health will be affected in turn. However, these substances also have direct adverse effects on foetal development and growth.

Clearly, giving up all your bad habits as soon as possible will give you a much improved chance of a better pregnancy and a better baby. (If you're not pregnant yet, then our recommendations for giving up all of these substances apply to both you and your partner for at least the four months preceding conception.)

WHAT SHOULD I GIVE UP WHEN I'M PREGNANT?

Smoking

There are over 4000 active substances in cigarette smoke. These substances can cause cancer, cause changes to DNA, retard growth and suppress immune function, and at least 20 of them are known to be mutagens, or substances capable of causing genetic damage. Do you need any more reasons for giving up? What's more there is absolutely no doubt that women who smoke have a much higher risk of experiencing all sorts of problems during pregnancy and giving birth to a significantly smaller, less healthy baby than non-smoking women.

Smoking increases the risk of stillbirths, miscarriage and maternal rejection of the foetus at all stages of pregnancy. Smoking increases the risk of bleeding which can be regarded as a threatened rejection. It also reduces the rates of cell replication and protein synthesis, so can have profound effects during the first trimester when the rate of cell division is very high. Smoking has been shown to cause an increase in all congenital malformations including hare lip, cleft palate and malformations of the central nervous system, heart and digestive system. As if this weren't enough, cigarette smoking reduces oxygen delivery to the foetus and this results in babies born prematurely (and with low birth weight). Further, since the mid 1980s, several retro-

> **ADVERSE EFFECTS OF SMOKING**
>
> Low birth weight
> Premature birth
> Stillbirth
> Spontaneous abortion
> Foetal malformation
> Poor physical and mental health in children
> Poor immune function

spective studies have reported an increased frequency of both physical and mental health problems among young children born to smoking mothers. Diseases of the respiratory system (including asthma) were most widespread, while hyperactivity and other problems linked to impaired mental development were more common in the children of smokers.

Passive smoking

Remember that passive smoke inhalation has been shown to be almost as damaging as active smoking, so it's important when you give up cigarettes that your partner gives them up too. (And a recent study has shown that men who smoke run a much greater risk of fathering children who develop cancer and who suffer from asthma.) It's important that your workplace is also a smoke-free zone. (Fortunately, most are these days.)

Alcohol

Alcohol is a social poison which is so widely consumed that its ingestion is rarely considered as drug use, and the insidious thing about alcohol consumption is that very few experts are prepared to come right out and tell pregnant women to avoid alcohol completely. The more usual approach is to condone one or two drinks which gives the green light to alcohol consumption in general. Most drinkers seriously underestimate the amount of alcohol they consume, and it's very easy to 'top up' your glass of wine 'just a touch' once or twice ... or several times, or to just 'have a taste' or a 'sip'.

Drinkers are deficient in nutrients

Nor do these modest cautions take account of the fact that a regular drinker may be seriously deficient in nutrients (B-complex vitamins and essential minerals such as chromium, magnesium and zinc are particularly affected by alcohol). Of course these nutrient deficiencies will have an adverse effect on the drinker's health during pregnancy and on the development of the foetus, quite apart from the direct harmful effects of alcohol on both mother and child.

The most common chemical teratogen

We've known for a very long time that alcohol has extremely damaging effects on reproductive health. There are references in the Bible, and the ancient Greeks and Romans banned the drinking of alcohol by young women and newlyweds. It's interesting to compare this with our present relaxed attitudes about alcohol consumption which persist despite increasing recognition that alcohol is the most common chemical teratogen causing malformation and mental deficiency in human offspring. One of the foremost experts and contemporary researchers in this field is Dr Ann Streissguth of the Department of Psychiatry and Behavioural Sciences at the University of Washington, who has researched, published and lectured widely on the teratogenic effects of maternal alcohol consumption.

Foetal Alcohol Syndrome and Foetal Alcohol Effect

While the adverse effects of alcohol on various body systems and on reproduction have long been recognised, the condition which results from alcohol abuse during pregnancy has only been given clinical status relatively recently. Foetal Alcohol Syndrome (FAS) is the term used to describe the cluster of ill effects seen in the child of a woman who drinks moderately to heavily during pregnancy.

The most common characteristics of children born with FAS are growth, craniofacial, musculo-skeletal, cardiac and nervous system abnormalities, and neuro-developmental delay or mental retardation. Moderate to heavy alcohol consumption can be likened to 'social drinking' one or two drinks on most days, or a binge drinking session of five drinks or more on any one occasion.

While the full Foetal Alcohol Syndrome only occurs twice in every 1000 births, the less severe Foetal Alcohol Effect (FAE) is seen in a much larger percentage of children. FAE may occur after much lower levels of consumption and the number of children affected is truly unknown. The characteristics of FAE children include poorer overall performance as newborns, lighter weight, difficulties with habituation, weaker suck, disrupted sleep patterns and abnormal reflexes. They may be jittery and tremulous. Some of the effects are very subtle and it may be difficult to ascertain whether they are due to the consumption of alcohol or to other lifestyle or environmental factors. However the effects are not transient, and overall school performance is affected and on maturation these children

> **ADVERSE EFFECTS OF ALCOHOL**
>
> Growth abnormalities
> Cranio-facial abnormalities
> Musculo-skeletal abnormalities
> Cardiac abnormalities
> Nervous system abnormalities
> Neuro-developmental delay
> Mental deficiency

show subtle and permanent neurobehavioural deficits, and IQ and achievement decrements.

What we are certain of, however, is that there is no threshold below which alcohol fails to affect the foetus. In other words, even the smallest amount of alcohol will have some effect. Knowing this, we have no hesitation in advising you to avoid alcohol consumption completely during your pregnancy (and while breastfeeding). Because alcohol is a low molecular weight substance it is quite capable of crossing the placenta and the level in the foetal circulation approximates the level in the mother.

If you consider the size differential between foetus and mother you might be less inclined to have 'just one drink'.

Caffeine

Caffeine, which is contained in tea, coffee, soft drinks, chocolate, some processed foods and some medicines (such as pain relievers and

> **ADVERSE EFFECTS OF CAFFEINE**
>
> Miscarriage
> Chromosomal abnormalities
> Congenital abnormalities
> Late spontaneous abortion
> Foetal growth impairment
> Increased excretion of minerals
> Impaired absorption of iron

antihistamine preparations), is another drug you should completely avoid during pregnancy. Like all drugs, it is capable of significant pharmacological effects. It raises blood pressure and has a diuretic effect, increasing the excretion of many minerals, particularly zinc. And caffeine taken at the same time as a meal inhibits the absorption of iron.

As well as playing havoc with your nutritional status, the consumption of caffeine during pregnancy has been linked to miscarriage, chromosomal and congenital abnormalities and Sudden Infant Death Syndrome. Caffeine affects foetal growth and impairs the utilisation of oxygen by foetal cells. Pregnant women metabolise caffeine three times more slowly than non-pregnant women, which results in caffeine being accumulated and the foetus receiving very significant caffeine exposure. So even a small amount of caffeine can be dangerous and it is best completely avoided.

Pharmaceutical drugs

Pharmaceutical drugs include those bought over the counter for the treatment of minor ailments as well as those prescribed by medical practitioners.

Pharmaceutical drugs affect nutritional status

Most pharmaceutical drugs interact negatively with nutrients, and consequently compromise your nutritional status and all aspects of your reproductive health. Just a few examples here will suffice. (See page 77 for what to do if you still need to take medication.)

Pharmaceutical drugs	*Nutritional interaction*
Antibiotics	Deplete B-complex vitamins and, due to alteration of normal gut flora, decrease synthesis of vitamins K and B-complex
Anticonvulsants (for epilepsy)	Decrease folate
Aspirin	Decreases blood folate, increases excretion of vitamin C
Diuretics	Increase excretion of essential minerals
Laxatives	Generally decrease nutrient absorption
Oral contraceptives	Alter the whole nutritional profile, with zinc levels particularly adversely affected
Ulcer treatment	Decreases mineral absorption

The mutagenic effect of pharmaceutical drugs

More serious than the drug–nutrient interactions, however, are the more direct ways in which your baby may be adversely affected by drugs. Mutagenic agents in pharmaceutical drugs may cause changes in your baby's genes or chromosomes, resulting in birth defects or miscarriage. Mutagenic substances should be avoided in *any* dose.

The teratogenic effect of pharmaceutical drugs

A teratogen is a chemical which affects the development of the embryo's organs. (This occurs particularly during the first trimester.) Most of you will remember the thalidomide 'disaster' which alerted the world to the teratogenic effect of that drug. An anti-nausea preparation, it was prescribed for morning sickness, but caused limb-reduction deformities in some of the babies born subsequently.

Interestingly, the ill effects of thalidomide may have been due to the fact that it resembled the vitamin B2 molecule. This resemblance meant there was competition for absorption at the B2 receptor sites and this effectively made a woman who was taking thalidomide deficient in vitamin B2. It is possible that other teratogens act by similar nutrient-related pathways. Fortunately, most pregnant women are now well aware that they must avoid drugs during the critical first trimester when there is the greatest potential for damage to the developing embryo. However, this awareness should extend beyond the first trimester and to pharmaceutical preparations of all sorts.

Other adverse effects of pharmaceutical drugs

There are still more reasons for avoiding pharmaceutical drug use of any kind during pregnancy, as many commonly used preparations have effects which are specifically contra-indicated at this time. Here are a few examples.

- *Aspirin* decreases the viscosity of the blood and will increase the tendency to bleed in both the mother and the newborn. This has serious implications in the later stages of pregnancy.

- Commonly used *migraine preparations* (such as Migral), which contain derivatives of ergotamine, will cause uterine contractions and can lead to premature labour or hypertonic contractions during labour.

- *Anti-inflammatory drugs* of the non-steroidal type (such as Brufen and

> **ADVERSE EFFECTS OF PHARMACEUTICAL DRUGS**
>
> Drug–nutrient interactions
> Mutagenic effects
> Teratogenic effects
> Disturbed electrolyte balance
> Depressed newborn respiratory function
> Increased bleeding
> Premature labour
> Prolonged labour
> Discoloured teeth
> Abnormally slow foetal heartbeat

Naprosyn) inhibit the synthesis of the prostaglandins which stimulate labour, and therefore have the ability to prolong it.

- All commonly used *diuretics*, which increase urine output (and may be prescribed to reduce oedema or swelling), enter the foetal circulation and cause disturbances to electrolyte (sodium/potassium) balance.

- Some *antihypertensive drugs* (which lower high blood pressure) cause the heart rate of the foetus or newborn to slow abnormally.

- *Antibiotics* of the tetracycline family affect the teeth during the period of mineralisation (that is during the second and third trimesters and during the first eight years of a child's life), leading to discolouration.

- Commonly used *tranquillisers* and *hypnotics* of the benzodiazepine class (such as Valium and Serepax), if used routinely during pregnancy, can lead to depressed respiratory function, low blood pressure and lowered body temperature in the newborn. Babies born to mothers addicted to benzodiazepine tranquillisers are more likely to be admitted to intensive care than those born to mothers who are heroin addicts, can experience withdrawal symptoms for up to three months after birth, and display negative effects to brain function which may only become evident during adolescence.

Street/recreational drugs

Any of the so-called 'street drugs' (marijuana, cocaine, heroin, crack, speed, ecstasy and so on) should be completely avoided. Drug use of this type during pregnancy has the potential for all manner of adverse effects on the mother's health and may cause growth retardation, miscarriage, malformation and stillbirth. There may be long-term effects on growth and behaviour if the baby survives. Even occasional use of

---

ADVERSE EFFECTS OF STREET DRUGS

Miscarriage
Foetal growth retardation
Stillbirth
Malformation
Infection
Prematurity
Jaundice
Respiratory distress
Prenatal mortality
Long-term effects on growth and behaviour

substances of this type can be very damaging and it may be necessary to enlist professional help in breaking this addiction.

HOW TO GIVE UP HARMFUL SUBSTANCES

You've never had a better reason than your pregnancy to give up your bad habits. Thankfully, this will be a very strong motivation, but make no mistake, some of these lifestyle factors are very addictive. You might need a bit of help to go with your motivation. Let's look at some of the things that can make breaking these habits a little easier.

Breaking away from alcohol, caffeine, cigarettes and street drugs

Bear in mind that smoking, drinking, caffeine consumption and 'soft' drug taking are all factors over which you have complete control, and which you can change in a very positive way. (In that they're different from environmental factors over which you may have a lot less control.) So look at this list of things anyone can do to break an

---

BREAKING ADDICTIONS

Eat regular nutritious meals and snacks
Have healthy food available at all times
Take your supplements regularly
Avoid sugary snacks and drinks
Avoid situations which call for coffee, cigarettes or alcohol
Avoid stressful situations
Use exercise, yoga, meditation to reduce stress
Keep busy
Get your partner to give up these habits too
Think positively
Say an affirmation
Do a visualisation

addiction and grab your chance really to clean up your lifestyle and take a very positive step towards a better pregnancy.

If all of this fails, and you still find it difficult and stressful to avoid these everyday drugs, or if the spirit is willing but the flesh is weak, we suggest hypnotherapy. At the Jocelyn Centre, Francesca finds that this is the most helpful support for those patients who are finding such lifestyle changes too challenging.

Reducing your need for pharmaceutical drugs

With careful attention to all aspects of your diet and lifestyle during pregnancy, minor ailments such as headaches, constipation and so on will be vastly reduced and this is also usually the case with chronic conditions. Obviously, in some instances, medication will still be necessary, but a practitioner who has training in nutritional and environmental medicine will be able to prescribe supplements to help make up for those nutritional imbalances which may be induced by pharmaceutical drugs. Your doctor may also be able to prescribe alternative drugs which are less problematic.

If you do suffer minor discomforts despite your best efforts, there are lots of natural alternatives to pharmaceutical drugs to try. Chapter 13 discusses lots of ways to treat both minor and not so minor complaints, without resort to pharmaceutical drugs.

HEALTH CONCERNS FOR THE TRAVELLER

While being pregnant means you should watch your diet and cut out those unhealthy habits you've meant to kick for years anyway, it doesn't mean you have to stop doing everything you enjoy. As we keep saying, pregnancy isn't an illness to be endured, it's a special time of your life to be relished and enjoyed. So don't mope at home feeling sorry for yourself—get on with your life as you otherwise would, holidays included! You may have to take a few extra precautions and forgo a few risky pleasures, but you can still have a great time.

We know that lots of you will see your pregnancy as the last opportunity for a holiday alone together for quite some time. You may also feel it's your last chance to take that much desired trip to some exotic and little-visited location. We hate to tell you but you're probably right (in the short term) on both counts!

Flying

We'll see in the following chapter that flying increases your exposure to radiation and should be avoided during pregnancy, and especially in the first trimester. Another problem with flying during pregnancy is one of miscarriage. Although statistics can be quoted (and they often are) to show that the two are not related, we have rarely met a medical or health practitioner who is not cautious about flights, especially those undertaken during the first trimester. Many of these professionals have at least some anecdotal evidence of a link. Many IVF clinics give explicit advice not to fly during the first twelve weeks. We are certainly aware of a number of miscarriages which seem to be related to flights, and because of our other concerns we reiterate our recommendation against flying throughout the whole period of pregnancy.

Vaccinations

Travelling to international destinations brings concerns other than flying if you are pregnant. Depending on where you're going, your doctor may advise that you need to be vaccinated. Some vaccinations and anti-malarial drugs are clearly contra-indicated during pregnancy and your doctor will advise you about this. However, like a number of health practitioners, we have some concerns about all vaccinations and their long-term effects on the immune system.

Short-term effects are of equal concern. For six weeks following vaccination, levels of T-helper cells (part of your immune system) fall below the levels found in AIDS patients. This is usually the time (particularly in the case of short-term travellers) when you are most in need of a strong, fully functional immune system.

So if you're pregnant and your heart is still firmly set on that overseas trip, then you need to weigh up carefully the actual risks of contracting a disease in the country to which you are travelling. We feel that vaccination for travellers is often a case of massive overkill. The general assumption seems to be that the benefits of vaccination outweigh any risks, and you may feel that too, if it is only *your* health at risk. Of course, the situation is quite different when your unborn baby's health is involved. We certainly question the widespread and blanket vaccination of travellers, particularly those travelling from five-star resort to five-star resort in air-conditioned comfort.

Of course, not everybody travels from luxury resort to luxury resort (impecunious authors certainly don't!). If you're of the impoverished or hardy breed who like to take their holidays in untrekked and out of the way places, you need to look at the infections to which you might *really* be exposed (you'll find details in Appendix 9). However, if you're serious about having a better pregnancy, then you might also seriously consider leaving any trip to an area where there is a risk of contracting a very unpleasant infection until a more opportune moment. Not only are you risking infection, but you'll have difficulty eating really well and you'll have trouble getting enough purified water. In fact you'll be exposed to more problems than those created by the odd mosquito or water-borne infectious agent.

Remember there are fascinating untrekked and unvisited areas in this magnificent country of ours (most within reach by car, train or coach, and all no more than an hour or two's flying time away if you must fly), which are also blissfully free of the health problems which plague many overseas destinations. Trust us, the Amazon will still be there, and we have seen intrepid parents with intrepid small children travelling far off the beaten track.

Alternatives to vaccination

However, if you're committed to that trip and if you've also carefully assessed your chances of infection and decided against vaccination and anti-malarials, then it is essential that you put other precautions in place. As well as stimulating your immune system with nutritional supplements and herbal remedies there are other choices, including homoeopathic nosodes (details can be found in Appendix 9).

We also offer the following recommendations for staying well while travelling.

- Take a course of *Echinacea*, an immune stimulant herb, for several weeks before departure, and during travel.

- Take your full complement of nutritional supplements as outlined in Chapter 4. Nutrients which are particularly useful are those anti-oxidants directly involved in the immune response such as *zinc*, *vitamin C*, *selenium*, *vitamin E* and *beta-carotene*.

- Maintain the dietary recommendations we've already outlined as far as possible. We realise that this can be difficult while you're travelling, but poor dietary habits can seriously compromise your immune response. Sugar is a particular problem, as are refined carbohydrates (including alcohol).

- Drink only bottled water, or water which has been boiled (for one minute for each 300 metres above sea level), and avoid ice cubes in areas where sanitation is poor. Use bottled or boiled water to clean your teeth.

- If it is not possible to use bottled or boiled water, use an *iodine* or *citrus seed* extract additive to kill bacteria.

- There are portable water filters available commercially that can be used by travellers. If you don't have one of these, at least filter water through a fine cloth or a coffee filter paper.

- Only eat vegetables that have been cooked, or fruits that you can peel.

- Wash your hands thoroughly before touching your face or mouth and always before eating. Avoid wiping your hands on any sort of communal towel.

- Avoid dairy products, and foods made from them, and, although this is not our usual recommendation, use canned milk rather than fresh.

- Be aware of the source of any seafood you eat. Avoid it if it's from a polluted lake, river or ocean. You should also avoid swimming in polluted water.

- Use *citronella* as a mosquito repellent. Rub it on your skin or put it in an oil burner, and always sleep under a mosquito net. Avoid rural areas, especially those near water, at night. Soak your clothes and nets in citronella.

Happy travelling!

A clean environment

chapter 6

Environmental pollution means you are constantly exposed to an extremely potent chemical cocktail. It is estimated that you may be in contact with as many as 800 chemicals every day! (That makes 4800 if you're a smoker.) Of course, many of these chemicals affect you adversely, not only individually, but possibly also in combination (though very few studies have investigated this phenomenon). Nor have many studies been carried out to look at the effects of long-term, low-level exposure to compounds such as pesticides and plastics. However there is increasing recognition that some of these effects may include endocrine (hormone) disruption with profound implications for fertility and other aspects of reproductive health.

Few if any, generational studies have been made. So we really have very little idea of what effects your exposure to agricultural chemicals and to chemicals in the home, your holiday flights and your computer use, all combined with a mouthful of mercury (in the amalgam in your fillings) may have on your children, your grandchildren or even on your great-grandchildren.

However, there is no doubt that the effects of some environmental pollutants are synergistic. This means that the ill-effects are magnified when the two substances are present together. This is certainly the case with the heavy metals. You must also remember that some ill-effects will be more pronounced if your nutritional status is very compromised. For example, diets which are low in calcium, zinc, iron and manganese may enhance lead uptake. Of course, fortunately, the reverse also holds true to some extent.

YOU CAN CLEAN UP YOUR ENVIRONMENT

We're sorry if this paints a very grim picture. Environmental pollution is certainly ubiquitous, and quite frightening in the extent to which it affects every one of us. But in making you aware of its extent we hope we've also made you aware of just how important it is that you take whatever active steps you can to reduce your total exposure. We don't want you to hear all of this and just throw up your hands and say, 'How can I possibly have a healthy pregnancy or a healthy baby?' The reality is you can, but you need to take some positive steps to clean up your environment. What we want to look at now are those pollutants which you must avoid as far as possible.

HEAVY METALS

The heavy metals include lead, mercury, cadmium, and aluminium. These substances have no role whatever to play in human metabolism, but may displace essential minerals from enzymes and hormones. This can affect your health at any time, but especially your health during pregnancy. Heavy metals accumulate in the body, particularly in the placenta, which will affect your baby's development.

As you can see, there are many sources of heavy metal contamination. These substances are ubiquitous in our environment and you may not be able to avoid them all scrupulously, but it's important that you avoid as many as you can. We particularly caution against the common forms of exposure to mercury and lead described below.

SOURCES OF HEAVY METALS

LEAD
Leaded petrol, exhaust fumes, food grown in contaminated soil, lead-lined cans, bonemeal, old paint, dust, water supplies, plumbing alloys, tobacco, cosmetics, hair darkeners, coal burning, printing processes, batteries, metal polishes, glazed pottery, solder, crystal, wine, electrical wiring, painted toys

CADMIUM
Cigarette smoke, water supplies, plumbing alloys, manufacturing processes associated with paint, batteries, electronic equipment, television sets, photography, burning plastics, electroplating, rustproofing, welding, solders, fungicides, pesticides, ceramics, shredded rubber tyres, processed foods, evaporated milk, phosphate fertilisers, shellfish

MERCURY
Dental amalgam, electrical appliances, laboratory measuring equipment, paint, fluorescent lights, batteries, felt, pesticides, fungicides, contaminated water supplies, bottom-dwelling fish, fish high in food chain, soft contact lens solutions, vaccine products, haemorrhoid suppositories, nasal sprays, vaginal gels, cosmetics

ALUMINIUM
Cookware, white flour, salt, baking powder, milk substitutes, processed cheese, food colour additives, preservatives, antiperspirants (especially sprays, which may be inhaled), toothpastes, antacids, water supplies, aluminium foil, 'tetra' packs, some brands of soya milk

If dental work is unavoidable during your pregnancy, ask your dentist to use composite resins instead of products containing mercury. If you need the name of a sympathetic dentist, you should contact the Australasian Society for Oral Medicine and Toxicology (see Contacts and Resources). Sympathetic dentists should be quite easy to find these days, since the National Health & Medical Research Council, in August 1997, withdrew its endorsement of the safety of dental mercury amalgam. Also remember to tell your dentist that you're pregnant and that you want to avoid X-rays. It's probably a good idea to avoid the injection of local anaesthetic as well. Take this opportunity to focus on your breathing instead of any pain you might be feeling—think of it as a little trial run for labour.

If you really must renovate
Pregnancy is definitely not the best time to renovate, since so many of the products used are toxic. However this seems to be the time when couples are most inspired to build an extension, rip out a wall or two and scrape off all the old paint, often lead-based. We know you want to create a pleasant environment for your new baby, but honestly, a baby takes up hardly any room at all, and will be much more enchanted by being physically close to you than having a freshly painted room to himself! In fact a baby won't need a separate room for a very long while (and we'll talk more of this in our next book). However, we do agree that the whole family will be much better off without the old flaking lead-based paint— just make sure you follow all the guidelines for its appropriate removal and disposal! We recommend that you contact the Environmental Protection Authority in New South Wales or the equivalent agency in your state for comprehensive guidelines and, if possible, have a professional company attend to the work on your behalf.

How to counteract heavy metals
Since the ill-effects of heavy metals may be more pronounced in those individuals who have compromised nutritional status or whose systems are too acidic, an organic whole food diet rich in alkali-producing foods such as vegetables, coupled with a comprehensive supplementation program, is going to boost your body's defences against these substances. Foods which are good at getting rid of heavy metals include *legumes* (lentils, chickpeas and all the dried beans), *garlic*, and *apples* stewed with their pips (which contain pectin). If you've been exposed to heavy metals in the past or if you think you're still exposed now, your nutritional supplements should include extra *vitamin C* (in dosages at the higher end of our recommended range) and extra *selenium*, *zinc* and *garlic*. While this will give your body the best chance of dealing with the toxic metals, you must avoid exposure to them as well.

If you are really concerned about exposure, test kits are available to detect the presence of heavy metals in urine. Although this test provides limited information on the degree of contamination and by which metals, it can be useful to indicate whether there is a problem or not (and when it has been resolved).

If this test is positive you may want further information so you can identify and exclude sources of contamination, and use gentle (nutritional) detox measures detailed in Chapter 7. The best test for this purpose is the hair trace mineral analysis (HTMA). (See Appendix 11 for details.)

CHEMICALS

Chemicals in the food supply

It has been estimated that as many as 20 000 chemicals are presently in use in food production and manufacture. About 4000 of these are added directly to the food supply, but only about 10 per cent of the 4000 are actually listed on labels. Almost every facet of our food supply is subject to some sort of chemical treatment.

First the seed is fumigated, then the plant is sprayed during planting, growing and harvesting and it is also fertilised a number of times. Further chemical treatment is carried out during storage or before transport. Then of course there is refining and processing, and finally cooking and serving (condiments, sauces, relishes etc.). Livestock may be fed antibiotics and hormones and will be dipped or drenched as well. In non-sustainable farming operations, something, mostly in the form of a chemical, is added to the original product at every step of the production process. We wrote earlier of the reasons for buying organically grown and fed produce. Not surprisingly, there is a significant reduction in chemical residues of all types in produce grown by sustainable or organic methods.

Chemicals in the workplace

Many individuals are constantly exposed to numerous toxic compounds (or radiation, which we will discuss shortly) in the course of their work, many of which may be harmful to their health. Some at-risk occupations include the following:

- Hairdressers
- Motor mechanics
- Auto manufacturers and repairers
- Dentists
- Hospital and healthcare workers
- Anaesthetists
- Radiologists
- Industrial cleaners
- Domestic cleaners
- Long-distance drivers
- Couriers in city traffic
- Builders and renovators
- Artists and jewellers
- Glass and pottery workers
- Electrical workers
- Food workers
- Electronic and semiconductor workers
- Chemical workers
- Clothing, textile and leather workers
- Factory workers
- Agricultural workers and farmers
- Printers
- Home handymen/women
- Lead lighters
- Plumbers
- Painters
- Pest controllers
- Flight attendants and pilots
- Smelter and foundry workers

Workers exposed to the following are also at risk:
- Intense heat
- Overhead cabling
- Dust
- Pollution
- Spraying
- Constant traffic
- Frequent flying

If you are exposed to chemicals at work you should seek expert advice about the harm they may cause to your developing baby or your reproductive health. People who work in the same industry may not be your best source of advice as they have a vested interest in playing down the risks to which you might be exposed. An independent body such as the Environmental Protection Authority, Worksafe Australia or the Toxic Chemicals Committee (see Contacts and Resources) may be a better source of information. However, it is important that you not only acquaint yourself with possible adverse effects, but that you take the potential threat to your baby's health very seriously. If you consider that the threats to your own and your child's health are too great, you should seriously consider alternative work arrangements during your pregnancy. Your employer is legally required to change your working conditions or hours, to offer suitable alternative work or to suspend you on full pay, if your health or safety is at risk.

Chemicals in the home

So much for the contamination of your food supply and your work environment. Don't think you're safe when you get inside your front door! When you open your kitchen, laundry or bathroom cupboards, or the door of the garden shed, you'll encounter a further assortment of products containing chemicals. Many of the most commonly used household chemicals (such as glues, paints, insecticide sprays, mould treatments, oven cleaners, ammonia-based cleaning materials and other products which contain organic solvents) have known adverse effects on human health, so there's absolutely no doubt at all that they will have adverse effects on the developing embryo and foetus. There are even problematic substances in floor coverings, furniture and building materials. Stanford University researcher Wayne Ott, who was with America's Environmental Protection Agency for 30 years, has likened your indoor environment, where you may spend up to 95 per cent of your day, to a 'toxic dump', and a study carried out by Dr Judy Ford, in Adelaide, showed a clear link between many of these substances and miscarriage or congenital abnormalities.

Kitchen, laundry and bathroom alternatives
In many instances you can reduce your exposure to chemicals when you're at home by re-educating yourself to use safer, less toxic

products. There are numerous environmentally and reproductively safe choices for use in the kitchen, the laundry and the garden. Health food shops offer ranges of cleaning products (and personal care products as well) which are non-polluting and pose no threat to your or your baby's health.

> ### SOME ALTERNATIVES FOR CHEMICALS USED IN THE HOME
>
> Sodium bicarbonate for stainless steel, chrome, enamel
> Borax for floors, tiled surfaces
> Salt for sinks, chopping boards, glass, marble, Laminex
> White vinegar in hot water for cork, slate, lino, tiles
> Lemon juice : Olive oil (1 : 2) as furniture polish
> Hot wash (65°C) + Sunshine for nappies
> Pot-pourri or essential oils as air-freshener
> Companion planting to deter pests
> Light a match to burn off methane, the offensive-smelling gas that emanates from faeces

The toxic metals and pesticides which may be tracked in from outside to reside in your carpet can be reduced by wiping your feet on a commercial grade mat or, better still, leaving shoes outside. An effective vacuum cleaner, used regularly, will remove many pollutants (and this is particularly important when small children are learning to crawl and walk). Of course your organic whole food diet and your antioxidant supplements can help your body deal with unavoidable exposure.

We've already mentioned the dangers of renovating during pregnancy. However, if you're still committed to adding that family room and decorating the nursery there's really not much we can say, so in Contacts and Resources, we have listed suppliers of alternative products which are friendly to the environment and to your reproductive health. You can now find many non-toxic paints, solvent replacements and other products to use in the home if you simply must undertake those renovations.

Alternative treatments for household pests

Similarly, this is not a good time to spray your home for pests. But there are some essential oils which can be used very effectively, either around the house or applied directly on your body. You're probably already familiar with *Citronella*, which can be used to repel mosquitoes. This can be used in an oil burner, you can sprinkle it around the room, or rub it directly on your skin. You can do the same with *Lavender*, or *Neem* oils (neem oil is odourless, can be easily mixed with other oils, and protects against all biting insects). *Lemongrass* and *Lavender* oils are similarly useful for repelling flies, and *Peppermint* and *Spearmint* are useful for getting rid of cockroaches. Dab some of the oil directly on the areas where the cockroaches live—they'll soon move out! Beetles and slugs dislike a mixture of *Eucalyptus*, *Peppermint* and *Rosemary*, and mice are discouraged by *Peppermint* and *Spearmint*, which can be grown around the house or used as an oil. *Peppermint* and *Lavender* both discourage ants, so sprinkle some near their entry spots.

> **ALTERNATIVE TREATMENTS FOR PESTS**
>
> Citronella, lavender deter mosquitoes
>
> Lemongrass, lavender deter flies
>
> Peppermint, lavender deter ants
>
> Peppermint, spearmint deter cockroaches, mice
>
> Eucalyptus, peppermint, rosemary deter beetles, slugs
>
> Rosemary, lavender, lemon, cloves deter moths, fleas
>
> Neem deters all biting insects

Moths and fleas have an aversion to *Rosemary* or *Lavender*, which can be used in your wardrobe, as can *Lemon* or *Cloves*. You can use sachets of the flowers, with extra essential oils added. Though your cats and dogs may not be as fond of the smell of *Rosemary* as you are, they'll tolerate it better than the fleas, or the toxicity of other treatments. Mix some of the oils in warm water (25 ml to 1 litre) and spray it over your carpets, and wipe the undiluted oil on window frames. *Lavender* is an all-round insect repellent. A few drops on a light bulb keep moths away, and when used inside cupboards it will also deter silverfish. Other natural remedies include *Nettles*, soaked in water for two weeks, boiled for half an hour and left to cool (useful as a general insecticide), and *Pepper*, to keep cats off flowerbeds.

Pennyroyal and *Rue* are two oils traditionally used for pest control, but both of these are also abortifacients. If you use either of these to rid your house of insects, you must also take care to avoid direct exposure to the vapour, and make sure to wash your hands after handling. (Of course essential oils should *not* be taken internally during pregnancy.) This natural approach to pest control will not only be much safer than using chemical treatments, but will have the added benefit of making your home smell quite delightful!

NON-IONISING RADIATION

The non-ionising type of radiation is pervasive. Radio frequency radiation, including microwave radiation as well as radiation produced in electro-magnetic fields, falls into this category. This means that exposure comes from computer monitors, microwaves, mobile phones, fuse boxes, transmitter towers, power lines, electric blankets, waterbeds, clock-radios and the like. Heat generated by this type of radiation can cause tissue damage, depending on several factors including the wavelength of the radiation. There is much public concern regarding the potential health risks of electro-magnetic radiation, but unfortunately results of studies are not always definitive and in some instances results are completely conflicting.

But it is clearly emerging that non-ionising radiation can lead to many ill-effects, particularly during reproduction, and that the effects may be more pronounced in individuals who are exposed to a variety of other environmental stressors, and in individuals whose nutritional status is inadequate or whose systems are acidic. A study conducted in Canada and the USA found that 62.8 per cent of all pregnancies of computer users were marked by abnormalities of some kind, including miscarriages, premature and stillbirths, congenital abnormalities and respiratory illnesses. Studies from Sweden, Japan and Poland returned similar findings and all confirmed the fact that increased exposure meant increased risk of poor reproductive outcome.

Therefore we recommend that you avoid, as far as possible, exposure to this type of radiation throughout your pregnancy. Ideally you should limit the time you work in front of computer monitors (which emit eight different types of radiation) to no more than four hours per day. If at all possible, avoid this type of work altogether during the first trimester. However, this is obviously a difficult recommendation to adhere to. These days, most of you will spend some time in front of a computer and some of you will spend the major part of your working day exposed to this type of radiation. Fortunately, there are some protective measures which you can take.

Protective measures for computer users

Although none of these measures can completely eradicate all risk, if you put as many of them into place as you can, there will be a significant reduction in exposure.

- Be aware that the sides and back of a monitor can emit greater amounts of radiation than the front, so be careful how your unit is positioned in relation to those of co-workers.

- If you have a separate monitor and disk drive, you can turn your monitor off when it is not in use—the harmful radiation comes from the screen. Your computer can continue to run.

- Move away from the monitor (at least 1.5 metres) if you are involved in other work.

- Anti-radiation screens are available, which are not the same thing as anti-glare screens. The more expensive ones are the most effective (ain't it always the way!). Protective clothing can also be worn, and some employers (notably those in Scandinavia and the USA) are using such methods to reduce their workers' exposure to radiation from VDUs.

- Some small anti-radiation gadgets, which can be worn by the user, are also available. Alternatively these can be attached to the monitor or inserted between the plug and the socket. Some of these devices change the frequency of the whole circuit that they are plugged into, protecting all the units running off that circuit. (You can find details of these in Contacts and Resources.)

- The newer the screen, the lower the radiation output.

- Laptop computers don't emit radiation, as they use an LED display, not a cathode ray tube, and are a much healthier alternative, as long as you don't actually place them in your lap. If you do, the electromagnetic field is much closer to your growing baby and your reproductive system.

- One or two packets of *Epsom salts*, placed in front of the unit, are supposed to absorb radiation. The best place to put the packets is

> **PROTECT YOURSELF IF YOU USE A COMPUTER**
>
> Position unit carefully
> Turn off/move away
> Fit anti-radiation screen
> Wear/use anti-radiation device
> Use Epsom salts to soak up radiation
> Position green plants around your computer
> Consume anti-oxidant nutrients
> Use herbs to strengthen your body's defence system
> Use homoeopathic remedies to desensitise

between the bottom of the anti-radiation screen, where some leakage will occur, and your lower body. Replace the Epsom salts when their crystalline appearance changes to that of a dry flaky powder. You can tell when this has happened by shaking the packet if you don't wish to open it.

- Green plants growing in the work environment are also supposed to help by absorbing the radiation. Peace lilies and sunflowers are particularly useful.

- Anti-oxidant nutrients, such as *vitamins A, C & E, zinc* and *selenium* can also have a protective effect, as can *vitamin B5. Reiishi* and *Shiitake* mushrooms (available as tablets) and the herb *Burdock* (available as a tea) have also been shown to help recovery from radiation effects when taken internally.

- Take flower essence (*Yarrow*) or homoeopathic phenolic desensitising remedies (ask your naturopath about these).

Avoid electro-magnetic radiation (EMR) in your bedroom

In their book *Perils of Progress* John Ashton and Ron Laura of Newcastle University look at the health problems that go with the technological society. They say that electric blankets and heated waterbeds are among the worst electrical pollutants and their use appears to result in increased rates of miscarriage and slower foetal development, so turn off your electric blankets and other appliances when you turn off the light. Better still, unplug them, or turn off at the power source, especially if the appliance has a standby light which is still drawing current through your bedroom walls. This way you can have at least six to eight hours of each day free from this type of pollution. Remember that clock-radios emit some radiation from their glowing numerals, and check too that your bed isn't on the other side of the wall from a fuse box. Of course, if you live near a transmitter, high voltage power lines or an electricity substation it may be difficult to avoid EMR.

Protective measures for mobile phone users

- Use your mobile phone as little as possible—it's better kept for emergencies, not regular use.

- Keep your mobile phone switched off when not in use. Remember, it attracts radiation even if you are not making a call.

- When it is switched on, keep your phone away (at least one metre) from your lower body—though there are health concerns for all parts of your body, your baby is particularly vulnerable.

- Use a hands-free model when making calls. An earpiece can keep the phone away from your body.

- Use the same natural remedies we've suggested for computer users.

> **PROTECT YOURSELF IF YOU USE A MOBILE PHONE**
>
> Restrict use
> Switch off
> Keep away from body
> Use hands-free model
> Use anti-oxidants
> Use herbs to strengthen your body's defence system
> Use homoeopathic remedies to desensitise

Avoid ultrasound

Ultrasound should also be avoided and certainly should not be used routinely during pregnancy. There are no advantages, nor improvements in the eventual outcome of the pregnancy, for the woman who has regular ultrasound scans of her foetus. We'll deal with this issue more fully in Chapter 11.

IONISING RADIATION

Ionising radiation, which is associated with nuclear weapons, cosmic radiation and X-rays, is extremely damaging, particularly to rapidly dividing cells. If the cell is not killed the DNA may be damaged, and this can be passed on to daughter cells as division takes place, spreading the possible ill-effects. These include broken and misshapen chromosomes, mutated genes and early cell death. Since your baby's cells are dividing at the greatest rate during the first trimester this is the time when X-rays are most damaging. But X-rays (to any part of the body) should be undergone only if absolutely necessary, and always with full protection to your lower abdomen.

Cosmic radiation

Cosmic radiation is a particular problem for those who fly frequently. You may not realise that each international flight (where the aeroplane climbs to more than 10 000 metres) exposes you and your baby to the same amount of radiation you would experience if you had an X-ray through your whole body (or two chest X-rays). Domestic flights expose passengers to slighly less radiation, as the planes generally fly lower, although levels of cosmic radiation fluctuate considerably.

The work of Dr Eugen Jonas, undertaken in the 1950s in Czechoslovakia, and reported by Sheila Ostrander and Lynn Schroeder in their book *Astrological Birth Control*, suggests that conceptions occurring at times of certain planetary configurations (known to coincide with sunspot activity and a greater level of cosmic radiation) are more likely to result in deformed or non-viable foetuses. These configurations include 90° and 180° angles between the larger planets and the sun. It may be especially important to avoid flying at these times. An astrologer can calculate unfavourable dates for you.

Protection from cosmic radiation is difficult to achieve. There are some gadgets on the market (often taking the form of a necklace or pendant) which claim to protect the wearer. It has also been suggested that sitting in the middle of the plane (as opposed to next to the window) can help. The nutrients, herbs and homoeopathic remedies we've mentioned can be taken during, and for some weeks after, the flight. Of course you could make a suit of Epsom salts (a bit crunchy!)

or lead (a bit overweight?). However, the only absolutely certain protection is not to fly during your pregnancy.

Checklist of additional protective measures

In Appendix 5 you will find a questionnaire which you can use to gauge the levels of toxicity to which you are exposed (it can give you an idea of how healthy your diet and lifestyle are too!). This questionnaire will alert you to those things which you need to avoid, and we suggest you use it and update it regularly. However there are some additional protective measures which we have listed below.

- Avoid tinned foods, especially unlined or old tins, and never leave tins open in the fridge (tranfer contents to glass or plastic containers).

- Avoid fish caught in contaminated rivers, harbours and lakes, bottom-dwelling fish, crustaceans and large fish such as tuna, shark and swordfish (high in mercury).

- Avoid aluminium and copper cookware and kettles, and avoid cooking or storing food in aluminium foil (use baking paper instead.

- Don't cook high acid foods (e.g. tomatoes, rhubarb) in metal or ceramic dishes. Use heat-proof glass instead.

- Avoid carbon tetrachloride, used in dry cleaning, as it damages the liver.

- Check all chemicals you are exposed to at work. Use whatever safety and protective precautions you can.

- Don't handle lead storage batteries.

- Close car windows in heavy traffic and tunnels. Put net curtains over windows facing busy roads and wash them frequently.

- Use unleaded petrol and make sure your exhaust system is intact.

- Don't stand by the photocopier for extended periods.

- Move your bed if it's presently near, or on the other side of a wall from, a fuse box.
- Consider moving if you live close to a busy highway, flight path, transmitter tower or power lines.
- Use your mobile phone as little as possible, and don't carry it next to your reproductive system.

We hope you're now inspired to reduce your exposure to harmful environmental pollution. That's great, but as well as reducing your exposure to these toxic substances it's appropriate that you undergo a gentle detoxification program to compensate for past exposure. We look closely at detoxification—which will boost your chances of a better pregnancy—in the next chapter.

Detoxification

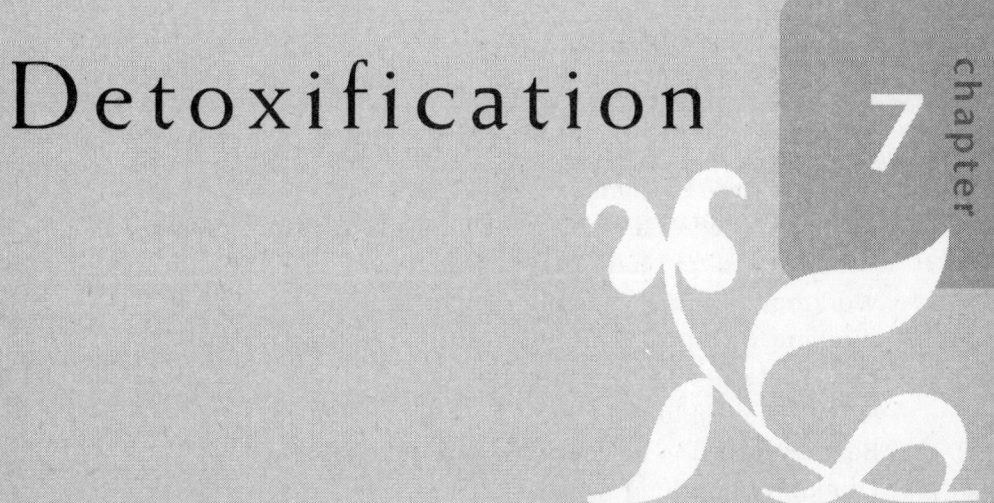

chapter 7

Continuing exposure to toxins is inevitable in today's society. Yet the optimal health of you and your baby relies on avoiding or eliminating them from your body as much as possible. (The easiest time to achieve this is before you conceive, and details are in Appendix 11.) While we don't recommend a rigorous detoxification program during your pregnancy, there are several measures which are still appropriate. If you cannot avoid doing any of the following (if you can you might let us know how on earth you manage it), it's important that gentle detoxification is carried out while you're pregnant.

ACTIVITIES WHICH MAKE 'DETOX' NECESSARY

- Using a computer
- Using a mobile phone
- Flying
- Living near power lines

- Sleeping near a fuse box
- Working with radiation (e.g. in hospitals and dental surgeries)
- Travelling through heavy traffic
- Living near a busy highway or under a flight path
- Being in close proximity to smokers
- Being exposed to agricultural chemicals or crop spraying
- Being exposed to industrial pollution
- Working with heavy metals, copper or iron
- Working with chemicals or industrial cleaning materials
- Living in a newly renovated house
- Being exposed to the fumes of paint, solvents or glues
- Being exposed to insecticides, garden sprays
- Drinking unpurified water
- Eating foods which are not organically grown, or which contain additives
- Getting stressed, sunburnt or exercising excessively (all cause oxidative stress or free radical damage)

As you can see, simply living in today's society makes it important that you protect yourself and your unborn baby from the ill-effects of lifestyle and environmental pollution.

Some of our suggestions for detox you can easily follow yourself, some are best carried out with the help of a practitioner; but none of them present a threat to you or your baby.

PURIFIED WATER IS THE SIMPLEST DETOX MEASURE

Drinking plenty of purified water is a simple and essential method of detoxification. The 8–12 glasses daily that we recommend will help detoxification by flushing toxins from your body via the kidneys. Most other drinks that you commonly consume are likely to contain caffeine, sugar, or chemical additives, and are better avoided.

Use only purified water

Make sure your drinking water is purified. Bottled spring water can be used as a substitute, though it may not be quite as reliably pure, and will definitely end up being more expensive in the long run. Unpurified water may be full of many of the toxins you are trying to avoid, such as agrochemicals, fluoride and heavy metals. Water may also travel through pipes made of copper or (less frequently) of lead, and can contain high levels of these metals too.

Toxins actually become concentrated when water is boiled, so boiling your water is not an alternative to purifying; indeed water that is used for cooking and hot drinks must be purified before being put into the kettle or saucepan. Vegetables also need to be washed and cooked in purified water, and if you add 25 ml of vinegar to 500 ml of water, this will help to remove surface lead. Soaking the vegies is not a good idea, as it will leach nutrients.

When buying a water purifier, ask for reliable information on how well it removes contaminants. You need to know that it will remove a very high proportion (95 per cent or more) of all heavy metals, copper and iron, pesticides, herbicides, chlorine (and its by-products) and parasites.

We recommend either reverse osmosis or block activated carbon purifiers with a long water contact time (with or without ion exchange) as the most effective. They can be fitted to your tap so you can easily switch from purified water to unpurified, for washing up. There is no significant problem using unpurified water for dishwashing, so you can extend the life of your filter by only using it when necessary. However, it is important to rinse detergent from all dishes and pans. In most cases, the jug-type purifiers are not sufficiently effective, though some of the clay models are relatively thorough. You will need to find out how often the removable filter needs replacing, and mark this in your diary. Never let the filter go beyond its use-by date, as it may dump trapped toxins back into the water. (In Appendix 10 you will find more guidelines on how to choose a purifier.)

DETOXIFYING NUTRIENTS

Consuming an organic whole food diet and taking regular supplementation as recommended in Chapters 3 and 4 are other simple avenues to detoxification.

Anti-oxidants

Supplements of anti-oxidant nutrients
These include zinc, selenium, vitamins C, E, and beta-carotene (or mixed carotenes) and are useful for helping to eliminate all kinds of toxins. Detox requirements are an additional reason why anti-oxidants are necessary during pregnancy. The dosages we have recommended in Chapter 4 will be sufficient in most cases, though extra emphasis may be required if you feel you are exposed to considerable levels of toxicity. Consult your natural health practitioner before increasing doses. It is preferable, during pregnancy to use beta-carotene rather than vitamin A, although there is absolutely no evidence to show that dosages of vitamin A up to 10 000 IU daily are any cause for concern.

Acidophilus and bifidus lactobacilli
These help to increase the healthy bacteria in the gut which control and decompose some of the precursors to oxidants which are so damaging to your baby's DNA, proteins and other essential nutrients. The lactobacilli are present in natural yoghurt or can be taken as a supplement.

Other foods which contain anti-oxidants
Foods such as fresh fruit and vegetables, garlic, onions, green tea, cold pressed olive oil, nuts and seeds, soya beans and other legumes, deep-sea cold-water fish, seaweed, apples and pears stewed with their pips (which contain pectin), and some common herbs such as *Marjoram* and *Rosemary* also work as detoxifiers, through anti-oxidant activity.

Other helpful anti-oxidant nutrients
These include *Co-enzyme Q10, pycnogenol* (from maritime bark), *grape seed* extract, *spirulina* and *lecithin* (which you can purchase in tablet form from a health food shop).

Some other detoxifying nutrients and foods
Listed below are the nutrients which your body uses to rid itself of heavy metals such as lead, mercury, cadmium and aluminium. (While

both iron and copper are needed by your body in small amounts, an excess of either can also be toxic.) From this chart you can get a really good idea of how environmental pollution adversely affects your nutritional status.

NUTRIENT/FOOD   HEAVY METAL DETOXIFIED

	Lead	Mercury	Aluminium	Cadmium	Iron	Copper
Calcium	Yes	-	Yes	Yes	-	Yes
Zinc	Yes	Yes	Yes	Yes	Yes	Yes
Chromium	Yes	-	-	Yes	Yes	-
Magnesium	-	-	Yes	-	Yes	-
Silica	-	-	Yes	-	-	-
Iron	-	Yes	-	-	-	-
Manganese	Yes	-	Yes	-	Yes	Yes
Selenium	Yes	Yes	Yes	Yes	-	-
Vitamin C	Yes	Yes	Yes	Yes	Yes	Yes
Vitamin D	Yes	-	-	-	-	-
Vitamin E	Yes	-	-	-	-	-
Vitamin B1	Yes	-	-	-	-	-
Vitamin B5	-	-	-	-	-	Yes
Copper	Yes	-	-	Yes	-	-
Molybdenum	-	-	-	-	-	Yes
Garlic/onions	Yes	Yes	Yes	Yes	-	-
Legumes	-	Yes	-	-	-	-
Algin	Yes	-	-	-	-	-
Citrus fruits	Yes	-	-	-	-	-
Black tea	Yes	-	-	-	-	-
Wheatgerm	Yes	-	-	-	-	-
Eggs	Yes	Yes	-	-	-	-
Asparagus	Yes	Yes	-	-	-	-
Brussel sprouts	Yes	Yes	-	-	-	-

You can see clearly why eating an organic whole food diet and taking your supplements is important. The essential nutrients they provide are necessary to rid your body of toxic metals. However, there are some further specific nutrients and foods you should know about which can protect you and your baby against other forms of pollution.

- *Selenium* is specific for general pollution detoxification (including heavy metals).
- *Vitamin B5* protects against radiation (and excess copper).
- *Vitamin A* activates the enzymes needed for detoxification.
- *Reiishi* and *Shiitake* (Japanese mushrooms) protect against the effects of radiation.
- *Citrus fruits* cleanse carcinogens and lead from the liver. (Citric acid aids excretion of heavy metals.)
- *Bananas* have anti-toxin qualities.
- *Apples* and *pears* (especially the pips) help to reduce absorption of toxins as well as aid detoxification through the action of pectin.
- *Cruciferous vegetables* (cabbage family) inhibit the carcinogenic effects of chemicals.
- *Brocolli* stimulates phase 1 and phase 2 (complete) detoxification processes in the liver.
- *Garlic* and *onion* are particularly potent detoxifiers of all pollutants.

A HEALTHY BOWEL AIDS DETOX

It's essential to have at least one easy, effective bowel motion daily to rid your body of poisons. If transit time is longer than this, toxic matter putrefies and ferments in the bowel. The motion should not smell foul, contain mucus or sink to the bottom of the toilet bowl. 'Fluffy floaters' are an indication of good bowel and liver function. Usually, if you're consuming a whole food diet, you shouldn't be troubled by constipation. But sometimes, despite your best efforts, you may need a little extra help.

Use dietary fibre instead of laxatives

Laxatives are not appropriate during pregnancy since they irritate the gut and impair absorption of nutrients. Fibre supplements can be very effective as they provide bulk and moisture for smooth elimination, help form soft, bulky stools which are easy to pass, are effective detoxifiers and act gently.

- *Oat bran* is preferable to *wheat bran* as a source of fibre, as quite a high proportion of people are wheat-sensitive and it can cause irritation in the intestines. The phytates in wheat can also reduce the absorption of iron and zinc which are both important nutrients during pregnancy.

- *Guar gum* is helpful and also keeps cholesterol levels down, as does *pectin*, which comes from apple or citrus fruits, and also has a special role in detoxification (as we've discussed).

- *Psyllium husks* are also a good source of fibre and are the active ingredient in many patent constipation remedies available from your health food shop or pharmacy.

Other remedies for healthy bowel function

Of course, as noted above, your diet should be an excellent source of roughage (fibre). Raw vegetables and fruits, brown rice, lentils, beans, peas, sprouts, seeds and nuts are all helpful. Dried fruits, especially figs and prunes, traditionally have been used to maintain healthy bowel function but these may be very high in sugar and may also contain chemical additives. Fresh figs (organically grown) are preferable.

You might also find the following hints helpful if you continue to experience constipation.

- The juice of a freshly squeezed *lemon*, taken in purified water, first thing in the morning before breakfast, aids healthy bowel function.

- Try *acidophilus powder* (or live natural yoghurt) which provides beneficial intestinal flora to keep the gut healthy.

- *Slippery elm* assists the smooth flow of the faeces.

- *Cold-pressed olive oil* cleans the gut and improves digestion and has been used traditionally for this purpose. It also stimulates bowel contraction, soothes the mucous membranes and promotes bile secretion in the liver.

- *Flax seed oil* (or seeds) has a similar action to olive oil.

- Adequate *purified water* will keep the faeces liquid. Remember to drink 8 to 12 glasses daily.

⚘ Good *zinc* status is important to reduce bowel toxicity—yet another reason to be sure you're getting enough of this valuable nutrient.

Exercise and massage can improve bowel function

Exercise can improve digestion and stimulate peristalsis (the motion of the large intestine as food passes through the gut). We look at exercising during pregnancy in Chapter 9. Massaging the abdominal region, especially in a clockwise direction, can have the same effect. Your baby will appreciate this hands-on attention too.

A HEALTHY LIVER AIDS DETOX

Your liver is the other important part of your digestive system that is involved in detoxification. A healthy and effectively functioning liver is essential to process any poisons you may have ingested. *Zinc, selenium*, the *B-complex vitamins* (especially *choline, folic acid* and *biotin*) and *vitamin E* all assist your liver to carry out this function, and there are also several very beneficial herbs and foods which can be used quite safely during pregnancy to boost liver function, and which are easily available.

Dandelion root is an excellent remedy for a sluggish liver and is used to make a coffee substitute, but take care that this contains no added sugar. *Globe artichoke* is a food which stimulates the liver, and so does the freshly squeezed *lemon juice* we recommended for constipation.

DETOX OCCURS THROUGH YOUR SKIN

As anyone who has suffered from pimples knows only too well, the skin is one of the body's channels for detoxification. Keeping your skin healthy and clean can assist this process, and make sure that unsightly blemishes don't result. The elimination of toxins takes place through the sweat glands, and the amount of waste cleared in this way has been estimated at half a kilogram a day!

Dry skin brushing can stimulate the circulation of blood and lymph, (which are the primary channels for removal of toxins from cells and tissue), open pores and remove the top layer of dead skin, dirt and acid, and deeply cleanse the pores without removing protective oils. Brush hard enough to produce a slight pink flush (but no harder). You may need a softer brush for your face than for your body.

Epsom salts baths will also draw out toxins and waste fluid through the sweat glands. Add half a kilo of Epsom salts to a warm bath and soak for 10 to 15 minutes.

EXERCISE, MASSAGE, DEEP BREATHING, AND SUNLIGHT HELP DETOX

We've discussed how exercise can encourage peristalsis and improve digestion. It also, through the pumping action of arms and legs, stimulates the flow of lymph around your body, which carries away toxins and debris.

Exercise will also help you to breathe more deeply and regularly. This is especially true of yoga, where breathing techniques are an integral part of the exercise process. This can help you to clean out the deeper recesses of your lungs (which are often untouched by the shallow breaths which most people take) and allow you to eliminate waste as you exhale.

Breathing deeply can become more difficult as your tummy expands in pregnancy, so it's useful to pay some attention to this process.

To practise deep breathing, place your hand on the top of your ever-increasing tummy, and feel it get even bigger as you pull the diaphragm down as far as you can as you expand your lungs, drawing in air. Then pull your tummy back in (comparatively speaking!) and feel your diaphragm push the air out of your lungs again. Breathe in through your nose and out through your mouth and, if helpful, imagine your lungs as two big balloons, inflating and deflating.

Of course, if the air around you is polluted, breathing deeply can increase your level of toxicity. Negative ionisers or air purifiers can improve the air quality in your home or work environment. Ionisers can also help to reduce stress by improving your mood. You probably know how tense you can feel as a storm builds (when positive ions are prevalent) and how your feelings of wellbeing increase after the storm, when this situation is reversed.

Speaking of wellbeing, lymphatic massage is a delightful way to achieve lymphatic drainage, which reduces toxicity and can be combined with essential oils which help this process. Of course essential oils can also be used for a number of other purposes, such as calming and relaxing. (We'll be giving more information on essential oils in Chapters 10 and 13.)

Sunlight has also been shown to help the removal of toxins, so don't shun it. Simply take care with extended midday exposure when UV levels are high, use hats in place of sunglasses (except in cases of high UV exposure such as the snow), and avoid tinted windows.

Of course, the best approach is preventative, and this means rigorously avoiding the harmful substances and conditions covered in the environment and lifestyle chapters. As this is very difficult to achieve in today's society, despite your best efforts, a gentle, ongoing detox through pregnancy will be important for most pregnant mums. It will, of course, also contribute to your feeling of wellbeing, as well as your baby's health.

Because a more rigorous detox than we've outlined here is difficult (and can even be dangerous) during pregnancy, we've included, in Appendix 11, some ideas on how a more extensive detox program can be achieved in the preconception months, for those of you who are able to take advantage of this easier approach.

Allergies and infections

ALLERGIES

Do certain foods bring you out in hives, give you catarrh, send you into paroxysms of sneezing or coughing, bring on diarrhoea or abdominal pains or simply make you feel decidedly 'second-hand'? If the answer is 'yes', then you're probably like a significant proportion of the population who have an allergy or sensitivity to a certain food or foods. Of course, some of the effects of allergy may be much more subtle and you may not relate the way you feel to something you've eaten. For example, some of those second-hand effects we talk about can range from feeling hyped up or irritable to feeling depressed and falling asleep after your lunch break.

Perhaps it's not foods that are a problem for you. It might be airborne pollution, dust mites, mould, animal fur or feathers, grass pollens, perfumes or chemical solvents that affect you. These offenders might make you sneeze, become wheezy and breathless, itch all over, develop migraines or exhibit any number of other symptoms. If this is the case, then once again you're in good company. A large percentage of the population also reacts adversely to substances in the environment. It's hardly surprising really when you consider the number of chemicals you're exposed to. Of course this brings us back to the reasons why you should avoid as many chemical contaminants as you can. In reducing the total toxic load on all systems you give your body—and your baby—a much better chance of being able to cope with those you simply can't avoid.

Why allergies are a problem

Allergic mother—allergic child
While your child shares your body, he also shares your allergic responses. The more frequent or severe these responses are, the more likely it is that your baby will be vulnerable to these same responses as a child and adult. Unfortunately, many people are unaware of their allergies and sensitivities; as the adverse response becomes chronic, it's accepted as 'just the way things are'.

If you have general feelings of malaise or fatigue (and you may have experienced these for years), then it's worth considering some of the approaches and diagnostic methods we outline here, or consulting with a natural health practitioner who specialises in allergy detection, as there are often non-invasive tests that can be carried out during pregnancy.

A practitioner may also be able to help you devise a realistic dietary plan, if you are having difficulty sorting it out yourself, but eating according to our recommendations and avoiding prolonged or frequent contact with allergens will make a considerable difference. However, total avoidance of the offending substances appears to be less effective in protecting your child than substantially reducing exposure.

Of course a strong immune system is your best defence against allergy, and good nutrition is an essential precursor to this, but ironically this is a chicken-and-egg situation, so the allergy must be effectively dealt with first.

Allergy means compromised nutritional status
Unfortunately if you have an allergic profile this means that your nutritional status is compromised. A food allergy can impair absorption of

essential minerals and vitamins, and other nutrients are used up as your body tries to restore itself to balance and good health. Obviously this can affect your health and that of your baby. One of the reasons we recommend nutritional supplements is to make up for the deficits which might be due to an allergic condition.

How to identify allergens

Some common food allergens include cow's milk dairy products, beef, wheat (and rye, oats and maize), eggs (and chicken meat), citrus fruits, pork, peanuts, yeast, cane and beet sugar, and food additives such as colourings and preservatives. If you suspect that food allergies or sensitivities are a problem for you, and therefore for your baby, there are several very simple tests which you can administer yourself to identify the culprits.

Which food do you crave?

First of all, you could ask yourself which food you crave. If you can identify a food which you believe you simply could not live without, then that food is frequently the offender.

Keeping a food diary

An extremely simple way to identify allergens is to start keeping a record of what foods you've eaten in the six-, 12- and 24-hour periods that have preceded adverse symptoms such as fatigue or hyperactivity. You might also note any unusual environmental circumstances.

The pulse test

The pulse test is another way to identify possible problem foods. You simply take your resting pulse rate then eat a normal size portion of the suspect food. After eating, you take your pulse rate again at 10-minute intervals for an hour, and if the rate is elevated or lowered by more than 10 beats per minute, that food is likely to be one which is affecting you adversely. Remember not to confuse an increased pulse rate with increased physical activity—make sure you stay relatively quiet while you're applying this test.

Kinesiology, or muscle testing

Another way to easily detect sensitivity or allergy, or even to determine if a food (or condition) is helpful or not, is through kinesiology, or muscle testing. This is best carried out by a trained practitioner, although you can learn to use a simple form quite effectively at home. It can also be used to suggest which treatment is most effective or which organ or system needs attention. You need to stand erect with one arm extended, level to the shoulder. The practitioner or 'tester' places one hand on your extended arm at the wrist and the other on your opposite shoulder. If you then imagine a strengthening situation (such as eating a bowl of green salad) followed by a weakening situation (such as eating a bowl of white sugar) and the 'tester' presses down firmly on your extended wrist after each visualisation, there should be a detectable difference in resistance.

These two baseline responses can then be used as a benchmark while you imagine (or affirm out loud) that you are eating/experiencing a certain food/situation. Even better, you might hold up the food, with your free hand, to your thymus area (at the base of your neck above your breast bone), or place a small amount under your tongue. This method of testing is remarkably accurate and generally as reliable as any other method of allergy testing, though much simpler and less expensive!

Dowsing

If your practitioner has experience in using a pendulum (dowsing), he or she may be able to obtain quite accurate clues as to which foods or conditions are affecting you. This can be done by swinging the pendulum over the food (or even over the written name of the food) while maintaining contact with you.

Both muscle testing and dowsing can also be used to ask questions such as, 'How often can I eat this food? Once a week? Every other day?' and, 'How long do I need to abstain from this food? A week? A month?' etc. This sort of testing can also be used to answer questions of dosage, duration and appropriateness of treatment.

Warning: Provocation testing (which involves introducing a sample of the suspected substance and observing the reaction) and elimination diets are *not* recommended during pregnancy.

Avoid problem foods/chemicals and take your supplements

Once you're certain that you're reacting adversely to something you eat, inhale, touch or are otherwise exposed to, there are several things that we recommend you do during your pregnancy.

- First of all you should avoid any foods which you know are definite problem ones for you. It's often more difficult to avoid airborne allergens such as pollen, but it's important that you do the very best you can. The total avoidance of many foods is extremely difficult, but don't panic! If you aim for total avoidance you'll probably end up with a very occasional exposure to, or ingestion of, the allergen—fortunately, recent research shows that this is even better, in terms of the outcome for your child and his allergic status, than complete abstention, as long as the exposure is infrequent and only to small amounts of the offending substance.

- Use our recommended doses of nutritional supplements throughout your pregnancy (and during the full period of breastfeeding as well).

- There are some useful herbs which act as immune system modulators, helping to prevent an over-reaction of the immune system, such as *Hemidesmus*, and reducing allergic response, for example *Albizzia*.

- Maintain a healthy diet and gentle detoxification program, and avoid pollutants whenever possible.

By doing all of these things you will improve your own general health because the total stress on your immune and other organ systems will be reduced. You'll also give your baby a better chance of nutritional adequacy, a better chance of an immune system which isn't compromised and consequently a better chance of being free from similar allergies and sensitivities.

Don't eat cow's milk products if you're allergic to them

We certainly don't recommend that you continue to eat an offending food, even if it's one which is generally considered essential for pregnant women. We mention this because many women have a morbid fear of going without cow's milk during their pregnancy—they imagine a child with brittle bones and teeth falling from its head. Since milk is by far the most common allergenic food (hardly surprising when it contains hundreds of very reactive phenolic compounds which we'll talk about in just a moment), many of you will be allergic to cow's milk and products made from it. Surprisingly, both you and your baby will actually be better off without these products, since constant consumption can lead to nutritional deficits and a very compromised maternal immune system (and probably a child with a similar allergy).

Now that we've hit you with an iconoclastic statement about avoiding dairy foods during pregnancy, our reputations will be mud in orthodox circles, but there are a few relevant facts which might help to reassure you about our recommendation. Minerals such as zinc and magnesium, and nutrients such as vitamin A, are as equally important as calcium in bone and teeth formation. Magnesium in fact is the only mineral which has been demonstrated to increase bone density.

Furthermore, calcium is actually very poorly absorbed from cow's milk, and if you're allergic to cow's milk, that absorption is even further impaired.

We'd also like to remind you that a significant proportion of the world's population cannot tolerate dairy foods, yet manage to obtain all the calcium they need from other sources. Remember too that weight-bearing exercise keeps calcium in your bones (we'll look at this further in Chapter 9).

Non-cow's milk sources of calcium

There are numerous foods which are good sources of calcium if you cannot tolerate cow's milk. Milk, yoghurt and cheese from goats or sheep, seaweed, collard leaves, beet, dandelion and turnip greens, parsley, watercress, broccoli, spinach, sesame seeds (hulled), tahini paste, almonds, brazil nuts, tofu, ripe olives, cooked soya beans, salmon and sardines (with the bones) are all good sources of calcium. Of course if there's still some doubt in your mind (and we understand this, given the pervasive influence of the dairy industry), a supplement containing calcium is always your insurance policy. Remember that such a supplement should not be taken alone (since it will inhibit the absorption of zinc and iron), but should only be taken as part of our full recommended supplementation program.

You don't need to avoid problem allergens forever

Once the offending substances have been recognised, it shouldn't be necessary for you to live on a totally restricted diet or in a sterile atmosphere. There is much that can be done using natural medicine to strengthen your immune, digestive and other systems. It should in fact be possible, with an improved diet and lifestyle, and generally strengthened systems to re-introduce the offending substances (dietary ones anyway) on a rotating basis. This is in fact preferable to total exclusion. Research shows that a child is less likely to be allergic to substances which have been eaten in moderation during pregnancy rather than totally avoided.

What if you can't detect or avoid the allergenic substances?

If you know that you're reacting adversely to foods, chemicals or other substances but aren't really sure just what the offenders are, avoidance is obviously going to be difficult, if not impossible, to achieve. However, you should be able to get at least some very good clues from the tests we've already described.

There is also a fairly new and innovative treatment for allergy or sensitivity which can be used during pregnancy, and this may be a treatment option for you. It is non-toxic and easily administered and can be used to treat multiple allergies safely and effectively, even during pregnancy. This technique, known as phenolic desensitisation using homoeopathic remedies, has the potential to make the treatment of all sufferers of these conditions much simpler and more effective.

Phenolic desensitisation using homoeopathic remedies

This procedure was pioneered by Robert W. Gardner PhD, biochemist and emeritus professor of Animal Science (Animal Nutrition) at Brigham Young University, Utah. Dr Gardner was motivated to explore this topic because he suffered from total food allergy himself. He was afflicted with a progressively worsening condition which meant that everything he ingested caused one or more adverse reactions. After undergoing conventional medical treatments to no avail, it was suggested that as a biochemist, he might be able to find answers that had eluded the physicians to whom he had looked for help.

The common belief has always been that allergies are caused by the protein fraction in foods and other substances. However, Robert Gardner found that only about 10 per cent of reactions are actually due to the protein fraction, and that about 90 per cent of sensitivities or allergies are due to the phenolic compounds which are found in food, perfumes, chemicals and drugs. Phenolics (or aromatics as they are also sometimes called) are compounds that colour, flavour and preserve foods and living organisms. They give you most of your sensory perception of your environment. They are the chemical codes, passwords and defences that all living organisms use to know their place in the world.

However, the breakdown of phenolics results in such pharmacologically active chemicals as histamine, serotonin, tryptamine, tyramine, and dopamine, to name just a few. Some phenolics are so abundant in nature as to be in virtually every plant source. While they are essential to life as we know it, when metabolised incorrectly, they can cause major and minor physical, mental and emotional disturbances in large numbers of patients.

Cow's milk is ranked as one of the most allergenic foods in the entire human diet. Up to 20 per cent of the forage in a cow's diet may be phenolics and when coupled with fermentation products from the rumen, milk becomes a composite of a large array of very reactive phenolic compounds. It is estimated that cow's milk contains 500 of these compounds, 200 more than the next most allergenic food.

Ironically, it has been proven that homoeopathic dilutions of phenolics, taken under the tongue, can not only immediately relieve symptoms, but over a period of time can permanently cure the allergy. In this procedure, several drops of a one per cent solution of the compound are placed under the tongue, and the reaction is observed. A positive response occurs when there is a change of pulse, blood pressure, symptoms begin or are intensified, or changes in handwriting or similar function are observed.

If the one per cent dilution gives a reaction, the number 2 dilution is tested. The number 2 is made of one part of the number 1 dilution and four parts of water. Progressively, more dilute solutions are tested until the patient reaches the dilution which reverses the symptoms, and this becomes the neutralising dilution. Because under the tongue testing is such a laborious method, many practitioners use electro-dermal testing, using a machine which monitors changes in electrical 'hot spots' on the skin (similar to acupuncture points). Both this method and kinesiology (muscle testing) can quickly ascertain the neutralising dilution.

Phenolic therapy seems to offer a wide array of options for the treatment of allergies and other health problems. Benefits of treatment by this means include the rapid relief of symptoms (unlike conventional injection therapy, which may take many years), good patient compliance and long-term tolerance to the allergens. Additionally, it's easy and safe and relatively cheap. The technique of rapid neutralisation with phenolics has the potential to become the preferred method of therapy for allergic problems. It can be used safely during pregnancy.

(As with detoxification, allergy treatments can be more easily implemented before conception occurs. See Appendix 11 for more details.)

CANDIDA

A very problematic infection which is common during pregnancy is chronic or intestinal candida. *Candida albicans*, normally a benign yeast organism present in the gut (and in all mucous membranes) but held in check by 'good' bacteria can, in some circumstances, proliferate and cause an invasive overgrowth. In many instances, chronic candida occurs together with other infections, particularly those of the genito-urinary type, and is a significant contributing factor in a vast range of different disorders (both physical and mental), and in a full range of compromised reproductive outcomes, which include infertility, miscarriage, premature birth and compromised health in the newborn. It can also adversely affect your ability to digest and absorb those oh-so-vital nutrients.

If ill-health is due to this condition, it is essential that once it is diagnosed, it is also properly treated, and that it is kept under control throughout the pregnancy (when it is likely to worsen, due to the high level of circulating hormones). Diagnosis and treatment will be most effective if supervised by a health professional, but will also involve you in many self-help measures.

Is it candida?

The first sign of candida is often an ongoing vaginal infection with discharge, a yeasty smell, intense itching or soreness. This is usually referred to as 'thrush', and is often what people mean when they refer to candida. If the vaginal condition won't go away, or keeps recurring, it is possible that your gut is also infected, and local treatment won't be effective.

You need to be sure you are suffering from candida and not some other infection so that you can be confident in your treatment. A lower vaginal swab, which can be performed safely during pregnancy (by a medical doctor) should reveal the presence of candida.

Local vaginal infestation is encouraged by:

- Hot weather
- Antibiotics
- Tight trousers
- Oral contraceptives
- Synthetic underwear
- Lack of acidity in the vagina (normal pH 5.5)
- Vaginal deodorants
- Intercourse (semen is alkaline)
- Soaps and detergents
- Wiping 'back to front'

If you suspect that you have candida, then you should avoid as many of these conditions as possible. Avoiding intercourse until the infection has cleared will also minimise cross-infection with your partner.

Intestinal candida is more difficult to diagnose, though your naturopath may have some suggestions, as there are various techniques and procedures which can help to identify this condition. You may be more likely to suffer from systemic candida if you have used antibiotics recently or frequently, taken the oral contraceptive pill or had a poor diet high in sugar and refined carbohydrates, as these will all act to disturb the delicate balance of 'healthy' bacteria and yeasts in your gut. Symptoms include:

- Fatigue
- Colic/abdominal pain
- Flatulence

- Food cravings
- Eczema/tinea
- Alcohol/sugar cravings/intolerance
- Dry flaky skin
- Digestive disturbances
- Rashes
- Depression/anxiety
- Difficulty concentrating
- Mood swings
- Muscle weakness
- Poor memory
- Nasal congestion
- Blurry vision
- Headaches
- Chronic respiratory infections
- Aches and pains
- Allergies (especially yeast and mould)
- Cystitis
- Itchiness (especially anal)

Treating candida

Since chronic candida is an indication of something much more fundamental amiss, the underlying problems must also be adequately addressed. An anti-candida diet must be rigorously followed. This diet excludes absolutely all refined carbohydrates and sugars, including alcohol, because they act as 'food' for the organism (which must be starved to be defeated). All products containing yeast (to which you may have become allergic) must also be strictly avoided, unless you are confident that they don't affect you adversely. The diet we have suggested, if followed assiduously, will address the problem, and you can assess your susceptibility to yeast products in the same way we have outlined for other allergies. (There are many good books on candida and its treatment; see Recommended Reading.)

The best local vaginal treatment of candida is with a tea-tree based cream used around the outer vaginal area, or acidophilus yoghurt (live culture) which can be very soothing internally. Treatment should be continued until symptoms have abated for several days, and/or you have a repeat vaginal swab which is clear.

Your partner may also need treatment. He can dunk his penis in a mixture of tea-tree oil (4 drops) and white vinegar (50 ml, or 2 tablespoons) in 2 litres of warm water (or use glycerine as a base). You may need to avoid having sex while treatment is carried out, since intercourse can cause the condition to flare up. Strictly speaking, candida is an infestation, not an infection, therefore it cannot be 'caught'. However it can spread to susceptible areas.

Treatment for intestinal candida requires action on several fronts simultaneously. You'll need to undertake all the following measures.

- Kill the yeast. This can be achieved through drugs such as Nystatin, which can be used safely during pregnancy. However, you may prefer to use gentle, natural remedies such as *Garlic, Citrus seed extract, Capryllic acid*, and herbs such as *Marjoram* (which can be used in your cooking). A garlic suppository (just a clove of garlic) can also be inserted anally.

- Starve the yeast. As we've already mentioned, you should eat no sugars (of any kind), no fruit (for the first month of the treatment and then re-introduce slowly), no refined carbohydrates (white flours/grains), and no alcohol. (Not that you'd dream of eating any of these things anyway!)

- Stabilise blood sugar levels. This is necessary to help prevent sugar cravings (which can be strong), since sugar feeds the troublesome yeasts. Here we would use *chromium*, and bitter herbs such as *Dandelion Root, Agrimony* and *Fringetree. Gymnema* (a very bitter herb) can be used to quell sugar cravings as they arise, as it neutralises the sugar receptors on the tongue. Put 1 or 2 drops in a little water, and swill around the mouth. Bitter herbs should be used with caution during pregnancy (i.e. as tea or as small doses of a fluid extract for a limited time only).

- Avoid allergens. This list is likely to include yeast-containing and fermented foods and fungi, but any food to which you are allergic can compromise your immune system, irritate your gut and undermine recovery.

- Boost the immune system. You can do this with herbs such as *Echinacea* and a full complement of nutrients, especially the *B-complex vitamins* and *zinc*.

※ Re-establish gut flora. These are beneficial bacteria which, in normal circumstances, keep the yeast under control. This healthy balance has to be restored, and you can achieve this with live *acidophilus* and *bifidus* (preferably in powder/tablet form, though live yoghurt is also useful as long as it contains no sugar or additives).

This treatment is likely to be required for two to three months in many cases before the problem is eradicated. Sometimes there can be an initial adverse reaction, called 'yeast die-off' as the yeast cells are killed and eliminated. This should be very temporary, and in most cases wellbeing will be quickly restored. In fact, as the candida infestation is brought under control, you should feel a lot healthier altogether, as a chronic problem can be very debilitating. Don't worry if it takes a while to complete treatment—it's important to persevere.

(The best time to diagnose and treat candida is, of course, before conception, when it will be much easier to get under control. It's also possible, at this time, to use more 'aggressive' treatments, which will also speed up the process. See Appendix 11 for details.)

GENITO-URINARY INFECTIONS

Genito-urinary infections (sometimes misleadingly called sexually transmitted diseases when many of them are not) are exceedingly common and very frequently undiagnosed, since you can be suffering from an infection of this type but still be relatively (or completely) symptom free. However, untreated genito-urinary infection can have severe effects on your general health and nutritional status, and also on foetal development. The consequences can be as severe as miscarriage, perinatal death, congenital abnormalities and severe health problems in the newborn.

Diagnosis and treatment during pregnancy

The offending micro-organisms are of an astonishing variety, (fungal, flagellate, viral, bacterial and mycoplasmal) and many do not show up in blood or urine samples. You will need to have a lower vaginal swab, while your partner will require a urethral smear and semen culture and analysis, unless you are tested clear before conception (for details of preconception tests and treatment, see Appendix 11). These tests *should* be performed even if there is no reason to suspect a problem—since many of these infections are subclinical—and will need to be carried out by a medical practitioner. However, if infection is present, complementary treatments can be very effective in eradicating the pathogens.

Herbs can be used to great effect to boost the immune system. The best herb to use during pregnancy is *Echinacea*.

Antibiotic therapy is, of course, usually contra-indicated during pregnancy. However, there are some antibiotics which are less problematic than others and your medical practitioner may decide that the infection presents the greater threat to you and your baby.

When using antibiotics *always* replenish the gut flora with *Acidophilus* and *Bifidus lactobacilli* to prevent an outbreak of candida. During pregnancy it is also possible to use the *homoeopathic nosode* for the disease or infection, coupled with the use of *Garlic*, *vitamin C* and *Echinacea* to boost the immune response. This may not result in the blood or smear test becoming negative, but should help to give protection against the disease. (Homoeopathic treatment is not recommended if the infection is of viral origin.)

Your partner should also be treated to prevent cross-infection, and unprotected intercourse should be avoided until treatment is completed. You may also want to talk to your health practitioner about the implications for your pregnancy of any diagnosed infection and, if you are at increased risk of miscarriage, put some of our recommendations in place to prevent this (see Chapter 13).

(Obviously it is easier both to diagnose and treat these infections before conception, so if this applies to you, see Appendix 11 for more details.)

OTHER INFECTIONS

Three other infections need to be screened for during pregnancy if you have not already had the all-clear prior to conception. These are rubella, toxoplasmosis and cytomegalovirus. Though these are better treated before pregnancy starts, there are protective measures that can be put in place at any time. We have found natural therapies very helpful in eliminating toxoplasmosis and cytomegalovirus. Rubella, if contracted, will run its course quite rapidly, though the immune-enhancing treatments we have already discussed will assist recovery.

Toxoplasmosis

Toxoplasmosis is a parasitic disease which can be contracted from cats, especially through contact with the excreta (so always use gloves when changing your cat's litter), or through eating contaminated raw animal foods. It can have extremely serious effects on foetal health, especially if contracted during the first trimester, although the disease is less likely to cross the placenta at this stage. If it does, however, it can lead to miscarriage or stillbirth. If infection occurs later in pregnancy, the chances of the baby being infected are greater, but the effects are not as severe. The child may be born alive, but with a high risk of hydrocephalus (excess fluid on the brain), brain lesions (scarring of brain tissue) and retinochoroiditis (damage to the retina). Overall, the chance of a child being infected through the mother is 40 per cent, with 10 per cent of these babies being seriously affected.

A blood test can show present infection or immunity (through past infection). If infection is detected during pregnancy, it can be treated with the *homoeopathic nosode* and immune supportive herbs such as *Echinacea* with *Garlic* and *vitamin C*, just as with the genito-urinary infections.

An existing infection does not pose as great a risk as one which is first contracted after conception. There are some antibiotic drugs which can be used for this condition even during pregnancy, though there may be some side effects. More information is available from the Toxoplasmosis Trust in the UK (see Contacts and Resources).

It is preferable to diagnose and treat this disease before conception, when herbal treatment can include remedies contra-indicated during pregnancy. It is usually then possible to avoid the rather aggressive antibiotic therapy otherwise required.

Cytomegalovirus

Cytomegalovirus belongs to the herpes family of viruses, but is not to be confused with genital herpes. It is often found amongst pre-school children, so if you are in contact with young children, keep up to date on the existence of any epidemic. It's useful, in these cases, to know if you are already immune. This is one advantage of preconception diagnosis. The other is that treatment is easier. Like toxoplasmosis, this infection can have severe repercussions for foetal health, but it can often be treated safely and effectively with *Lemon Balm* and *Echinacea* during pregnancy, in conjunction with *vitamin C* and *Garlic*.

Rubella

Most of you are probably aware of the ill-effects of rubella on pregnancy, and a test for antibodies will be part of your first medical check-up once you have conceived. Again we would like to suggest that diagnosis and treatment are better carried out preconception, as your options are limited once you are pregnant.

The best approach, if you find out you are not immune, is to boost your immune system with *Echinacea*, *Lemon Balm*, *vitamin C* and *Garlic*, and to avoid contact with any possible source of infection.

CONSEQUENCES OF INFECTION DURING PREGNANCY

Testing for these infections may, of course, generate some unwelcome news as well as heart-searching about hard decisions. However, unlike other antenatal tests (covered in Chapter 11) which also look for risk factors, these tests and the possible treatments carry no additional risk to the pregnancy. Although we've offered some remedies to ameliorate the effect of these infections if diagnosed when you have already conceived, we certainly can't guarantee that these treatments will ensure an absence of repercussions on the health of your pregnancy or baby, though the ill-effects of any infection will lessen after the first trimester.

Some women or couples may decide that the possibility of problems poses too severe a threat to their baby, and may decide to terminate the pregnancy. We recommend that before making any decision you access as much information as possible on the ill-effects, and only come to a decision after much discussion between yourselves, supported by professional counselling. Your doctor may be able to help you, as may support groups (see Contacts and Resources). This is not a decision that should be taken, or influenced, by anyone except yourselves.

chapter 9

Exercise

There are three sorts of exercise to consider during your pregnancy—aerobic exercise, muscle strengthening exercise and stretching exercise for flexibility.

AEROBIC EXERCISE

First of all let's define what we mean by 'aerobic'. It's probably a term you've heard before but you mightn't be sure exactly what it means. Very simply, when you exercise aerobically your body uses up oxygen. 'Aerobic' literally means 'in the presence of oxygen'. Aerobic exercise also utilises fat as its energy source. So it's the huffing and puffing sort of exercise like power walking, jogging, rowing, cycling and swimming, as well as some types of 'aerobic' classes. Of course the amount of huffing and puffing that you do during pregnancy should still allow you to hold a conversation comfortably.

The benefits of aerobic exercise during pregnancy

There are lots of benefits to be had, particularly during pregnancy, when you exercise aerobically.

Better delivery of oxygen and nutrients

First of all, your lungs and heart will work more efficiently, and your whole body, particularly your uterus and placenta, will benefit from the improved function of your circulatory and respiratory systems. There'll be a more efficient delivery of oxygen and of essential nutrients to all your tissues and to your developing baby as well.

More efficient circulation, lower blood pressure

Because of the improvement in your circulation, you'll be less likely to suffer from haemorrhoids and varicose veins. We think that avoiding these two conditions, which plague countless pregnant women, should be enough to get you started on an exercise program without delay!

Moderately strenuous aerobic exercise has also been shown to have a significantly lowering effect on elevated blood pressure which may be important in the prevention of toxaemia. Toxaemia is the high blood pressure which affects 10 per cent of pregnant women.

Better bowel and kidney function

Aerobic exercise also improves peristalsis (that's the movement of your gut) which means you'll be less likely to suffer from constipation. Of course, while you're exercising you'll also be drinking lots of purified water, which is a simple way to flush toxins from your body.

Calcium retained in your bones

Aerobic exercise will also help your body to use up any excess calories and if the exercise is weight-bearing—like walking, jogging, cycling or 'aerobic' classes (but not swimming)—this will mean increased bone density because more calcium is retained by your body. This means a reduced risk of osteoporosis later in your life (long after your childbearing years are over), but for now it's important that the maximum amount of calcium is retained in your bones because the foetus can obtain its calcium requirements from your skeleton if there is any nutritional shortfall.

More energy, sounder sleep
Regular aerobic exercise means you'll have improved stamina and endurance. This is a great bonus when you're carrying around an extra 10 kilograms (or thereabouts) by the end of nine months. You'll experience less fatigue, you'll feel less stressed, and you'll also sleep better.

Benefits of aerobic exercise at birth
The benefits of a regular aerobic exercise routine will extend beyond your pregnancy to the birth of your baby. Labour is hard physical work, and it's been calculated that the energy that you will need is similar to that used up during a brisk 6 kilometre hike. Women who continue to exercise right through their pregnancy usually have a shorter, easier labour. Your increased stamina and endurance mean that you'll tire less readily. They also mean that you'll be much more likely to participate actively in the birth, particularly if you've practised all the appropriate stretches (see below). This active participation means you'll have a much more fulfilling birth experience, and a good level of fitness also means that you will make a rapid recovery after the birth.

There's absolutely no doubt that a regular program of aerobic exercise has lots of benefits for both you and your baby. But before you start, there are a few things to think about. Of course if you have any questions or specific health concerns you should consult your nearest fitness centre, personal trainer or health practitioner.

How much aerobic exercise should you do and how often?
To get all those benefits from your exercise you must elevate your resting heart rate to no more than 140–150 beats per minute and keep it there for not longer than 15 consecutive minutes. (The table with which you might already be familiar, giving age vs. maximum heart rate to aim for during aerobic exercise, is not appropriate during your pregnancy.)

We suggest that your regular aerobic exercise routine should involve a minimum of 30 minutes of aerobic activity at each session, but remember that no more than 15 consecutive minutes should be at your maximum heart rate (140–150 beats per minute). You should try for at least three sessions per week. Some of you will probably do more exercise than this, but if you do, remember to keep very well hydrated (see 'Staying cool' later in this chapter), listen very carefully to any signals of discomfort that your body may be sending, and heed those signals.

When should you begin your exercise program?

If you are already physically fit when you conceive, then your body will have developed physiological responses to allow your baby to cope well with the circulatory and respiratory changes which occur during exercise. However, these mechanisms won't be quite so well adapted if you've never exercised at all, and any strenuous activity to which you are unaccustomed could put stresses on your baby. Therefore, if you're pregnant and exercising seriously for the first time, check with your health practitioner first and take things very gently to begin with. But the sooner you get started the better, as it is then more likely that you'll be motivated (and able) to continue to exercise aerobically right up to the time of your baby's birth.

Getting started, staying motivated

During the first 12 weeks of your pregnancy the embryo is growing at an extremely rapid rate and your body is also undergoing great physical changes. Hormone levels are high, you may be experiencing some nausea and you will probably feel less energetic than normal. Therefore you might not feel very enthusiastic about undertaking any physical activity. Even if you were a regular exerciser before your pregnancy, you may find during these early weeks that you don't feel quite so motivated. Don't despair. This period of having less energy will pass.

Strangely enough, if you do begin (or continue) your exercise program now you'll probably find your energy levels pick up quite a lot. Your circulation will improve and the better delivery of nutrients will make you feel more energetic. The endorphins which are produced will give you a general feeling of wellbeing, and you'll sleep more soundly too. But whether you decide on a swim or a walk or a bike ride, just start off gently and, over the coming weeks, gradually build up to a more sustained level of activity.

Get some extra sleep and remember there's no need to push yourself to achieve a pre-pregnancy level of training. Even if you are a regular exerciser, don't let your heart rate rise above 140–150 beats per minute during exercise. Your resting heart rate normally rises during pregnancy, but this does not mean you are becoming less fit.

Staying cool

It's best to exercise during the coolest part of the day and sensible to avoid extremely prolonged or sustained exercise during the early weeks of pregnancy. At all times, it is absolutely essential that you keep well hydrated. This is important because overheating during the first trimester can cause damage to the developing brain of the embryo. This means that your body temperature shouldn't rise above 38°C during pregnancy. Theoretically, this type of overheating could occur if you are unused to very strenuous exercise, although regular exercisers should also take care not to become too hot if the activity is sustained. (For instance, we don't think biathlons or triathlons are wise in the early weeks, and would have to question such sustained activity at any time during your pregnancy.)

Keeping well hydrated means that you must drink plenty of purified water, and drink before you actually become thirsty. (Of course consumption of 8–12 glasses of purified water daily is also a very effective detoxification measure.) You should increase the level of intake on very hot days. Unfortunately, we don't have a solution to what this level of water intake is going to do to your bladder which already needs much more frequent emptying, due to the increasing pressure of the uterus. But you could try drinking most of your water before mid-afternoon, which at least should keep nocturnal waking to a minimum.

While on the subject of staying cool we also recommend that you avoid saunas, spas, very hot baths and solariums during the first 12 weeks of your pregnancy, as these high temperatures can adversely affect embryonic development.

Which type of aerobic exercise is best?

Of course the changes that happen to your body during pregnancy will inevitably affect the type of exercise you prefer to do, and probably also the rate at which you do it.

Walking

If you were a jogger before your baby was conceived, you might find that as your pregnancy advances, jogging loses some of its appeal. However, you don't need to be afraid that your baby will 'fall out', particularly during those very early weeks. While it's still a tiny embryo, it's no more likely to become dislodged than your kidneys. As the size and the weight of the foetus increases, however, power walking may be a much more comfortable choice than jogging. Your baby still won't fall out, but jogging can certainly make it feel as if it might. During a power walk you can still get your heart rate into that target zone by walking briskly with your arms swinging and your stride lengthening.

Aerobic classes

If you were passionate about aerobic classes before your pregnancy, you may now find your baby turning somersaults in response to the loud insistent music. Both of you might prefer something a little less jarring to the body and the eardrums. On the other hand, Janette found her first baby quite soothed by the strains of 'Saturday Night Fever', which was a soundtrack much favoured by aerobic instructors when she was pregnant, and one of the naturopaths at Francesca's clinic has just given birth to a John Lennon fan!

Swimming

Swimming is undoubtedly one of the best forms of exercise while you're pregnant. The water acts like a great big cushion which gives your body total support. The jarring which you experience when jogging isn't an issue, and you really don't need to make any allowances for your changing size and shape. That 'beached whale' feeling which you might experience on land will disappear once you're in the water.

There are some minor drawbacks to swimming, however. First, non-weight bearing exercise like swimming does not help to keep calcium in your bones, and swimming in a pool which is treated with chlorine and copper-based chemicals is not ideal for you or your baby. Unfortunately, the best way of ridding your body of these chemicals is through sweating. However we've just mentioned that excessive heat should be avoided during pregnancy, especially during the first trimester, so saunas and steam baths are definitely not recommended as a means of working up a sweat. A saltwater or ocean pool which is not treated with toxic chemicals is the best place to swim, or you could simply swim in the sea itself.

Rebounding

Rebounding on a mini-trampoline can be enjoyed in the privacy of your lounge room, so it's easy to fit into a busy schedule. You don't need to go anywhere or even get changed (although we'll leave that decision up to you). Rebounding, like aerobic exercise, will improve your circulation and lymphatic drainage as well as 'toning' your reproductive organs. It also avoids the jarring to your skeleton which can be experienced with some other forms of exercise.

But to experience all the other benefits of aerobic exercise obviously you need to do more than bounce up and down on the rebounder. You need to run, do 'knees-ups' and move your arms in a pumping motion to elevate your heart rate (but not to more than 140–150 beats per minute). You will still need to keep your heart rate elevated for at least 30 minutes on at least three occasions per week.

Francesca, whose desire to exercise is limited by an aversion to indoor gymnasiums and any activity which involves multiple changes of costume, is a dedicated rebounder. She has found that many of her patients, while finding it difficult to fit other forms of exercise into their already over-busy schedule, can usually manage 20 minutes per day on the mini-trampoline. One other advantage of this form of exercise is that the motion is transmitted to every cell in your body, including those in your reproductive system (which is often stationary or jarred during other forms of exercise).

On the down side, however, Janette fell off one of these devices while exercising at her favourite gym. Her concentration had wandered to the legs of the young man who was instructing her class. We suggest you concentrate on the task at hand and definitely leave the TV turned off. Another problem with rebounders is the risk of twisting your ankles, especially while carrying the extra weight of a baby.

MUSCLE STRENGTHENING EXERCISE

The second type of exercise which is important during pregnancy is the type which will strengthen specific muscle groups.

Strengthen your muscles to avoid discomfort

Strong back, buttock, and abdominal muscles are particularly important for prospective mothers. These muscles form a supporting and protective girdle around your lower body. If all these muscles are strong, the increasing size and weight of your baby will be far less likely to cause backache which is frequently due solely to weak muscles. The yoga exercises we suggest later in the chapter are good strengthening exercises.

Sometimes the abdominal (rectus) muscle separates during late pregnancy or in the postnatal period. While this is a reversible condition, it's not an attractive look, as it allows the abdominal contents to bulge through. So if you want to avoid this happening (we're sure you will!), you'll need to strengthen your abdominal muscles too.

You need to be strong to carry your baby

If all your muscles are strong then obviously you will be better equipped to tolerate physical stress and better able to carry loads without tiring. Make no mistake, these are important factors to consider. You may be surprised at how much extra physical work, particularly of the lifting and carrying variety, you will be required to do once you become a mother. In our subsequent books we'll talk about the importance of always carrying your baby close, particularly in the early months, so don't say we didn't warn you! Small babies are happiest when they are carried close to your body. Strong muscles are a necessity if you are going to be able to carry your newborn in some sort of sling (or an older child in a backpack) for a considerable part of the day.

And, trust us, the need to be strong doesn't stop once your baby becomes mobile. The extra lifting and carrying continues for years (probably forever—we'll let you know). First it's your baby, who turns quickly into a very heavy toddler, after that it's probably another baby. Then there's the shopping and the washing, then there are the toys and the books and later the school bags to lift, carry and set down somewhere else. Then you'll have to haul bicycles and boogie boards, bags of roller blades and helmets, cricket stumps and cricket bats. Maybe there'll be drum kits and double basses? Perhaps it will be trail bikes and horses? Ever heaved a couple of saddles into the boot of a car?

Even if you think your children can, will (and should) manage it all by themselves, they will inevitably surprise (or disappoint) you. Janette remembers a seven-year-old who happily walked eight kilometres uphill to the top of Mt Kosciuzko, but spat the dummy on the downhill walk and finished the hike on his mother's shoulders. She also remembers a 12-year-old who insisted on carrying his own pack on the first day of the Milford Track walk. That pack had lost all of its appeal and had become strangely heavy by lunchtime, despite the consumption of all the lunch and most of the water. Janette finished the day carrying a pack both front and back. Francesca's (now grown-up) son has an attraction to futons, but an aversion to bed-making, and sleeps in an inaccessible loft. Need we say more?

Finally, after years of picking up after them and lifting and carrying for them, your children will eventually leave home and with any luck they'll take all their paraphernalia with them—but we guarantee you'll still be there to help them move it all! Message—you need to get strong now and stay strong!

Set an example to your children

Of course you should also consider our version of an old saying: 'The family who plays together stays together.' This means being more than just the spectator on the sidelines. This means keeping your children company at some of their sporting activities; it also means introducing them to the ones that you enjoy. This is what family life is all about. Janette goes rock-climbing with her boys, and Francesca plays tennis with hers. Pretty soon they'll be much better than we are, but in the meantime we're strong enough and fit enough to be there with them. While climbing in the Blue Mountains with your children or guiding them to Wimbledon may be the furthest thing from your mind when you've only just conceived, believe us, it all happens far too quickly.

If you get into the habit of regular exercise now, it will be much easier to incorporate that habit into your life when you actually have small children. Finally, it's a very positive example to set those children.

Strong muscles won't just happen

If you are thinking, 'Well, women from traditional societies manage a baby strapped to their body while they work in the fields—I'll be OK, I'll just get used to it as I go,' then also think of the regular exercise these women get every day of their lives. You probably usually travel by car or take public transport and have a host of labour-saving devices in your home. The levels of fitness which women from traditional societies enjoy, and which were once commonplace in Western society, you can now only obtain with conscientious effort. And we say that in spite of the vastly increased level of activity which is coming your way when you become a parent!

If you jog or cycle you might consider that is sufficient exercise for you, but remember these exercises primarily strengthen your leg muscles. Conversely, swimmers frequently have very well developed muscles in their arms and upper body but less well developed muscles in their legs. So if you swim, jog or cycle, make sure that your exercise program includes some specific exercises to strengthen all the other muscle groups.

PELVIC FLOOR MUSCLES NEED STRENGTHENING TOO

Have you ever wondered why women who have had children prefer walking to running and why they always choose the 'low-impact' aerobic classes? Chances are it's because their pelvic floor muscles are very weak. These muscles, which were probably weak when these women gave birth, were further traumatised by their baby's entrance into the world, and have been sadly neglected ever since.

A weak pelvic floor simply means incontinence. Incontinence means that you will wet your pants every time you jump or run (and sometimes even when you laugh or cough or sneeze). This is definitely not a good look! Strong pelvic floor muscles mean that you will avoid this embarrassing (and very debilitating) condition. But you need to know how to strengthen them, and you need to work at strengthening them (along with your abdominals, buttock and back muscles), all the way through your pregnancy, and after your baby is born as well.

How to strengthen your pelvic floor

Your pelvic floor muscles form a sling-like band which surrounds and forms the base of the vagina, anus and urethra. The muscles support all the abdominal contents and your baby will pass through them as he is born. It will help you to identify them if you try this exercise.

Next time you urinate, try to stop the flow in mid-stream, then, after a moment or two, relax the muscles—you have just exercised your pelvic floor. We don't recommend you do the exercise each time you urinate—just until you get the hang of contracting and releasing. Now that you are familiar with the sensation, you can repeat this exercise whenever you like. This is one of the few exercises that you can do any time, any place. Just think, no-one need ever know! Try to increase the number of times you contract and release your pelvic floor, and also increase the time for which you hold each contraction. Repeat the exercise at least five times every hour and hold each contraction for at least five seconds.

You can try another version of this exercise. Think of the pelvic floor muscles as a lift. Take the lift up several floors and be sure to stop at each floor. Then take the lift down, stopping again at each floor. When you reach the ground floor, continue to the basement. To do this you must release your pelvic floor muscles completely. This is what you do when you urinate or empty your bowels. This is exactly how you will use those muscles in the second stage of labour.

You can give these muscles a further workout when you're making love. Contract and relax them rhythmically—your partner's sure to enjoy this exercise—and these muscles will soon be so strong that you'll be able to jump and run to your heart's content after your baby is born.

Dads, don't drop out!

Prospective fathers who think they've done their bit just because their partner's pregnant need to hang in there and begin, or (better still) continue, their regular exercise routine. Improved cardiovascular fitness as well as muscular strength are going to benefit fathers as well. While these days they may not be sent out to fetch buckets of boiling water while their partner's in labour, there'll be other things they'll be required to do which will make them glad of their aerobic conditioning.

They shouldn't exempt themselves from those muscle strengthening exercises either. If their abdominal muscles are weak their bellies will sag, if their back muscles are weak, they'll be candidates for back pain. If they really want to take their turn at carrying and caring for their babies, then they'll need to work at strengthening all those muscle groups too. Remember, you're in this venture together! Fathers will need to heft a few baskets full of washing and to load those bikes into the back of the car too. Maybe one day they'll coach the soccer or the netball team. Or they might decide to take their kids sea-kayaking, cross-country skiing or bungee jumping. Who knows what their mid-life crisis will bring?

STRETCHING EXERCISE FOR FLEXIBILITY

Finally, the third sort of exercise you need to do during pregnancy is the sort that improves your flexibility. We have included below some stretching exercises for your whole body. You should do the appropriate ones at the end of every aerobic exercise session, but feel free to do them all (perhaps you could also learn some others) more frequently. Doing these stretches regularly means that your muscles will be supple and ready for activity and movement. If you increase your flexibility you will be able to experience the full range of motion for which your body was designed without experiencing tension or stiffness. Improved flexibility also means it is much less likely that you will sustain an injury when you exercise. Stretching is also a great way to relax and reduce tension. Just be careful to avoid any stretch which involves your head being lower than your heart (a traditional caution given to pregnant yoga practitioners).

Stretching for an active birth

Exercises to improve your flexibility are the ones which will really affect the ease with which you give birth. There is now no doubt, even in the minds of the most conservative obstetricians, that moving

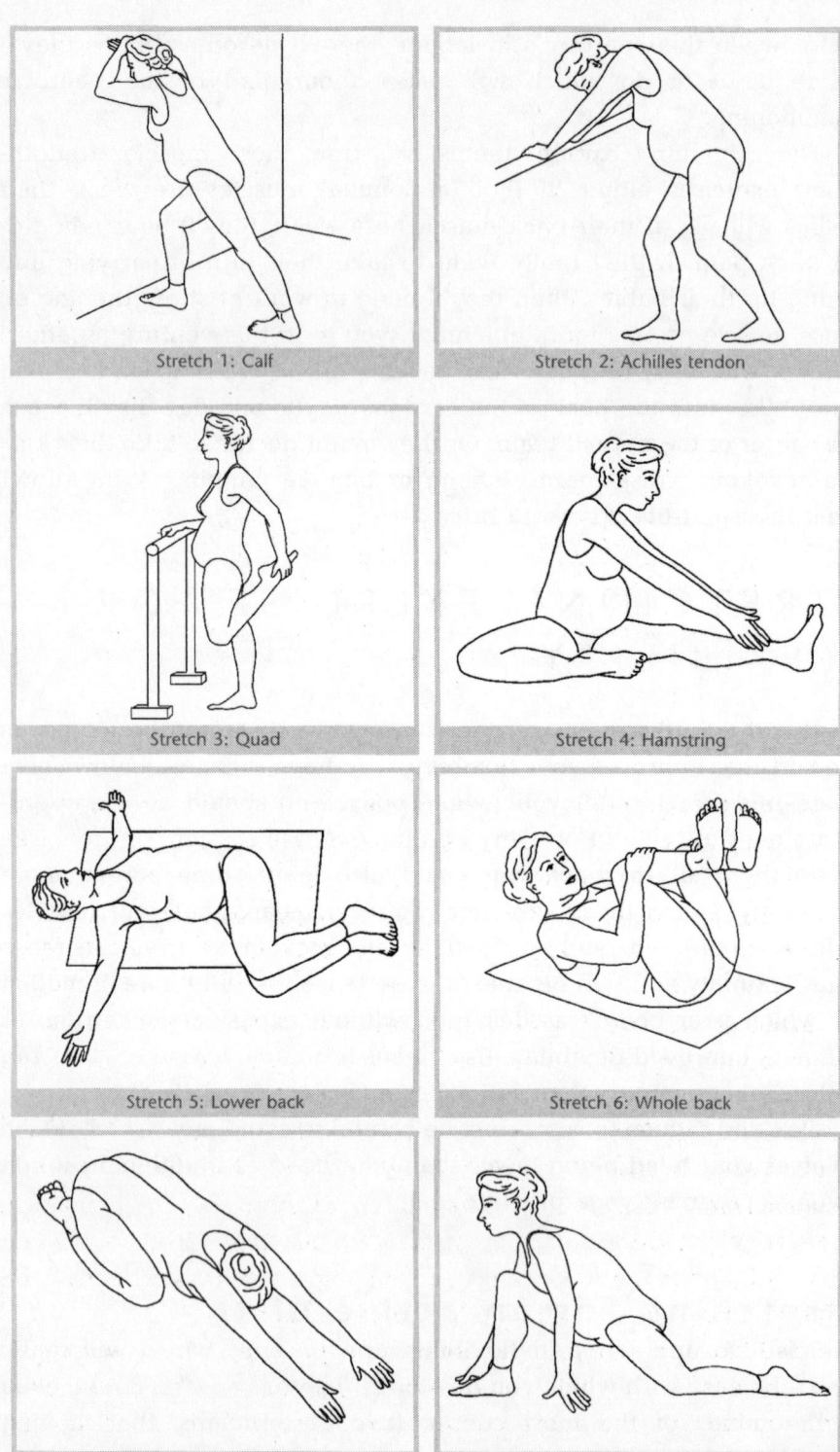

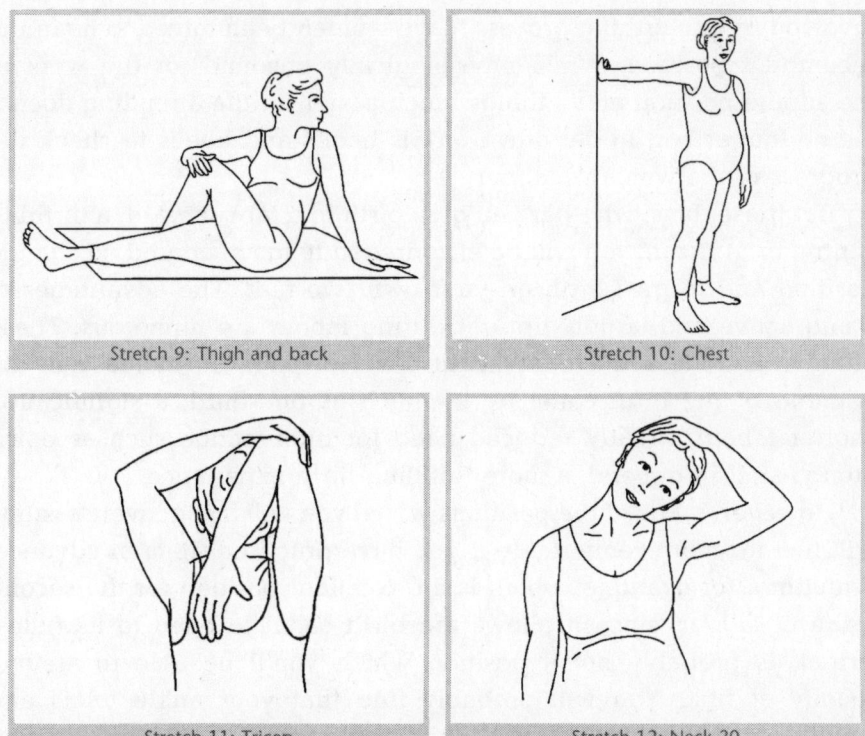

Stretch 9: Thigh and back

Stretch 10: Chest

Stretch 11: Tricep

Stretch 12: Neck 20

around and maintaining an upright position during labour are beneficial. In other words, though once women were confined to the supine, or worse, lithotomy position (feet up in stirrups) during labour, you are now actively encouraged to walk, lean, sit or squat; in other words, to assume the positions which are most comfortable for you during your labour and birth.

In an active labour, you'll find that you instinctively assume the position which gives you most relief from the pain of the contractions and the one which most readily assists the passage of your baby down the birth canal. The positions that you take up will vary, and they will change as your labour progresses, but you'll be able to get into those positions more easily, and maintain them for longer, if you've practised them regularly during your pregnancy. In our next book we will deal more fully with the importance of remaining upright and active, but what you need to know now is really quite simple.

Traditionally, women have always given birth in an upright position, as this gives them the assistance of gravity in birthing their baby. Only since the mid-seventeenth century, when men first became involved in the birthing process, have women been forced to lie in the recumbent position. While physiologically unsound for the woman, the supine position made things much easier for the attending doctor. He no longer had to get down on his hands and knees to check the progress of the woman's labour!

But these days, whether you give birth in a labour ward, a birthing centre, or at home, you will be encouraged to move around, to change position and to give birth on your own two feet. The advantages of being active and largely upright during labour are numerous. These benefits include a decrease in the level of pain, an increase in the opening of the birth canal by as much as one-third, a significantly shorter labour, greatly reduced need for intervention such as episiotomy, and, in general, a more fulfilling birth experience.

However, many of the positions which you will instinctively assume will feel far more comfortable if you have practised them in advance. Squatting, for example, which is an excellent position for the second stage of labour, since it allows the birth canal to open to its fullest extent, is probably not a position which you'll be able to assume readily at first. You will probably find that your ankle joints and Achilles tendons are quite stiff. While women from more primitive societies spend a good part of each day squatting, it is unlikely that you will feel really comfortable in this position until you have practised it for several months prior to the birth. Maybe even then you'll still feel more comfortable in a 'supported squat'. This position should be practised too, then your partner, who will support you, will realise the importance of being fit as well.

Yoga during pregnancy

Many of the stretching exercises which will facilitate an active birth are very similar to a number of yoga poses, and in fact many pregnant women find the calm, inward centred approach of yoga much more appealing than the running/jumping types of exercise. Regular yoga practice confers other significant benefits on both mother and baby. One of the most important of these is the ability to put the body and mind into a very relaxed state. Yoga exercises also make the pelvic joints very supple and will help strengthen back, abdominal and pelvic muscles.

If you're a complete novice, you would probably benefit from attending yoga classes where a qualified yoga teacher can guide you. In a structured class, the correct postures can be easily learnt, and the teacher can advise you of those poses which are not suitable during pregnancy. Specific instruction can also be given which will take into account previous experience, how advanced your pregnancy is and any other limitations or considerations.

However, we describe below some simple yoga poses which anyone can do with complete safety. All of these poses will be of benefit during your labour as well as during pregnancy. When you're practising at home it is wise to build the time spent in each posture gradually. Even if you don't hold the posture for the maximum time, any time spent will still be very beneficial. Daily practice is recommended for best results.

Baddha Konasana (Supta): The cobbler pose

Sit on the floor with the soles of your feet together, heels as close as possible to your perineum (that's the area between your anus and vulva), with a folded blanket under your feet. Press your toes open against a wall. Then lie back with a folded blanket supporting your head and neck if you wish. Initially, you should try to hold this pose for 2 minutes, building to 5, 10, then 15 minutes. This posture is great for creating internal space within the pelvic cavity which can facilitate labour and birth. When you're ready to get up, use your left hand to manually lift the left knee over to the right knee and allow your body to roll to the right, finally coming up on your hands and knees.

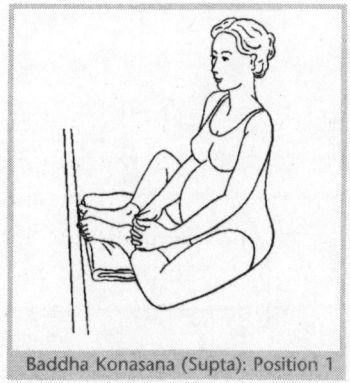
Baddha Konasana (Supta): Position 1

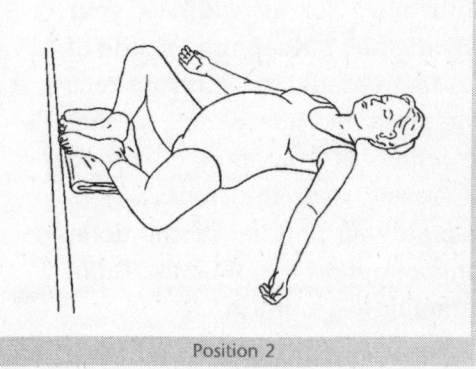
Position 2

Virabhadrasana II: The second warrior pose

This is a standing posture and very useful for increasing strength that will be helpful when you're giving birth. Stand with your back against a wall for support. Place your feet about a metre apart, pointing your right foot away from you and with the left turned in slightly. With your right knee in line with the second toe of your right foot, slowly bend the right knee until it forms a right angle. Hold your arms out straight against the wall at shoulder height, and keep the back leg strong with the knee pulled up. Build to 30 seconds. Come up slowly, keeping the right knee in line with the second right toe on the way up to avoid knee strain. Repeat on the other side.

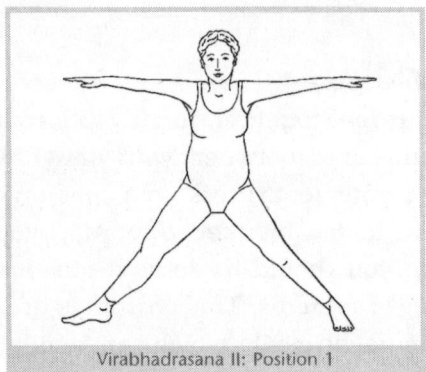
Virabhadrasana II: Position 1

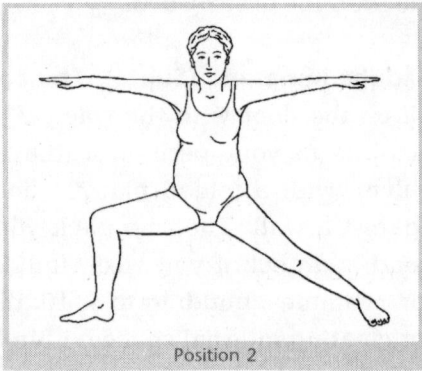
Position 2

Squat (supported)

Squat with your feet about hip width apart (or as wide as your belly dictates). Keep the outside of your feet parallel, stretch your toes wide open and heels back, so that the whole of your foot is spread generously over the floor. Squat, keeping your feet flat on the floor, using a support to hold onto. Build gradually to 1 minute.

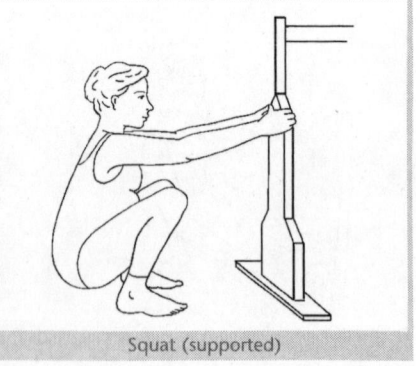
Squat (supported)

Upavista Konasana

Position a chair in front of you, then sit on the floor, with straight legs open comfortably (but not as wide as they will go). Press your heels away, push into your feet, keep your toes turned up. Use the chair to lift your body up. Aim to get your thigh bones closer to the floor. Build up to 3 minutes.

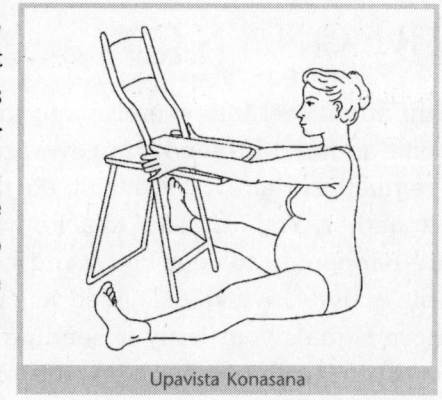
Upavista Konasana

Virasana (Supta)

Kneel with your feet apart, sitting between your feet with a folded blanket under your buttocks. Make sure your feet are facing straight back. When this posture becomes comfortable, lean back, either against a chair, or on folded blankets, bolsters or supportive cushions. Build gradually to 10 minutes. Come up slowly.

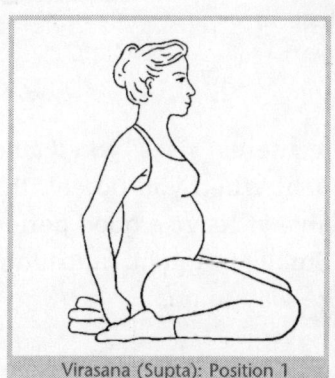
Virasana (Supta): Position 1

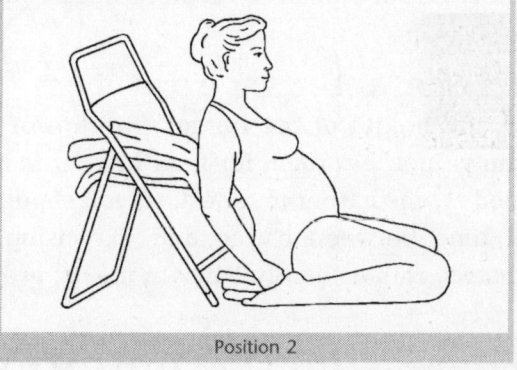
Position 2

EXERCISING IN LATE PREGNANCY

You might feel that exercise and the latter stages of pregnancy really don't go hand-in-hand. However, getting bigger and more noticeably pregnant certainly doesn't mean that you need to give up exercise altogether. You just need to acknowledge that quite profound changes are happening to your body, and be prepared to take up a more suitable activity. We've discussed lots of options already. Simply listen to those signals your body is sending you. This is a really good time to focus on all those changes—the increasing size of your breasts and belly are only the most obvious ones.

There's more blood for your heart to pump

Your blood volume is increasing (by about one-third). This means that your heart is going to work harder to pump all that extra blood, so you probably won't be able to run as fast or work out as hard. This definitely doesn't mean that you're becoming less fit.

There's less room for food

As the height of the fundus (the top of the uterus) rises, you'll find you've got less room for food in your stomach. When you do eat, the food seems harder to digest, so you should always leave a good period of time between eating and exercising. Small, frequent, nutritious snacks, rather than full-blown meals, are the way to go.

There's increasing pressure on your bladder

You'll experience increasing pressure on your bladder, and you'll feel that whether you're exercising or not. Because of that extra pressure, not to mention all that extra water you've been drinking, even sneezing or coughing can make you wet your pants. Running and jumping can be an unmitigated disaster, especially if your pelvic floor muscles are weak (so keep up those pelvic floor exercises).

You'll need to lie on your side
Any exercise which involves lying on your burgeoning belly is obviously impossible. Lying on your back for any period of time isn't recommended either. This puts pressure on the vena cava, which is one of the two major veins which carry blood back to your heart. Compression of this vein will reduce the blood flow to the placenta, and to your baby. So if an exercise involves lying down, only do it if it can be performed while lying on your side.

Your ligaments are softening
Your body produces a hormone called relaxin during pregnancy. This softens all the ligaments and by doing this it gives the pelvis extra flexibility to allow your baby to pass more easily down the birth canal. However, it is not just the ligaments attached to the pelvis which soften. Relaxin affects all the ligaments and this increases the instability of all the joints—so there is an increased risk of injury during exercise and stretching. Be aware of this and be extra careful, particularly if you are doing high-impact exercise, and when you are stretching try not to go much beyond your normal range of movement.

Hopefully we haven't made it sound as if exercise during pregnancy is fraught with things to beware of. It isn't. All you really need to do is tune in, adjust to your changing size and shape, and always listen to your body's signals. Then you should be able to keep your exercise program going right up to the time of the birth, and resume it shortly afterwards as well. Janette did her last aerobic classes a few hours before she went into labour and was back in the gym after a few weeks. (She's been there ever since!) And remember, exercise is great for your mental as well as physical health—more of this in the next chapter.

chapter 10
Reducing stress and thinking positively

Pregnancy is a time of great joy and wonder at the miraculous processes taking place right there inside you. The feelings involved in recognising the growth of another being inside your body are profound and intense and, for those who have such beliefs, quite spiritual. It's also an experience that most women will only have a very few times in their lives, so it's important to get the most out of it. If this is your first pregnancy it will also be an incredible adventure into unmapped zones.

However it may feel at the start, pregnancy does not last forever, and those nine months will slip by quite quickly. So, to get the most out of this short but event-packed experience, you need to be well prepared and have ways of dealing with any stress as it arises.

THE EFFECTS OF STRESS

Some of the potential stress during pregnancy may arise from normal daily life, which is likely to make new demands on you at this time, and some may be due to the processes of pregnancy itself. It's helpful to be able to identify the source of your stress and have appropriate strategies to deal with each situation, as stress can have several repercussions on the healthy progress of your pregnancy. Although there is often dispute about the extent of the role of stress in causing physical or mental health problems, there is no doubt that it is a significant cause of poor nutritional status, as it disrupts both the absorption of nutrients and the rate at which you can use them up. It is also a factor in adrenal, immune system and hormonal dysfunction, all of which can affect your pregnancy adversely.

Stress will also, of course, disrupt your sleep pattern, and if you believe in emotional awareness and communication between yourself and your unborn child (and we've never met a mother who doesn't), it will affect that too. It has certainly been implicated in both miscarriage and poor health in the infant, with a clear link to small, low birth-weight babies and all the problems with which this condition is associated. Although there is some dispute as to whether stress can actually cause miscarriage, it can certainly affect the states, systems and processes which may be involved in pregnancy loss.

Of course, different people have different levels of stress tolerance, and what will cause one person much anguish can leave another quite sanguine. It's how well you cope that is critical. You might ask yourself, 'Am I getting on top of the stress—or is it getting the better of me?' Once your coping mechanisms no longer deal with the level of stress you are experiencing, then the ill-effects can start to become evident. Coping mechanisms may include self-help processes and techniques you can apply in your daily life, you may rely on groups of friends or more formal associations, or you may seek the help of a professional. We will explore stress management techniques later, but let's start by looking at some possible reasons why you might be or become stressed, how you can tell if it's getting out of control, and how you might resolve stressful incidents and episodes.

HOW DO YOU KNOW IF YOU'RE TOO STRESSED?

Some level of stress is inevitable. Stress may even be associated with pleasant, much anticipated events. This is particularly true in pregnancy, when the happiness you experience may co-exist with psychological or physical demands that present new challenges to be met. Even in normal day-to-day existence it would be unrealistic and undesirable to eliminate stress altogether, as it provides that frisson of excitement as well as motivation and challenge. This aspect of stress is sometimes called 'eustress' (*eu* being a Greek prefix meaning 'good', as in 'euphoria'). It may be helpful to use the term 'distress' for unhelpful stress, to be more specific.

What symptoms might you experience?

Some symptoms are common to both eustress and distress. These include an increase in the rates of heartbeat, pulse and breathing. Other common symptoms of *distress* include:

- Insomnia
- Anxiety/irritability
- Mood swings
- Fatigue
- Eating disorders (too much, too little, or inappropriate foods)
- Digestive disorders
- Headaches
- Inability to concentrate
- An increase in inflammatory conditions (such as dermatitis)
- An increase in allergic conditions (such as asthma)

There may also be an exacerbation of more serious problems or disease states, and in pregnancy one obvious vulnerable area is your blood pressure. Clearly, it's important to resolve or control stress.

Before you jump to conclusions, remember it's quite normal to feel a little more tired during pregnancy, but if any of the above symptoms are becoming debilitating then you are probably too stressed and will need to look at where the problem is coming from.

REASONS FOR STRESS

As we've said, there are plenty of reasons—inherent in the demands of daily life today—why anyone, pregnant or not, might find it difficult to cope.

Daily life stressors include:

- Heavy workload
- Career path/job change
- Conflict at work
- Conflict with partner/relationships
- Change in partner/relationships
- Change in residence (amazingly common in late pregnancy!)
- Renovation of residence (not advised, due to the toxicity of paints, solvents etc.)
- Holidays
- Financial problems
- Long-term illness in family
- Death of family member/friend

And then pregnancy brings its own challenges. Once pregnant, your energy may follow different patterns, and you may need to adapt by changing your normal responses to demands on your time and energy, and by reassessing priorities. This will obviously apply to areas such as work commitments, the care of existing children and domestic duties.

Of course, pregnancy is not a static condition, and your concerns will change as your pregnancy progresses.

In the first trimester you may worry whether the pregnancy will hold until 12 weeks. Typical thoughts such as, 'What is that blood spot/cramp?', 'Is it normal not to be nauseated?', or 'Why is my heart racing?', may be rushing through your brain.

In the second trimester, when you are considering (or having) some (or all) of the possible testing procedures, your thoughts may turn to, 'Should I have them?', 'What will happen if I don't?' and 'Am I neglecting my baby's welfare?' In Chapter 11 we will try and give you guidance so you can resolve these issues in your mind and in your partner's mind.

At this time, women who have careers may well have to come to terms with the loss of any feelings of self-esteem that are bound up in their working lives, learn to surrender to motherhood, and give this new role the space and time it requires in their lives in order to flourish.

In the third trimester you may start to fear the impending birth or the pain of labour, or be concerned that you may not be able to give birth naturally. You may even feel that you could 'fail' as a mother, or that you won't be able to cope with the demands and responsibilities of caring for a child.

RESOLVING STRESS

So stressors can range from the practical to the emotional. Let's look at some potentially stressful problems you might encounter at this time and see what you can do to resolve them. Later we'll look at some specific remedies and treatments for stress.

Overcoming tiredness

You can make a lot of difference to your energy levels if you are eating well and supplementing along the lines we suggest. It is, however, quite a normal response to feel a bit more tired than usual—there's a lot of work going on in there! This is particularly true for the first trimester when your body is manufacturing the placenta, and in the last when your size is a factor. However, all through your pregnancy you are providing nutrients and energy to make another human being, and this is one of the most extraordinary things you will ever do, and a great achievement all on its own.

When you're feeling really tired and in need of more energy try telling yourself a positive affirmation, such as, 'I'm building/growing/creating some more skeletal/organ/muscle/brain cells for my baby.'

Make sure you get plenty of rest. This may mean being a little less scrupulous than usual about housework, getting some extra help or support from your partner, family and friends, cutting back on your social engagements, and perhaps reassessing job commitments, if this is a flexible arrangement. You're going to need to figure out how to adapt work to the demands of birth and early childhood anyway, so it may be that this adjustment needs to start now.

Young children in your family can perhaps spend some extra time with support people (if you have any), while your time with them can be spent doing things which provide rest and relaxation for both of you, such as reading or gentle activities, indoors or outdoors.

Take a nap in the middle of the day if you need to; even a short sleep can help. Full body relaxation and visualisation (see 'Visualisation and affirmation' later on in this chapter for ideas) can be even more refreshing than sleep. Either way, you may get more benefit if you lie down and put your feet up. You may also benefit from more sleep at night. Make a rule to turn the TV off at a certain time so you don't get hooked into nodding off in front of the late night shows.

Dealing with insomnia

Sometimes, despite putting aside more hours for rest, sleep just doesn't come. In pregnancy this can be a particular problem either in the first trimester if there is any nausea, or more commonly in the last when size becomes an issue and it can be difficult to find a comfortable position. There are also theories being advanced that the baby's metabolism may be a factor, as this doesn't slow down at night but places constant demands on the maternal supply of nutrients, and therefore on the mother's metabolism. In 'Specific natural remedies for stress reduction', later on in this chapter, we'll give you some helpful hints for dealing with insomnia.

Getting comfortable

The same discomfort that keeps you awake at night may be a problem during the day, adding to your stress levels. Now may be the time to invest in a good fan if heat is a problem, and you need to make sure your clothes are comfortable. A word of warning here from two experienced mums—don't spend a fortune on maternity clothes. Adapt any loose clothes you already have, and share with friends. Although it may feel as if pregnancy stretches ahead interminably, it really is over quite fast, and you'll be stuck with an investment that is likely to be out of fashion next time you're pregnant. Of course, you deserve a couple of really stunning outfits to make you look as beautiful as you feel!

Enjoying your body

In fact you *do* look beautiful and the naked pregnant woman has to be one of the most sensuous shapes around. Since Demi Moore made this a fashion statement we hope that even more women feel positive about their body image and attractiveness during pregnancy. It's important to continue to pay attention to your appearance and feel proud of your shape. However, some women, typically those for whom weight has previously been an issue, may become depressed about their looks. This you don't need!

If normal reassurance doesn't help, and it becomes a serious issue, you may be tempted to eat less. This is *not* a good idea (unless you're eating excessive amounts already!) and counselling may be necessary. Choose a therapist who has experience in eating disorders (hypnotherapy can be very useful; see Contacts and Resources).

Eating and supplementing well

The nutritional demands on you at this time are very high. Unless you pay attention to replenishing your stores you can become depleted and this can certainly affect your moods and stress tolerance. Later on in this chapter we'll discuss specific nutrients that may need to be increased if you feel overcome by stress.

Evaluating medical intervention

While everybody needs to make up their own mind on whether or not to have antenatal tests performed, this decision-making process—and the pressure from those who feel they have the answers—may cause you anxiety. You need to make a choice that feels comfortable and right to you. Trust your intuition, rely on your burgeoning maternal instinct! It's your body, your baby and your life. Try not to make your decisions based on fear.

Coping with fears

All prospective parents have some experience of anxiety about whether their children will be healthy, and all mums-to-be feel some concern about how that large bump in their belly will get out! For some women, however, this can become obsessive or all-consuming and may be associated with a previous bad experience or be based on other people's negative stories. Some of you may also worry how you will cope with being a parent—emotionally, physically or financially. In the 'Being prepared' section we give you some more tips to help you feel ready for your baby's birth and infancy, and in 'Visualisations and affirmations' there are some ideas for those who have had a previous trauma. Some doctors offer an ultrasound as reassurance. We would prefer to recommend counselling and remind you that following our suggestions on health care will reduce all risks substantially. Most good antenatal organisations will be able to offer or recommend a good counsellor (see Contacts and Resources).

Coping with rampant hormones

Your hormones are rampant during pregnancy, and anyone who has suffered from pre-menstrual tension knows what that can mean. The depression, anxiety and mood swings some women experience at this time may well have their origin in a purely physiological hormonal process.

So don't make it worse by feeling guilty! Tell yourself (and your family and friends!) that you will probably feel quite different very soon, and that this is part of a normal process. This should help to take the edge off the experience, and reduce the stress involved. This is a very profound and intense time you are going through and your feelings are bound to be strong and powerful. Cherish this opportunity to explore your emotions; it's an experience you'll never forget.

Riding rollercoaster feelings

Pregnancy is a time when one minute you feel like a queen and every seat you sit on enthrones your marvellous secret, and the next you feel completely out of control, prey to the inexorable march of your bodily changes—onward, like it or not, to birth. Luckily, for most of us the positive feelings outweigh the bad, but it's certainly true that if you're not used to dealing with deep emotions, this can be a challenging, though an immensely fruitful, time.

Being able to share this time with your partner, your friends, your midwife or perhaps your own mother will be good. Sometimes you'll want to shout your exhilaration and excitement to the rooftops; other times you'll want reassurance that millions of women have trodden this path before you. You'll notice babies and children in the street and marvel at the thought that you'll soon be sharing your life with another tiny being. You'll wonder what it will be like to have another person with you all the time, and how you'll cope with the commitment. You'll start to notice and feel great empathy towards other mothers and their children, a section of society which may have made little impact on you previously. The next minute the whole world is forgotten as you focus intently on an internal psychic conversation with your unborn child. You'll devour baby books, books on birth, books of names and in the next hour wonder if you'll ever have time to read good literature again.

You'll feel huge surges of positive energy, have creative thoughts, rearrange your entire house (this is 'nesting') and then collapse at the thought of how little energy you have for all that remains to be done. You'll dream vividly of your new child and your shared bliss, and the next night your present child or your partner will appear in your dreams to haunt you with accusations of neglect. You'll have a heart to heart with your mother that brings you closer than you've been for years, and the next day wonder if she'll ever leave you alone to make your own mistakes. You'll feel confident and excited about the home water birth you've just arranged, and then terrified that it'll all go wrong and you and the baby will both die as a result of your unorthodox choice.

You'll feel incredibly warm and loving towards your partner for his support and within minutes wonder how he can possibly be so insensitive and not understand your needs. You'll want to let him know every little detail of what's happening to you and then marvel at how he'll never come within cooee of understanding something so integral to being a woman. You'll look fondly at him and imagine him dandling the baby on his knee, and the image will turn to that of him abandoning you for someone slim and unencumbered.

You'll have daytime fantasies about the glories of motherhood, and then your nightly (oh-so-vivid) dreams will be full of your anxieties about your inadequacies, or losing your baby or mistreating it in some way. One minute you know your baby will be the most beautiful in the world, the next you imagine that it will be born with gross congenital defects. The image of breastfeeding your baby after the birth will give way to fears about pain in childbirth. Your dreams may even be extra-sensual, owing to the extra circulation in your reproductive system. If you have unusual sexual fantasies in your dreams don't feel guilty, it's all quite normal!

We've all done it, we've all been there, done that. That's what you need to hang on to. It's part of being, or becoming, a woman. Revel in it if you can, and affirm your right to your place in Mother Nature's realm, your right to be the way you are, and to be loved for it.

Staying relaxed

There's no need for concern about any of your feelings unless the bad start to outweigh the good. That's when feelings become stress. However, the last thing you need is to worry about being worried. If you feel things are getting out of control, put into practice some of the self-help remedies we suggest below or seek help. If you're someone who finds that difficult, remember you're a mother now, and responsible for your chid—it's your baby you're asking assistance for. If you're relaxed, so is your baby (and so is your partner—it's good practice for family life!).

Becoming a family

There's a big change going on. You and your partner are being transformed from a couple to a family. You are becoming a mother, he is changing into a father. It's a miracle, it's bigger than both of you and sometimes it's overwhelming. However it doesn't need to be hard, and the process is less likely to be problematic if you are both aware of the implications of the changes in your relationship. Growing through changes such as these is what life's all about. You will need to learn to see your partner in a new way, a different light, and a changing role. You will need to talk to each other about how you see parenting, how you see your respective roles in childcare, and how you see your relationship to each other absorbing these new demands. It's a lot better to sort things out now. Trying to demand that your partner change nappies at one o'clock in the morning when you're both dead tired is not likely to be successful if you have no prior agreement.

Fathers get pregnant too!

We've said a lot about how the mother feels, but now is the time to find out how the father copes with pregnancy and impending birth. He may not be prey to rampant hormones (well, that's probably disputable, and sex in pregnancy is something we'll get around to—even if you don't!) but he's certainly also experiencing some emotional and psychological conflicts. Whether or not he was as keen for a child as you were, he's now fluctuating between pride and anxiety about responsibilities; between the comfort of an imminent family, and his potential lack of freedom.

He's wanting to help, and not sure how to; wanting to be involved, but feeling excluded; wanting to express tenderness and love, and feeling jealous of all the attention and care you're receiving. He's probably got a lot of the same worries as you, but may feel less entitled to talk about them. He may feel worried about his role in your life when all your maternal love takes over. He's probably scared about the birth too, and unsure of what he will be called upon to do. Since the labour is unlikely to be a time when anyone gives him very much attention, it's important to address his concerns *now*, so he can give you the support you need, and feel confident himself.

All of this is normal in a committed, caring relationship. It may be compounded by unresolved issues that preceded the conception, or by the casual nature of a relationship where the baby wasn't planned, or agreed upon. It's an important time for him—for both of you—to clear the air, make plans together and clarify his role in the birth, the baby's care and in your relationship. Not that you can anticipate all the situations you are likely to face, but starting off with a sense of agreement, even if there's been a bit of give-and-take, will give a strong basis to all that follows. One area you need to discuss is money—who earns it, who spends it, and on what. Another is your ideas of how to feed a child, treat a child, educate a child, and talk to a child. For example, two issues that will come up fairly soon are circumcision and immunisation. In other words, you'll need to think about and talk about what becoming parents, and a family, means to each of you.

But of course you already *are* a parent. Your unborn child is conducting a secret life in there. You can both share this with your baby. Talk to your child, massage it through your tummy, play it music. It's amazing how responsive your child will be. It's clear, from the actions and movements involved, that your child is affected by all sorts of external stimuli and by your moods, so nurturing and parenting have already begun.

Being prepared

One way to stop feeling stressed is to feel in control. There are practical things that you can do that will help you feel prepared. These can vary from reassuring yourself that, at worst, you can turn out your underwear drawer and use it as a crib, to buying up the whole baby gadget shop. We recommend something in between.

Too much 'stuff'?

It's really unnecessary to have endless paraphernalia for your baby. Few couples go overboard the second time around, partly because there's nothing left to buy, partly because they have no money left and partly because they've learnt that not only does the baby not need, or use, a large proportion of what's on offer, but also that the baby grows up very fast and there simply isn't time to get involved in it all.

Recycle, be creative

Now is the time to reaffirm our need for loving relationships, not our need for material goods. You'll find many friends and members of your family willing to pass on equipment to you—stuff that was new and has hardly been used—or you may be lucky enough to have a family crib that gets passed on from generation to generation. It may be a time to hone those carpentry skills and produce something unique, or scour the second-hand shops, classified advertisements and shop windows. You will need a car capsule (if you have, or travel in, a car), a sling to hold your baby close, some nappies, shawls, cotton wool, baby sponge or face cloth and a pram or convertible stroller. If you have neither a car capsule nor a convertible stroller, you may need a carry-cot. And we probably don't need to mention baby clothes—you're likely to be inundated with these as gifts. A baby bath and a changing table are useful, but not essential. However, the only thing that is really important is to create a space for your child, wherever that may be. Hopefully it's as close to you as possible, with access to the family bed.

Make space for your child

As well as a place in your home, your baby needs a place in your life. You'll feel less anxious if you've sorted out your work commitments, your support groups and how you're going to pay for everything. If you don't have the luxury of certainty in these major areas, you'll still be able to feel a lot more optimistic and in control if you get the small details sorted out. Now is also a good time to work out how you will cope with the nappies, and whether your washing machine will be adequate. (We don't recommend polluting disposables, or nappy services that use bleaches.) There are some marvellous environmentally friendly alternatives to detergents and bleaches—try in your health food shop. If you have a freezer, stock up on some ready made dishes, and enlist the help of family and friends. The more prepared you are, the less stressed you'll feel.

The other thing you should have organised before you progress too far in your pregnancy is the kind of support you want for the birth, where you want to be for it, and what kind of preparatory guidance you require. We'll look at this further in Chapter 12.

Coping with other people's reactions

Whatever choices you make, someone will disapprove. Remember this is your baby and your birth, but also be aware of how these events affect your other relationships, and that others also have their hopes and dreams for this child. This is especially true of prospective grandparents, or most of them.

Your family

Your parents or parents-in-law may seem indifferent and unhelpful, and this can be a cause of stress. Or they may be over-protective or over-prescriptive, or even feel left out and concerned that their relationship with you will suffer. In most cases there will be a profound shift in your relationship with your mother as you start to share the experiences that she probably remembers vividly from her own time, and this may forge new and stronger links between you. This may also be true for your partner and his father. Pregnancy and parenting can be an experience shared with many members of your family and can bring you much closer together.

However, if your relationships with your parents or in-laws aren't working well, it would be good to talk it through so everyone can understand each other's feelings and work to improve things. It's certainly not going to help anyone if misunderstandings cause rifts. Apart from the stress this will cause you, it can be devastating for the grandparents too, and of course it would be a shame if bad feelings now jeopardised your child's relationship with his grandparents later. Try and establish some guidelines with your parents-in-law so they can feel as connected with the whole process as your own parents, without invading your privacy. Remember that all relationships are fluid, and that most people prefer, and are willing to work towards, a positive outcome, even if there are fundamental disagreements.

Your other children
If you already have children, then your pregnancy and the impending birth of a new sibling will pose challenges for them too. Try to involve your children in all aspects of the pregnancy and give them hands-on experience of the baby's movements. If older children will be affected by changes to domestic arrangements which are made to accommodate the baby, minimise their feelings of displacement by getting these in place well before the birth. Good antenatal classes can help you with this. Decide now whether your children will be present at the birth, and make sure they understand what may happen if they do attend. Try not to take out your feelings of fatigue or anxiety on your children, but let them know that you have needs and that they can help.

Other mums
Now is also the time to develop your support group, arrange to meet with other mothers and, if necessary, choose someone to help out at the birth—this is particularly important if you are a single mum. Don't be afraid to ask, most people will be flattered to be chosen.

One thing all new mothers comment on is how they feel in communion with all other mothers; how they notice other mums on the streets, and give that 'I-know-how-it-is' smile; how they help out when they see another woman struggling with her stroller and shopping bags up some steps; how they have lots to say to people that they would never have spoken to before. It's a great leveller, this thing called motherhood, it elevates us all to the same giddy heights and brings us all down to earth together.

Maintaining your sexual relationship
We've talked a bit about your relationship with your partner—one thing that may need to be discussed is how you feel about sex and how to go about it. Most women feel extremely sensual when pregnant, possibly because of the high level of circulating hormones. Although all your erogenous zones may become more sensitive, you may feel less like penetrative sex in the first trimester (when you may be quite tired) and the third, when your body becomes awkwardly large. This doesn't mean that this type of sex is prohibited, but

different positions may need to be explored to accommodate your shape.

Orgasm can exercise the uterine muscles, and may even cause contractions in the latter part of the pregnancy. These should last only a few minutes and are not dangerous. Sex should not, however, be over-athletic, and certainly you should avoid sex with a partner who may have an infection. Though the cervix is sealed and the baby protected in the amniotic bag, infections can be transmitted during delivery, so you should not put yourself or your baby at risk.

However, sex may be better avoided, on the advice of your midwife or doctor, if you have placenta praevia, have any breakthrough bleeding, if either of these problems occurred during previous pregnancies or if there is a history of threatened, or actual, miscarriage.

SPECIFIC NATURAL REMEDIES FOR STRESS REDUCTION

Now we need to look at some specific remedies and techniques for managing stress. Some of these are best supervised or initiated by a professional, others are self-help techniques, and quite a few are inherent in the advice we've already given. Into this category fall practices that should be part of your everyday life, like maintaining good nutrition, getting plenty of exercise and sleep, and gathering support from family and friends.

Nutrition for stress reduction

If you have a well-nourished body you will not only cope better with all aspects of your pregnancy, but you will also automatically reduce your stress levels. In addition to following our overall recommendations set out in Chapters 3 and 4, if you are still feeling distressed or anxious you could try increasing your *calcium* and *magnesium* (in a 2:1 ratio). Both these minerals are in great demand during pregnancy and can easily become depleted. They are also nature's sedatives and their lack can contribute enormously to anxiety, irritability or nervousness. Clues to magnesium deficiency include leg cramps and chocolate cravings (as chocolate is quite rich in magnesium but is not the source we recommend!).

The *B-complex* vitamins are also reduced by stress, as they are in greater demand at this time. They are also part of your body's coping mechanism, so you may need to temporarily increase your input. The same goes for *vitamin C*.

Fluctuating blood sugar levels can cause extreme fatigue and lead to stress. To stabilise them, eat little and often, especially light proteins such as nuts (particularly almonds) and whole grains and seeds, and you won't need to reach for the sugar bowl in a desperate attempt to increase your energy. Chromium can be helpful if sugar cravings continue to be a problem, and you may need to temporarily increase your dosage to the upper limit of our recommendations in Chapter 4.

Adequate sleep is essential

We've already looked at some of the reasons why sleep may be difficult during pregnancy. We just want to stress (there's that word again!) that adequate sleep is fundamental to getting through pregnancy in a relaxed and comfortable manner. Sleep should be undisturbed if possible, in a darkened room, and on a supportive mattress, away from technologies, telephones, intrusive noises and electromagnetic fields (especially electric blankets or water beds).

Here are some helpful hints for dealing with this situation. There's more on which herbs, essential oils, flower essences, homoeopathic remedies and acupressure points to use in the following sections.

- Don't drink too much too late in the evening. We encourage you to drink lots of fresh, purified water, but if you need to get up too often in the night, try to do most of your hydrating earlier in the day.

- Don't eat too fast or too late. Indigestion is a common complaint in pregnancy (you can find some remedies in Chapter 13), and can certainly keep you awake. Eat slowly, chew your food well, and have your dinner at least 4 hours before bedtime. This is good practice for family life and also good advice for non-pregnant people, as digestion is very inefficient once you are in bed. You might consider making lunch your main meal. It is, however, quite helpful to have a small snack of some light protein (e.g. almonds, other nuts, whole grains, seeds) last thing at night to keep your blood sugar levels stable. If they fluctuate too much, you will feel fatigued but restless, and are more likely to suffer nausea.

- Avoid watching disturbing shows on TV which can get your emotions churned up and your mind racing.

- Use relaxation techniques to get off to sleep (or back to sleep). Later in this chapter we'll give you some suggestions for visualisations and affirmations. You could try plain old counting sheep, which is really just a form of mantra meditation, or a favourite relaxation or music tape. Sometimes focusing on your own regular breathing pattern is sufficient.

- Have a warm (not hot) bath before bed, with some relaxing essential oils (see later on for specific remedies). These can also be used in a burner in your room, or sprinkled on your pillow. It's actually quite dangerous to let your body temperature rise above 38.9°C for sustained periods during pregnancy, so spas and saunas are not recommended as aids to relaxation at this time.

- Flower essences or homoeopathic remedies can be taken to help your mind stop spinning and assist relaxation, and some herbs are helpful too (though you should seek professional advice on herbs that are safe during pregnancy; see also our list in Appendix 6). Herb teas can be drunk cold as well as hot, so can be left by the bed for use in the middle of the night, and there are herbal pillows which you can take to bed with you. (See later on for specific remedies.)

- Calming nutrients such as *calcium* and *magnesium* can be absorbed really quickly if taken as celloid/tissue salts just before retiring. These work even better if combined with sedative herbal remedies.

- The acupressure points we recommend later on can be used at night to relax you and help get you off to sleep.

- Make sure you're comfortable. There are two issues here—size and heat. Try placing extra pillows under your tummy (you'll be better off on your side) and between your knees, and say a quick bedtime prayer of thanks that you're not this size all the time! You are also quite a bit hotter than usual during pregnancy (all that progesterone), so make sure you have plenty of cool fresh air in your bedroom.

- If you wake in the middle of the night and the measures we've suggested don't work, your wakefulness may be due to your baby's activity. If you get up and walk around for a while, this may help to calm him down. It's also good practice for after the birth! If all else fails, you could read for a while. You could try this book, though we quite resent our own suggestion that it might put you to sleep!

Exercise will help too

In Chapter 9 we talked of the helpful effects of exercise as a de-stressor. The endorphins released during normal exercise will help you to feel positive, and studies have confirmed that moderate exercise can increase the effectiveness of other treatments for depression.

During pregnancy we've advocated a more gentle approach to exercise, without sacrificing effectiveness, and all the recommendations in Chapter 9 will be effective in combating stress. Yoga, however, stands out in this regard, whether you attend a class or simply follow our suggestions at home. Integral to yoga are breathing techniques which are very calming and centring, and will be taught in any yoga class you attend.

Breathing, music, water and light therapies

Breath therapy, where breathing is used to release tension and psychological blocks, is part of many stress management programs. It can be part of yoga, meditation or visualisation, though some practitioners use it by itself. One form, commonly called rebirthing, often makes use of water immersion, and the calming and supportive qualities of water are also the basis of float tank therapy, where highly salted water facilitates effortless floating. If you enjoy this it may encourage you to consider a water birth for your baby!

Ambient or relaxation music is often played as you float, combining subtle and gentle musical compositions with natural sounds, at a relaxed pace. Music is uplifting and inspirational as well as relaxing, and you may prefer the classical variety, which could be acoustic or choral, secular or sacred. Your baby will enjoy it too.

Lighting also deserves a mention. There are studies which show increased levels of stress, agitation and health problems in people who spend a significant number of hours each day under artificial fluorescent light. Full spectrum light (as in daylight or special fluorescent tubes) is essential for the healthy functioning of the endocrine system, and there are ways of optimising the 'health' of your lighting systems. (For information about full spectrum lighting, see Contacts and Resources.)

For example, you should try to use incandescent bulbs rather than fluorescent, and full spectrum tubes where fluorescent lighting is unavoidable. (Unfortunately the new environmentally friendly fluorescent 'bulbs' are not full spectrum, and neither are those sold for growing plants.) Above all, use daylight wherever possible and try not to shade it out with over-enthusiastic use of sunglasses, tinted optical lenses or windows. Deal with the UV threat by wearing a hat or staying in the shade whenever possible, and limit exposure to the sun to short periods in the early morning and late afternoon.

Massage—way to go!

Massage is a favourite way to relax, and is particularly appropriate during pregnancy when posture problems can create back pain. Professional massage can be a real treat, but even massage exchanges between friends and family can be very effective. If a full body rub isn't appropriate, neck, head and shoulder or foot rubs may help to release tension in a most enjoyable way.

Of course a tummy rub is practically mandatory and we've yet to see a pregnant woman who doesn't automatically rub her growing belly. The touch here should not be too heavy-handed—imagine it's the baby you're massaging. Indeed it's often the case that the baby will move in response to the movements and touch of the masseur's hands. There's a growing trend to teach prospective and new mothers the art of baby massage, which is the natural extension of antenatal massage once your baby has been born. Massage of the lower back requires a firmer pressure, and there are quite a few practitioners who specialise in pregnancy massage.

Massage can be combined with other special techniques, such as acupressure, reflexology and aromatherapy, which can make it even more effective in relieving stress.

Acupuncture, acupressure (shiatsu) and reflexology

These techniques use specific points to trigger the release of stress and muscle tension. These points can be stimulated by pressure, laser beam, electric current, needles or heat (an acupuncturist will use a burning 'moxa' stick made of aromatic herbs). The theory is that energy flows through the body on certain pathways, and when blockages occur, disease results. The treatment is focused on releasing the blockage, and allowing the life force or 'chi' to flow freely. Whether these pathways correlate to Western understandings of physiological structures, such as nerve pathways, is not proven.

To use laser beams, electric current, needles or heat, it's best to attend a clinic (see Contacts and Resources), but acupressure is easy for anyone to use.

How to stimulate an acupressure point

First, find the point as accurately as you can. Then apply calming pressure by covering the point with the palm of the hand, or by gently stroking, for about 2 minutes.

Stomach 36: Bend your leg at a right angle (90 degrees). Measure four finger widths below the knee, on the outside of the tibia. Stomach 36 should be calmed for stress reduction but this point should *not* be used in the ninth month of pregnancy.

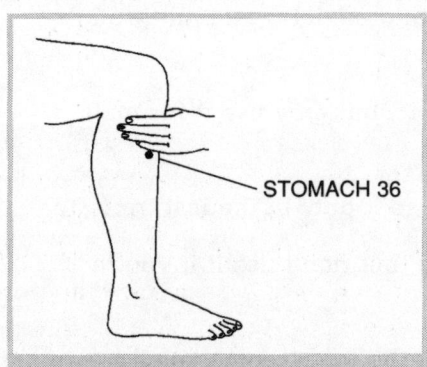
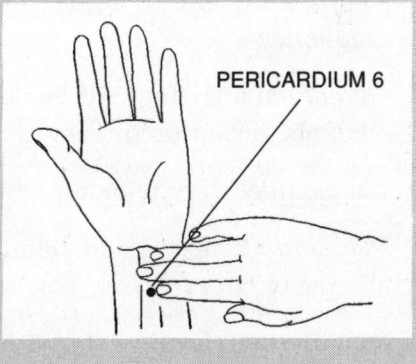

Pericardium 6: This point is three finger widths up the inside of your arm from the wrist crease, between the two tendons (third finger finds the spot). It should be calmed to help overcome insomnia. This point should *not* be used in the fourth month of pregnancy.

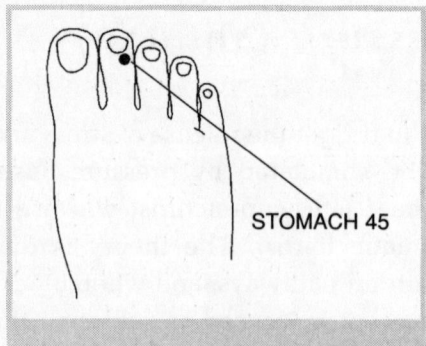

Stomach 45: You'll find this point on the bottom outer corner of the nail bed of the second toe on the side nearest to the third toe. It should be calmed to help overcome insomnia. This point should *not* be used in the sixth month of pregnancy.

Aromatherapy for relaxation

Essential oils can be used during massage, in your bath or in an oil burner to great effect. Calming oils that are appropriate for pregnancy include:

- *Lavender:* Anti-depressant and calming, but use it only in small doses (by this we mean keep the smell subtle, and don't use it all day and every day), and not in first trimester

- *Neroli:* Excellent for depression and anxiety, safe all through pregnancy

- *Geranium:* Relaxing and analgesic, but only use it in small amounts during pregnancy

- *Chamomile:* Very relaxing, but use it only in the last trimester

- *Mandarin:* Relaxing and calming, but don't use it if you're allergic to citrus

- *Sandalwood:* Sedative, but it may be too strong a smell if you are nauseated; use it only in small amounts during pregnancy

- *Rose:* Calming, cheering and very feminine, but only use in the last 2–3 weeks of pregnancy, as a preparation for labour

    (You'll find more details on the use of essential oils in Chapter 13.)

Flower essences for your emotions

Flower essences shift emotional blocks and transform negative feelings into positive. They work in such a subtle and gentle way that often people can't really remember why they started to take them! 'Stress? What's that? I'm sure I don't need to take anything!' The original and most famous are the *Bach Flower essences*, the discovery of Dr Edward Bach, who worked in England in the 1930s and whose remedies are used worldwide. Many countries have now developed their own ranges using native flowers. In Australia, Ian White, a health practitioner, has created the Australian Bush Flower essences.

Bach Flower essences recommended for use during pregnancy include:
- *Aspen:* For vague fears of unknown origin
- *Cerato:* For those who seek advice and confirmation from others
- *Clematis:* For lack of interest in present, inattentiveness
- *Elm:* For those overwhelmed by responsibility
- *Gentian:* For discouragement
- *Heather:* For self-centredness, self-concern
- *Hornbeam:* For weakness, doubting strength to cope
- *Larch:* For lack of confidence
- *Mimulus:* For fear of known things
- *Olive:* For complete exhaustion
- *Vervain:* For tension, hyper-anxiety
- *Walnut:* For protection from change and outside influences
- *White Chestnut:* For unwanted thoughts, mental arguments

The Australian Bush Flower essences appropriate for this time include:
- *Billy Goat Plum:* To accept changing body shape
- *Five Corners:* As above
- *Wild Potato Bush:* To accept difficulties of increasing size in the last trimester
- *Dog Rose:* For niggling fears, sense of insecurity about being pregnant, and fear of labour
- *Fringed Violet:* Especially in the last trimester to protect against the negative influence of other people's experience, or the shock of unwanted or unplanned pregnancy
- *Grey Spider Flower:* For terror about coming birth process: encourages calmness, courage and faith

- *Flannel Flower:* To help the prospective father express his emotions and communicate
- *Red Helmet Orchid:* To help a man bond to the baby during the pregnancy
- *She Oak:* For balancing hormones early in and after the pregnancy
- *Illawarra Flame Tree:* For feeling overwhelmed by responsibility
- *Sturt Desert Pea:* For any crying or grief which is experienced during pregnancy

Homoeopathy in pregnancy

Homoeopathy uses minute dilutions of mineral and herbal remedies which trigger the body to create its own responses. It's not appropriate to list specific remedies here, as treatment is usually restricted to one remedy at a time, which is prescribed by the homoeopath after he or she has assessed the whole picture of mental and physical health. These are very appropriate remedies for stress in pregnancy, but should be administered by a trained practitioner.

Herbal remedies for emotional states

Herbal remedies are extremely effective treatments for stress, anxiety, insomnia and depression. However, some of them are not safe in pregnancy, and you should consult a medical herbalist if you are interested in these treatments. See also the list of herbs contra-indicated in pregnancy in Appendix 6, if you are buying through a health food shop. Herbs can be taken as a tea, used as a fluid extract, or taken as capsules or tablets. They can even be stuffed in a pillow (for insomnia).

Unless the herb appears on the contra-indicated list in Appendix 6, you can safely drink it as a tea. As teas are a relatively weak form of the herb (compared to, say, a fluid extract), there are several herbs which have a caution attached to them in Appendix 6 but are still safe in occasional, small doses, as a relatively large amount would need to be ingested before there need be cause for concern. By 'occasional, small doses' we mean that 1–2 cups of tea daily, at a time of need, will be absolutely fine, but it might be better not to exceed this dose or continue to drink it every day in the long term. Use the following herbs as occasional teas only, and if in any doubt consult a medical herbalist.

Herbs to calm you
- *Valerian:* An excellent sedative, but use only small doses during pregnancy; particularly useful for insomnia, when it combines well with calcium and magnesium phosphate tissue salts
- *Lemon Balm:* Especially useful for anxiety, insomnia, nightmares; use only small doses in pregnancy
- *Motherwort:* Calming (though not causing drowsiness) and helpful with palpitations. Use small doses only in pregnancy
- *Skullcap:* Calming and helpful for deep refreshing sleep. Use small doses only in pregnancy
- *Hops:* Not during the first trimester and not for regular use in pregnancy, but excellent for occasional calming and insomnia
- *Zizyphus:* A safe, effective sedating herb, also useful for insomnia
- *Cramp Bark:* A safe, effective sedating herb, also useful for cramps
- *Lime Flowers:* A safe, effective sedating herb, also useful for hypertension
- *Catnip:* A safe sedative herb useful for mums (and children, as well as cats!); also full of helpful minerals

Herbs to lift depression
- *St John's Wort:* Shown in studies to be more effective than medical drugs in lifting depression. Use only in small doses during pregnancy
- *Damiana:* Lifts your energy. Use only in small doses during pregnancy

Herbs to help stress
- *Oats:* Can also be eaten, as porridge or muesli
- *Withania:* A traditional and wonderful tonic in pregnancy, helpful both to raise energy and calm simultaneously

Leisure and pleasure

Of course, one obvious way to reduce stress is to indulge in pleasurable leisure activities. At this time when you are, perhaps, at your closest to Mother Nature, you might find contact with natural environments helpful to lift your spirits and soothe your soul.

Talking through your problems

Talking through your problems can be very therapeutic. Remember the old saying, 'A problem shared is a problem halved'? You can ease your problems by talking with friends and family, your partner, or with a professional counsellor. You might feel that you need to seek help if the self-help remedies we have suggested don't relieve acute anxiety or depression, or if fears become phobic. There is a wide range of psychotherapy modalities available, and practitioners may use a combination of techniques, such as counselling, hypnotherapy, body-centred or breathing therapies, or energy balancing. There's also the chance to talk things through with your midwife, or the teacher at your antenatal class, who may well be qualified and equipped to meet your needs.

Hypnotherapy

Hypnotherapy is a particularly useful form of therapy for the kind of fears and anxieties that often beset the pregnant woman. This is essentially a very deep state of relaxation in which you can release negative emotions that have become locked into a subconscious pattern. Contrary to common belief, there is no loss of control in hypnotherapy, and you are not prey to suggestions that you don't feel comfortable with or would not welcome in your fully conscious state. You can stop a hypnotherapy session at any time. It's a very useful way to help you stay motivated if you are tempted to smoke cigarettes, drink alcohol or indulge in other unhelpful or unhealthy habits.

Meditation, contemplation, prayer

Meditation is similar to hypnotherapy in that it aims to clear your mind, allowing it to reach a state of absolute calm. One way it achieves this is by focusing on a word known as a mantra. Meditation is usually self-induced (as is self-hypnosis). It can be learnt from teachers or therapists (see Contacts and Resources). Meditation can also be part of religious practice, and for those who are of a religious or spiritual persuasion, contemplation and prayer may also be good supports. Churches, ashrams and other congregations may also be able to offer you support.

Visualisation and affirmation

Visualisation is very similar to meditation, and can help create a confident and relaxed state. You can create your own images, or listen to a recording on which someone else describes a picture of a positive outcome or a calming circumstance. Affirmations are motivating statements that you can repeat to yourself or in your own mind, to help change your negative beliefs or fears to positive emotional states.

We'd like to offer you here a visualisation and some affirmations that you might find helpful, and which can be used at any time you feel in need.

Images of fertility and abundance

See yourself lying under a tree.

All around you there is luxuriant growth. Plants and animals are healthy and abundant. The tree above you filters the light from the sun, and patterns of light and shade dance over you.

Feel the tensions being washed from your body.

Your mind and body are clear and relaxed. Relax from your toes to your head with each breath. Feel each part of your body sink down into the soft bed of grass, and let the tensions drain away into the earth below.

Take three deep breaths.

Send the first to your head, to clear your thoughts. Imagine that you ignite there a spark of warmth and light. Send the second breath to your heart, to bring commitment, joy and strength. Ignite another spark. Send the third breath to your womb, to bring health and fertility, warmth and light.

See all these sparks of warmth and light start to glow.

They spread and join until they fill your head and body, and you feel wonderful.

Tell yourself that you will do this visualisation any time you are in need.

This could be whenever you need a boost in confidence, or when you have a choice to make.

See yourself rise.

Look around at the lush vegetation. Everything is growing and fertile, drawing nutrients from the soil. Mother Nature has blessed this place. You are part of this place, you are fertile and healthy. If you have a partner that you wish to include in this visualisation, see him rise also and take his hand.

Move to the start of a pleasant pathway.

Look along the path. There is a golden thread stretching from one end to the other. One end of this thread is attached to you, to the centre of your belly, your navel. At the other end is your child, smiling, healthy and happy.

Walk towards your child, one step at a time.

Each step accomplishes something on your journey:

With your first step—confidence and motivation.

With the second step—healthy habits.

With the third step—pollution free environment.

With the fourth step—nutritious diet.

With the fifth step—optimum health (general and reproductive).

With the sixth step—healthy eggs and sperm.

With the seventh step—conscious conception.

With the eighth step—normal full term pregnancy.

With the ninth step—easy birth and delivery.

With the tenth step—take your beautiful, healthy child in your arms, or put it to your breast.

Come back to full wakefulness.

Retain the feeling of joy, anticipation and confidence.

Affirmations for positivity

Sometimes, to finish a visualisation, or to take its place, you may like to use affirmations of your beliefs and intents. Here are some possibilities.

'I am bringing my body and mind back to health, harmony and balance.'

'As my baby grows so do my health and energy.'

'I am filling my body with nutritious food for the sake of my health and that of my child.'

'My pregnancy is unfolding, day by day, exactly as nature intended.'

'I can positively affect my pregnancy, and the health of my child.'

'The love that I share with my child succours and supports us both.'

'My child and I are growing together, and will do so for the rest of my life.'

'Life and love are growing in me day by day.'

'I am in control of my own life, health and pregnancy.'
'I am finding it easy to do all that is necessary to achieve a healthy pregnancy and birth.'
'I am making room in my life for my baby.'
'I am relaxing more and more easily and deeply every day.'
'As I relax more each day, my confidence grows.'
'My baby and I are sending and receiving love all the time.'
'My child is drawing closer and closer.'
'I can, and will, give birth to a very healthy baby.'
'I am honoured to be carrying my child.'
'I am joyfully anticipating the birth of my child.'
'The miracle of life is inside me.'
'I am confident in my ability to give birth easily and successfully.'
'I am confident in my ability to breastfeed my child successfully.'
'I am confident in my ability to care for my child.'
'My child and I will bring each other great joy.'

If you have had previous experience of trauma in pregnancy, or you have special concerns, you might like to use some of these affirmations.

'My pregnancy and baby are progressing exactly as they should.'
'My child is healthy and will survive.'
'My cervix is firm and closed and my baby is safe in my womb.'
'My baby is growing well and will continue to do so until we share the experience of a very easy and successful birth.'
'I will give birth to my baby just as nature intended.'
'My baby and I have great faith in each other.'
'Life is good—and giving life is even better.'

You may find it helpful to imagine a protective shield of white light or a glowing net around your baby, and across your cervix. Energetic or spiritual healing may also be appropriate. This can be done through techniques such as Reiki, a form of laying on of hands (see Contacts and Resources), or through your church or spiritual group. It is also believed to be possible to transmit such healing in absence.

We hope that in this chapter we've described enough natural, non-invasive methods and remedies to make it possible for you to stay relaxed and comfortable throughout your pregnancy and look back on it as one of the most joyful and rewarding experiences in your life.

Chapter 11

Antenatal testing

NON-INVASIVE TESTS

In the previous chapters we have mentioned some of the diagnostic tests which can be carried out to assess nutritional status and presence of infection. In this chapter we give you a comprehensive list of those tests (and of others) which can be performed to give you important information about the healthy progress of your pregnancy.

Zinc taste test

Since zinc is probably the most important trace element during pregnancy it's important that your zinc status is always adequate. The zinc taste test is an easy way to monitor zinc status. To administer this test you'll need to obtain a solution of zinc sulphate from your pharmacist or your local health practitioner. There are several proprietary products available, but your pharmacist can easily prepare some in the dispensary. The solution should contain 590 mg of zinc sulphate septahydrate in 100 ml of purified water. If, after taste testing, it's shown that you need to use the liquid form of zinc supplement, you can ask your pharmacist for a larger bottle to be prepared.

The liquid zinc is better absorbed than a zinc tablet. Ironically, good absorption of zinc depends on adequate zinc levels, so to break a vicious cycle of poor zinc absorption/low zinc levels use of the liquid zinc preparation is necessary.

Alternatively, there are some more concentrated liquid products available, which also contain the co-factors required for proper zinc absorption. This is important since zinc is best taken separately from food (the normal way to ensure the presence of co-factors), because many nutrients compete with zinc for uptake. However, these concentrated zinc drinks cannot be used for the taste test.

How to administer the zinc taste test

The administration of the taste test is absolutely straightforward and, even though it's a very simple test, it has been found that it correlates well with zinc status throughout pregnancy. You should *repeat the test every two months*, even if you had adequate zinc levels at the previous test. The levels may not remain the same, and it's very important that they stay within normal range.

To administer the taste test you take 5 ml of the zinc sulphate solution into your mouth and swish it around. The taste will determine the dosage and form of the zinc supplement you require (see table).

TEST RESULT	SUPPLEMENT DOSAGE & FORM (To be taken separately from food & other supplements)
If the taste is strong/prompt (and was also at the last test)	One zinc tablet daily of 20–25 mg elemental zinc
If the taste is strong/prompt (as a result of building zinc status since last test)	Two zinc tablets daily of 20–25 mg elemental zinc
If the taste test is medium strength/slightly delayed	5 mL twice daily
If the taste test is slight/very delayed	10 mL twice daily
If there is no taste	20 mL twice daily

N.B. The liquid measures we give here are only appropriate for the preparation we describe above. Other commercial preparations may be more concentrated, and an equivalent smaller dose can be used.

While taking the higher doses (of liquid zinc) you should administer the zinc taste test more frequently (for example, weekly) so you can adapt the dosages as required. One reason for a low zinc level, or for one which repeatedly falls away once the dosage is lowered, is a high body burden of heavy metals. If this happens, you may want to test for these also.

Tests for heavy metals

One possible reason for a repeated decline in zinc status and taste sensation is a burden of heavy metals. Your practitioner can use the urine test described in Chapter 6 to test for these, and if this is positive you may wish to have a hair trace mineral analysis performed. Details of this test can be found in Appendix 11.

Full blood count

Your doctor or midwife may take a blood sample to obtain a full blood count. This will show any abnormalities in red or white blood cells and whether there is an active allergic response. At the same time your blood can be tested for other factors, such as: thyroid and liver function; rubella, toxoplasmosis, cytomegalovirus and genito-urinary infections; iron stores; and the Rh factor.

Rubella

If the full blood count shows that you have no immunity to rubella, you may prefer to strengthen your immune system with herbal remedies and nutritional supplements rather than expose your developing baby to rubella immunisation.

Toxoplasmosis and cytomegalovirus

Both infections should be tested for, and treatment is discussed in Chapter 8.

Genito-urinary infections

As well as those GUIs tested through vaginal swab (see next section) if may be necessary to do blood tests for HIV, Hepatitis B and C and Syphilis, if your clinical history indicates any risk factors.

Iron stores (serum ferritin)
Several studies have shown an association between iron levels during pregnancy and an increased risk of prematurity, low birth weight and perinatal mortality. The preferred test is serum ferritin (iron stores), and these levels should be monitored at the end of each trimester, although levels fall during the last two trimesters due to expansion of plasma volume. The dosages of supplement that you may need will depend on the levels. If your iron stores are low it's important that you take only *organic iron* (such as iron chelate) because inorganic iron (such as ferrous sulphate) will compete with zinc for uptake and absorption, destroy vitamin E and may cause constipation. Inorganic iron (the type which should be avoided) is found in many commonly used iron supplements.

It's also very important that you don't take iron supplements unnecessarily. It's common for pregnant women to be given routine iron supplementation and we deplore this practice. Apart from the adverse effects of inorganic iron on zinc and vitamin E, your body has no mechanism for excreting excess iron (apart from menstrual losses, and of course you won't be experiencing any of these for a while).

Rhesus factor
Determining the rhesus (Rh) factor of both parents' blood is important. Problems only arise if the father is Rh positive and the mother Rh negative, and the baby inherits the father's rhesus factor. In this case, some of the baby's blood may enter the mother's circulation via the placenta and her body will start to make antibodies to the 'foreign' blood. This doesn't usually affect the first child, but subsequent children can be harmed unless they can be given a complete blood exchange soon after birth. If you fall into this category, ensuring that your nutritional status is adequate can also ensure optimal capillary strength with less likelihood of any blood leakage occurring.

Vaginal discharges and infections
If you have a vaginal discharge in pregnancy, it is probably thrush (Candida). To be sure, ask your doctor to take a low vaginal swab, and if confirmed there are numerous natural remedies which you can use (see Chapter 8).

Unless you have had a full GUI check-up before conception, we suggest that further swabs are taken to check for the following infections. It's wise to also check your partner (through urethral swab) so he cannot be a source of infection for you. The full list of infections is as follows:

Gonorrhoea	Strep. millerii
Herpes	Enterococcus
Ureaplasma	Haem. influenza
Staph. aureus	Anaerobic bacteria
Gardnerella	Klebsiella
Mycoplasma	Chlamydia
E. coli	B. strep
Candida	

If a positive result is returned, the infection must be treated as soon as possible. Antibiotic therapy might be the only option since some of these infections are very stubborn. It is important that acidophilus and bifidus lactobacilli are given concurrently and that naturopathic immune support is implemented as well. Antibiotics such as the tetracyclines should be avoided since they have an adverse effect on your developing baby's teeth, and unprotected intercourse avoided until a negative (clear) test result is obtained.

Dental check-up

We've talked about the importance of a dental check-up in Chapter 6.

ROUTINE ANTENATAL CHECKS

As technology advances, the simple tests, which your GP or midwife once carried out, have been replaced by a battery of sophisticated screening and diagnostic procedures.

There is no doubt that good antenatal care is essential to ensure that your pregnancy is progressing normally and remains free of complications, but despite what you might think, this does not depend on high technology procedures. There are several simple tests which will be carried out at your first antenatal visit, while at each subsequent visit your carer will carry out some further simple, non-invasive tests.

Blood pressure
Your doctor or midwife will check your blood pressure, and this will be monitored regularly to ensure that there is no hypertension of pregnancy (toxaemia).

Urine tests
Using a dipstick method, your urine will be tested for glucose (sugar) and albumin (protein). This simple test can be used to reveal a pre-diabetic state (glucose) and pre-eclampsia (albumin).

Your baby's size and position
Abdominal palpation or manual feeling of your belly will be performed to assess the height of the fundus and the size of the uterus. From this type of examination an experienced doctor or midwife can check both the size and position of your baby. You will be weighed to assess adequate weight gain (this should total about 13 kilos by the end of your pregnancy), to reveal if you are suffering from any fluid retention and, of course, to confirm the growth of the baby.

Doppler ultrasound
This instrument is able to detect the foetal heartbeat from 12 weeks, but, like the better known ultrasound scan, it employs sound waves or non-ionising radiation, which may not be without risk to your baby. From 24 weeks, your doctor or midwife can safely detect the foetal heartbeat with a stethoscope.

Cardiotocograph (CTG)
This is also called the non-stress test. It is used to assess foetal well-being by monitoring the foetal heart and is often used if your pregnancy continues past 40 weeks. Kick charts, which are a simple way to monitor your baby's movements, can sometimes be just as helpful, and more importantly their use can encourage you to tune in to your baby and to trust your intuition and judgement.

Be an active participant
During these regular check-ups it is important for you to ask questions and ascertain that all is proceeding well. If there are any uncertainties

about the test results you must be sure that you understand any implications for your health as well as for the health of your baby. This pregnancy is happening to you and it is wise for you to find out as much as you can about it. Don't be intimidated by medical specialists and their jargon. Don't feel that they have control over your pregnancy and don't feel obliged to agree to procedures or treatment about which you feel in any way uncertain. You should also remember that if any problems develop, there will be a lot that you can do to help in their management.

If, for example, your blood pressure is high, you may be able to lower it simply by resting, or by reducing your stress levels. There are also many natural remedies which can be useful. Other problems may be manageable by dietary manipulation, or by the judicious use of gentle herbs and vitamin and mineral supplements. Still others may respond to meditation, visualisation, osteopathic treatments or acupuncture. It is important that you explore treatment options in which you are the active participant rather than the passive recipient. If you respond to your baby's and your body's signals in this way, you are gaining trust in both. You will find that your confidence in your body's ability to make a healthy baby is enhanced and you will find too that you feel increasingly positive about your ability to give birth without the help of technology. Of course, we are not suggesting that you disregard your doctor's advice, merely that you enter into a dialogue with her/him, and explore other options.

ANTENATAL SCREENING PROCEDURES

There are numerous screening tests which you might be offered during your pregnancy. Some, such as the ultrasound, are now almost routine; other tests may be offered, depending on your age and your past history. These screening tests have been designed to help women have the 'perfect product'. However, despite all these tests (and the constant development of newer, more sophisticated ones), the accuracy of prenatal testing is still only approximately 60 per cent. Let's consider the tests you might be offered as your pregnancy progresses.

Alpha fetoprotein (AFP) test
An elevated level of alpha fetoprotein (AFP) can be detected by a blood test at 16–18 weeks and may indicate the presence of a neural tube defect such as spina bifida. However, a multiple pregnancy, uncertainty about dates and a threatened abortion are just some of the conditions which can lead to false positive AFP results. For every 25 women with elevated AFP, only one will actually have a baby with a neural tube defect. A low level of AFP can suggest a Down syndrome baby, although most babies with Down syndrome are not detected by the AFP test. It is chastening to reflect on the fact that more than 95 per cent of women who have an AFP test which is outside the normal range have a perfectly normal baby.

T-test
The T (triple) test measures AFP, conjugated oestriol and human chorionic gonadotrophin and relates those measurements to those of age, weight and length of gestation. It is performed at 15–18 weeks and will give an estimated risk for Down syndrome. However, only 1 in 57 women under the age of 37 who test positive will actually be carrying a Down syndrome baby.

b-hCG and PAPP-A test
The markers used in this test are beta-human chorionic gonadotrophin (b-hCG) and pregnancy associated plasma protein (PAPP-A). Though the accuracy of this screening test is just the same as the T-test, it has the advantage of being performed at 10 weeks gestation. If diagnosis with CVS or amniocentesis confirms the results of the screen, a woman can, if she so chooses, terminate her pregnancy much earlier.

Glucose tolerance test (GTT)
You may be offered this test at about 28 weeks. It involves ingesting 50 g of glucose drink. The excessive sweetness can often make a woman feel dizzy and nauseous. We wonder how that huge load of glucose makes her baby feel? You will remember that we talked about the importance of the baby's blood glucose levels being stable at all times! A high result on this initial test will see you sent off for a formal GTT which will take two and a half hours. A positive result puts you

in the category of 'high risk' for gestational diabetes and, as Enkin, Keirse and Chalmers, in *A Guide to Effective Care in Pregnancy and Childbirth* state, 'on the conveyor belt for an extensive and expensive program of tests and interventions of unproven benefit'.

Biophysical profile (BPP)

This test involves assessment of five biophysical variables:

- Foetal movement
- Tone
- Reactivity
- Breathing
- Amniotic fluid volume

They are assessed by studying serial ultrasounds and antenatal cardiotocography in high-risk pregnancies. Combining these to give a score is believed to indicate foetuses which are 'at risk' if the pregnancy continues. However, only two controlled trials of BPP testing have been carried out and their use does not result in any improvements in outcome for the baby.

Group B Haemolytic Streptococcus

This test determines the presence of an organism which may live in the female genital tract or rectum and occurs in 10–20 per cent of normal, healthy, pregnant women. However, no harm occurs unless the woman becomes very run down or clinically ill, and then the organism may proliferate and cause problems such as pre-term delivery or stillbirth. We feel that if you follow all of our recommendations throughout your pregnancy, proliferation should not occur. But you should be aware that if this routine swab (taken at 28 weeks) shows the presence of the Strep B organism, some hospitals make an antibiotic drip during labour compulsory. This means unnecessary administration of antibiotics to a high proportion of normal, healthy, pregnant women, since there's only about 1 per cent chance of the baby being infected. Most of these cases (of neonatal sepsis) are associated with one or more clinical risk factors—preterm labour, prolonged rupture of membranes or maternal fever.

Think carefully before you agree to screening

Some of these tests are designed to screen for neural tube defect and Down syndrome. But remember that these two conditions are by no means the only ones to cause serious disability. Remember too that there is significant potential for false positive and false negative results. We suggest you think very carefully about what you would do and how you would feel if your test result was positive before submitting to any of them.

ANTENATAL DIAGNOSTIC PROCEDURES

Ultrasound scan (USS)

The most popular of the diagnostic tests is the ultrasound scan. Sound waves are bounced off your baby to produce an image on a screen. Ultrasound waves are certainly not without risk, particularly when this procedure is carried out in the early weeks of pregnancy when the developing embryo is most vulnerable.

Subtle adverse effects on the foetus

Enough studies have now been conducted to establish conclusively the potential for a variety of adverse effects, which have been well-documented in Lynne McTaggart's excellent and highly recommended book *What Doctors Don't Tell You* (see 'Recommended Reading'). Many of these effects are very subtle, involving neurological deficits and developmental delays which may not be immediately apparent upon the birth of your baby, although a direct link has been established between ultrasound and low birth weight. Some of the other effects which have been reported include an increased incidence of miscarriage, lower Apgar scores (the measure of your baby's health at birth), left-handedness, delayed speech, dyslexia, damage of the central nervous system and changes to DNA and cell growth.

McTaggart records that as long ago as 1982, the following statement was made in a report published by the United States agency, the National Centre for Devices and Radiological Health, which is a part of the Food and Drug Administration: 'We can be reasonably certain that acute dramatic effects are not likely . . . But studies have not been made to detect less obvious effects, and the question of subtle, long-term or cumulative effects remains unanswered. The potential for acute adverse effects has not been explored and the potential for delayed effects has been virtually ignored.'

The International Childbirth Education Association (ICEA) has maintained that ultrasound is most likely to affect development (behavioural and neurological), blood cells, the immune system and a child's genetic make-up. Robert Bases, chief of Radiology at New York's Albert Einstein College, speaks of the 'bewildering array of ultrasound bioeffects described in over 700 publications since 1950'.

Alternative ways to assess foetal size

Why then would you submit your baby to this sort of screening? What do you hope to learn or to gain? An ultrasound scan obviously confirms your pregnancy, but then so does a urine or blood test. Confirmation of the presence of more than one foetus, or adequate foetal growth are other reasons given for performing a scan, but experienced obstetricians and midwives can assess the presence of a multiple pregnancy and the size of your baby by manual palpation. Scans are often used to assess 'dates', that is, the gestational age of the foetus as guaged by its size. Depending on the skill of the technician (and remember that training is not mandatory with the purchase of the scanning equipment), this assessment may not always be accurate and may therefore be in conflict with the dates you have calculated. If this is the case, the uncertainty which is aroused may undermine your confidence in the pregnancy. The performance of the scan for this reason will not influence the end result, which is a baby who will be born when it is ready.

False negatives/positives

A scan may also be performed to detect the position of the placenta. Using ultrasound diagnosis, a rate of placenta praevia of 64 : 1000 births has been found, yet the incidence of this condition at term is only 1 : 1000, which seems to indicate that 63 women may have been unnecessarily alarmed. Ultrasound can also be used to detect malformations and abnormalities, but according to Chitty, Hunt and Moore only 74 per cent of anomalies are actually detected. Despite this less than adequate success rate, ultrasound could be a less invasive way to check for some abnormalities (including Down syndrome) than CVS or amniocentesis, which can also give uncertain results.

Adverse effects of ultrasound on the mother
Reports have been published on the ability of ultrasound to damage maternal erythrocytes (mature red blood cells) which carry oxygen to all parts of your body (and to your baby). Ultrasound has also been shown to have an effect on human chorionic gonadotrophin (which is the hormone which maintains the pregnancy). What this means in real terms is not yet clear, but we think it better that you and your baby aren't part of the data bank which might allow researchers to find out.

Ultrasound will not improve the outcome of pregnancy
In 1984 the American College of Obstetrics and Gynaecology issued the following statement: 'No well controlled study has yet proved that routine scanning of prenatal patients will improve the outcome of pregnancy.' There is now consensus amongst doctors and researchers in both the UK and the US that of eight major studies (conducted since this statement was issued) attempting to evaluate the effectiveness of ultrasound, 'None has shown that routine use improves either maternal or infant outcome over that achieved when diagnostic ultrasound was used only when medically indicated.' All the pertinent US regulatory bodies now urge obstetricians not to use ultrasound routinely.

Before you agree to a scan, therefore, you should make sure that there is a very good reason for its performance (for example, to confirm placenta praevia if there is bleeding late in pregnancy). This is particularly important if your doctor wants to carry out more than one ultrasound scan. There are studies which clearly show that various adverse outcomes are more likely to occur in children born after even one scan was performed during pregnancy.

Chorionic villus sampling (CVS)
This test is performed at approximately 9–12 weeks of pregnancy to rule out chromosomal abnormality, sickle-cell anaemia and sex-linked abnormalities (such as Duchenne's muscular dystrophy and haemophilia). The advantage of CVS is that it can be performed relatively early in a pregnancy (as opposed to amniocentesis which cannot give results until about 20 weeks gestation). If there is to be a therapeutic termination then the earlier you have the results, the less traumatic (theoretically) that may be.

Risks include miscarriage

To perform the CVS, an ultrasound scan is carried out at 7–8 weeks to confirm the pregnancy and another scan is performed at the time of the biopsy. This involves taking a sample of the chorionic villi, the initial tissue of the placenta. The biopsy may be carried out through the walls of the stomach or through the vagina. The immediate complications can include perforation of the amniotic sac, bleeding which may be mild or severe, or infection. The stress on both mother and foetus may be considerable. In up to 45 per cent of cases, depending on the experience of the technician, there is failure to obtain a tissue sample. The procedure is said to carry a 1–10 per cent risk of miscarriage, again the rate depends on the experience of the technician. In 2–10 per cent of cases there is failure to produce a result. These are hardly statistics to instil confidence!

A further scan must then be performed at 16 weeks to confirm that the pregnancy is continuing normally, and of course three scans performed relatively close together may not be without further risk to the foetus. Apart from the risk of bleeding, infection and miscarriage, not to mention the need to repeat the test and the ultrasound effects, reports are now appearing of limb abnormalities in babies whose mothers had CVS. But it appears that limb abnormalities may be just the tip of an iceberg. In one study of 75 mothers who had undergone CVS, every single one had produced a baby with some birth defect, ranging from lost limbs to damaged nails!

False negatives/positives

Unfortunately false positives and false negatives are also common with CVS. It now appears that the genetic material found in the chorionic villus may not always be identical to that of the foetus. In other words, the chorion may contain abnormal chromosomes, yet those of the baby may be perfectly normal. This leaves open to question the entire theory upon which CVS rests.

Amniocentesis

Amniocentesis is performed at 15–17 weeks and is also used to detect chromosomal abnormalities and sex-linked diseases. An ultrasound scan is performed to locate the position of the baby and the placenta prior to a needle being inserted into the mother's abdomen. About 15 ml of amniotic fluid is withdrawn for testing.

Risks include miscarriage
This procedure obviously carries a risk, since the needle may pierce the foetus or infection may be introduced. This can lead to foetal death, miscarriage and stillbirth. This risk is increased if the practitioner is not highly skilled. Statistics generally rate the procedure as bearing a 1–2 per cent risk of spontaneous abortion, and 1–3 per cent of babies will exhibit evidence of being touched by the needle. In 1978 the British Medical Research Council also reported a 3 per cent increase in neonatal respiratory distress (which may be due to the amount of fluid withdrawn) and a 2.4 per cent increase in congenital dislocations of the hips and feet.

Some of Francesca's patients have chosen to have an amniocentesis (although many more do not). Of those who did, a significant number have miscarried (often after taking years to achieve conception). Of these, several have been told, despite the miscarriage happening within hours of the amniocentesis, that the procedure was not responsible. This certainly makes us wonder how the statistics on miscarriage are assessed, and whether the rate may be much higher than actually admitted.

A termination means a labour and birth
There is also little doubt that this test is extremely stressful for both mother and child. The results can take up to four weeks to be determined. Should an abnormality be detected the foetus is then at about 20 weeks gestation and already active in utero. If a termination is decided on at this stage in the pregnancy, it will involve a labour and birth. There are also plenty of false positives with this test, despite its claims for accuracy.

X-rays
X-rays can be used to assess the size and shape of your pelvis and the size and position of your baby. They are often used to determine whether vaginal birth is possible especially if the baby is breech or if you have had a previous Caesarean section. Unfortunately, X-rays cannot take into account the movement and relaxation of your pelvic

bones during labour or the way the baby's head moulds to help it pass through the birth canal, which makes the use of X-rays for this purpose of very dubious usefulness, and of course exposure to ionising radiation of any type is extremely damaging. This is especially so in the case of cells which are dividing rapidly (such as those of your baby).

CAN YOU JUSTIFY ANTENATAL SCREENING?

Why not trust your instincts?

We feel that the use of antenatal screening and diagnostic procedures may undermine your confidence in your pregnancy. Because the use of these tests is so routine, you may feel that without them you cannot be confident that your baby is healthy and is growing normally. Your reliance on these procedures may also set the stage for further reliance on technological intervention during the birth. Certainly in a low-risk pregnancy which is progressing normally the use of a test such as ultrasound scan may not only be unnecessary, but there are no studies which show that its performance makes any appreciable positive difference to the final outcome of pregnancy. It should be stressed too that the results of ultrasound and other diagnostic procedures are in no way a guarantee of a perfect baby. They simply exclude the presence of neural tube defects, of some chromosomal abnormalities such as Down syndrome and of sex-linked diseases. In view of these considerations, it is questionable whether it is worth exposing you and your baby to the possible negative effects of these tests.

Results cause needless concern or give false reassurance

There is also the real and very significant possibility of both false negative and false positive results. This means that you may be needlessly worried that your perfectly healthy baby is suffering from some congenital abnormality. Natalie Angier, writing in November 1996 in the *International Herald Tribune*, recounts her own traumatic pregnancy. At 20 weeks a 'routine' ultrasound scan detected a possible clubfoot. This diagnosis was confirmed by two subsequent scans performed by doctors with extensive expertise in ultrasound diagnosis. The latter half of this woman's pregnancy became a nightmare. She writes:

> We wept and wept. We offered up our own body parts in exchange: eyes, arms, feet. I became obsessed with clubfeet, medically and culturally. I learned that for several months to a year our daughter would have to wear a thigh-high cast designed to twist her foot gradually into a normal useable position. I learned that the cast would have to be changed every week, that casting alone might not work, and that she might require one or more operations. As for the asymmetry of her calves, that would be untreatable and permanent.
>
> Finally toward the end of the pregnancy I began to relax. In late August I gave birth to a healthy daughter with a set of lusty lungs, a full head of black hair—and no clubfoot.

For other women, given the diagnosis of disabilities much more serious than a clubfoot, or for women in search of an absolutely 'perfect product' the results can lead to the termination of a completely normal pregnancy. Conversely, the tests do not always detect an abnormality, and in the case where you have undergone the test for 'reassurance' you may be misleadingly 'reassured' when, indeed, there is a problem.

Male or female—do you really want to know?

Of course antenatal screening can also tell you whether your baby is a boy or a girl, but revelation of the sex of your unborn child by these tests may actually remove some of that special mystery from your pregnancy and may perhaps detract from the anticipation and excitement of the birth.

Do these tests help you bond to your baby?

A woman who has had routine ultrasound scans will frequently tell you, 'I certainly felt more comfortable after seeing him on the screen. I think it helped me bond to him.' If this woman's baby has no obvious abnormalities, she is unlikely to think that there were any physical or mental ill-effects from the exposure to ultrasound scans. But just remember—some of the adverse effects of the scans are extremely subtle and some of the neurological deficits may not be apparent for quite some time. As for the 'buzz' women get from seeing their baby on the screen and the thrill of having their 'first baby photograph', do these women ever stop to ask how the bonding process happened in the millennia before the technological marvel of ultrasound?

Do you need the doubt and uncertainty?

We recommend that you do your own reading and we have suggested some titles in Sources and Recommended Reading. Find out all you can about the procedure without simply relying on what your doctor tells you. Remember that screening and diagnostic testing equipment represents a multi-million dollar business, which is growing exponentially. The major beneficiaries of this business are the manufacturers of the equipment. However, the real and undisputed benefits to the consumers, the absolute advantage to those who are subjected to the screening and diagnostics, are much less clear.

There is no doubt that many women who fail to do any 'homework' and who put themselves trustingly in their physician's hands find themselves on a conveyor belt of one test after another. They find that what seemed to be a good idea at the time turns (particularly after a positive or uncertain result is returned) into a nightmare of doubt, questioning and uncertainty, followed by more tests and more doubt, and so on. Little counselling is given to women about how unnecessarily traumatic a positive result on a test can be. Natalie Angier considers the path of medical testing and retesting (and the corresponding doubt and ambiguity) as the contemporary version of consulting the Oracle of Delphi. This doubt and uncertainty obviously causes a lot of emotional and mental distress, but what about other ill-effects?

The adverse physical effects are real

While you are consciously avoiding smoking, drinking, drug-taking and environmental pollutants and their adverse effects, it's easy to forget that there may be adverse effects involved in the use of various diagnostic procedures. These procedures, originally designed for use in high risk pregnancies, have now become routine. In many instances they are used without consideration for their possible side effects, and in many instances they bypass non-invasive procedures which may give information which is just as reliable.

The risks which are inherent in these procedures may in fact outweigh the benefits. In general the technology has been introduced on a wide scale, but very few studies (if any) have been done to determine the long-term effects. As well, if the procedure is stressful for either you or the foetus, there will undoubtedly be ill-effects. These effects may be subtle and subjective and therefore not readily measurable, but you should remember that they are ill-effects nevertheless, and certainly have the potential to contribute to compromised maternal and foetal health. Quite simply, they will significantly reduce your chances of a better pregnancy and a better baby.

Is your age a consideration?

Of course some of these diagnostic tests are necessary if there is a history of hereditary congenital abnormalities or gene-linked conditions in your family. Diagnostic screening is also now considered the norm for women over 35, for whom it seems there is an increased risk of bearing a child with a chromosomal abnormality. However, it appears that the previously accepted concept that 'tired' eggs are the reason for the increased incidence of conditions such as Down syndrome in older mothers may be seriously flawed. Studies conducted at Freie University in Berlin discovered a direct link between Down syndrome (which increased sixfold in the city in January 1987) and the Chernobyl nuclear reactor accident which happened nine months earlier. These effects were not age-related. This study and several others appear to validate outspoken US medical critic Dr Robert Mendlesohn's long-held views that a woman's chances of having a Down syndrome child increase with the amount of accumulated exposure to X-rays, not with her age per se. There are also studies which link nutrient deficiencies—and not age—with an increased risk of Down syndrome.

REASSURANCE—YOUR RESPONSIBILITY

All of the foregoing should leave you in little doubt that during your pregnancy both you and your baby could be subjected to a number of screening and diagnostic procedures which may be unnecessary. These tests all have the potential for false positive and false negative results and also have some risk inherent in their use. These procedures may be both emotionally and physically stressful. It is important, therefore, that you always question their use in a healthy pregnancy which is progressing normally. While the use of these procedures may offer some benefit (and reassurance) for women in a high risk category, their routine use in uncomplicated pregnancies should certainly be questioned since they may have possible long-term health effects which are only belatedly being clearly defined.

> **QUESTIONS TO ASK WHEN TESTS ARE PROPOSED**
>
> Is there another way to determine what we want to know?
> Are there any risks involved? (You may need to do your own research on this.)
> What is the likelihood of false positives/negatives? (Again, do your own research.)
> What will we do if the test is abnormal/inconclusive?
> If further testing is necessary, what subsequent risk is involved?
> How skilled/well trained is the operator?
> Is the equipment regularly checked for accuracy/safety?
> Can we use an earlier test result?
> What is the real risk of my baby suffering from the condition for which we are looking?

Remember

- The rate of false positives with these screening and diagnostic tests is high, and could lead to the abortion of a perfectly healthy child.

- The risk of miscarriage with CVS and amniocentesis is high, and could also result in the loss of a healthy baby.

- Even if you 'pass' all the tests, this does *not* mean you are guaranteed a perfect baby—many quite severe problems cannot be detected.

- If you have been assiduous with your nutrition and avoidance of toxins (especially if this care was commenced before conception) your chances of having a baby with a congenital abnormality are extremely low.

- Are you sure you need to know? Would you terminate this pregnancy if you were told of an abnormality? All studies show that mothers of children such as Down syndrome babies have no regrets whatsoever about going ahead with the pregnancy.

Chapter 12

Choosing your carer

If you're in any doubt at all about how you personally perceive your pregnant condition, just remember that the World Health Organization (WHO) has made its position very clear. It states that 'Pregnancy and birth are not illnesses.'

DOES PREGNANCY NEED 'TREATING'?

Despite the stance of the WHO, the medical model is the one which currently governs reproduction, and many orthodox medical practitioners consider pregnancy a 'condition'. While strictly speaking a 'condition' is not the same as an 'illness' the tendency is for it to be treated as such and, at best, in need of constant monitoring and surveillance and, very frequently, a condition in need of medical treatment. Therefore the decision you make when you choose someone to care for you during your pregnancy and at your baby's birth will have profound implications. The choice you make will determine whether your pregnancy and labour are viewed as normal healthy functions or as pathological conditions which will require screening, diagnostic testing, intervention and treatment.

Unfortunately, if you embrace the medical model of conception, pregnancy and labour, you may lose your belief in your own ability to conceive, bear and give birth to your child without outside help. The innate certainty that you were designed for these things may be undermined, and the technological procedures employed during pregnancy and medical treatments prescribed for 'symptoms' may simply reinforce your dependence on medical and pharmaceutical approaches to perfectly natural functions. There is also the potential for inappropriate procedures to damage your self-confidence and your self-esteem.

This damage can be transmitted to every aspect of your life with particular implications for your child-raising skills and your relationships with your children. As you become detached and disconnected from the conception, bearing and birth of your child, you are denied the personal transformation which is an integral and necessary part of these major life events. Sadly, for many women today, pregnancy and the birth of a child have little more significance than the acquisition of a new home or motor car.

DOING IT 'YOUR WAY' EMPOWERS YOU

However, you can recover some of the power and wisdom which is yours when you carry your baby to full term without excessive medical 'surveillance' or 'treatment', give birth without intervention and nurture your child without outside interference. When you do this you will feel an enormous sense of achievement and empowerment which will affect every aspect of your parenting.

Doing it 'your way' allows you to grow in ways which can only enhance the rest of your life, and your family's life as well. In having a 'better' pregnancy and a birth without medical intervention there are opportunities for you to experience new and ever greater levels of self-determination and self-awareness.

TAKE YOUR TIME TO CHOOSE YOUR CARER

The decisions and choices you make regarding your care will affect your health, your baby's health and the whole family's health. Therefore, you must give yourself plenty of time to think about what you really want. You should read appropriate books and seek out relevant facts and figures. You need to talk to as many people as you can, including friends and acquaintances who have recently been pregnant and given birth. You must also talk to some of those prospective carers. This isn't a decision you should make in a hurry.

THE CHOICE MUST BE YOURS

But the choice must be yours! It is important that you personally take the responsibility for choosing the person who will care for you. Don't let the decision be taken out of your hands because you delayed too long, or because it was all 'too hard'. Don't rely on someone else's assessment of your needs, hopes and desires either. Make the decision for yourself, based on what *you* want. If you are content to rely on what your doctor tells you, if you select your carer without any forethought, if you aren't prepared to do some 'homework', you may find yourself going down the road of the high-tech pregnancy and birth before you are even aware that there is another way to go.

Maybe your partner will have very different views from yours about the best type of care for your baby. If you find your views diametrically opposed, with no possible compromise in sight, it's still important that your final decision is one with which *you* feel absolutely comfortable. Making this decision can be challenging, especially if you favour midwifery care while your partner likes the idea of an ultrasound picture of his son and heir at every antenatal visit.

Janette knows all about such challenges. Her partner was initially aghast when she informed him that she wanted no ultrasound, CVS or amniocentesis during her first pregnancy, despite the fact that she was nearing the grand old age of 38. We won't tell you what he said when she told him she wanted a homebirth as well. Since both were strong-willed and opinionated individuals, some heated discussions ensued. But Janette finally had both her pregnancies without screening or diagnostic tests, and she gave birth to their sons at home, with the total support of her partner. This change of heart was only achieved after much deliberation on his part and an eventual realisation that antenatal screening gives no guarantee of a perfect baby, that the risks of diagnostic tests outweigh any benefit, and in the case of a baby born at home all the benefits far outweigh any risks.

YOU MUST MAKE AN INFORMED CHOICE

But Janette's partner only came to his decision after fully informing himself of all the facts, and it's very important that you make a similarly informed choice. To do this you must seek out the appropriate information. This means that you must look beyond any medical dogma which your doctor may dispense. For example, you should question reassurances that routine ultrasound is 'as safe as watching television'. (We recommend keeping a good 1.5 metres away from the television, anyway, to avoid radiation effects.) You don't need to be a radical feminist, a confrontationist or a stirrer to question some of the 'routine procedures' which are part of pregnancy and giving birth today. After all, of the hundred or so common procedures carried out by obstetricians and midwives, about 20 of those are actually harmful. Being informed also means finding out about the false positive and false negative results which go hand in hand with all the latest diagnostic tests. Of course when you make the decision to be fully informed, what you find is often far from reassuring.

But once you're fully aware of the risks, of the potential for adverse effects, of the chance of being needlessly alarmed or wrongly reassured, and fully understand the possible repercussions for your physical, mental and emotional health and for your baby's wellbeing, you can weigh the odds. You can decide whether any possible or perceived benefits from the procedure or test can be balanced against the potential negatives. Lots of women who have been on the merry-go-round of screening and diagnostic tests say they would never have begun had they been fully aware of all the pros and cons. You may, of course, after due consideration, still choose to undergo the procedure(s), but at least your choice will be informed.

TYPES OF CARERS

The most common choice for Australian women is a specialist obstetrician/gynaecologist who will deliver your baby in a hospital, but if you make this choice your chances of a completely non-technological pregnancy and birth are small. Many doctors only have experience of a 'medically managed' birth and with a society increasingly tending to litigation when things go wrong, doctors may also favour the technological approach simply to avoid any criticism of negligence.

Less commonly, a local GP may be your choice, but GPs who deliver babies are an increasingly rare breed. They too have been seduced by the belief that pregnancy and labour are only safe when handled by the 'experts'. You might be lucky enough to have a hospital or birthing centre in your area, where a team of midwives will oversee your pregnancy and the birth as well. You may decide to be cared for by an independent midwife who will perform the appropriate antenatal tests and also be present during the birth in your own home or alternatively in a birthing centre where you can give birth in an environment which is more like home, but has ready access to medical facilities.

When you make your decision about medical or midwifery care, it might also be worth thinking about the option of a 'water' birth. Even if you don't actually give birth to your baby in water, the pain of labour can be significantly reduced if you're in a birthing pool, so it's a good idea to find out if the centre of your choice has this option available.

WHAT TO LOOK FOR IN A CARER

While it might seem like a pretty straightforward choice for you, particularly if you want to avoid the high-tech approach, there are some further factors which need careful consideration. First of all, you need to choose someone with whom you feel absolutely comfortable. Your pregnancy is a time when feelings and emotions run high, and a time when you will also have doubts and worries. It is inevitable that you will want to share some of those feelings, and to confide some of your hopes and fears to your carer.

You must feel confident and comfortable

It's no good being in someone's care if you don't feel completely at ease with them. During the labour and birth you are very exposed and vulnerable—probably as never before. Giving birth is an extraordinarily intimate experience. If you feel at all inhibited or uncomfortable in the presence of your carer then chances are it will be a long labour, simply because you will find it really difficult to 'loosen up' and let go.

It's also very important that you feel confident that your carer will make appropriate decisions on your behalf, as these may need to be made at a time when you're preoccupied and unable to pay full attention. The births of Francesca's two sons were complicated to some extent by a pelvis which had previously been broken, making it more difficult for the baby to travel down the birth canal. Her two birth experiences were very different. With her first, her carer was a doctor committed to a gentle birth, but with whom she had little contact and whose stance on more complex issues was unknown to her. The second time around she chose differently, and had much more confidence that the decisions taken were those she would have made herself. Even if your birth experience isn't quite what you hope for or dream of, you should be free of regrets about the way things were handled. After your baby's born, you need to be able to focus your full attention on the job of parenting, rather than reliving what might have been done differently during your labour and birth.

Your questions deserve answers

You need to feel free to ask questions of your carer. This is really just another aspect of feeling comfortable, of course. If you're too stitched up or inhibited to ask a question—because you might be thought silly or because you're afraid of taking up too much time—then you need to let go of those inhibitions and ask about whatever it is that's bothering you.

If you ask a question and your carer fobs you off, or is dismissive, then you need to find someone who will listen attentively and who will take the time to answer, no matter how trivial the question. You must be sure that your worries and concerns and your desire to be informed about all aspects of your pregnancy and birth are respected.

Make sure this carer is right for *you*

Obviously you must feel confident that the person you choose to care for you during your pregnancy and labour has all the necessary skills to help you and your baby achieve the sort of birth you desire. You must also be sure that person has a really serious commitment to the approach you have chosen. Usually, you will need to ask a lot of questions but don't be afraid to do this—even if the practitioner has been recommended by someone you know well, you need to feel certain that this carer is right for you. What your friend wanted may have been quite different from what you want, so don't take anyone's recommendations as gospel. Make your own enquiries and then make your own decisions based on those.

If you're looking for an obstetrician it might be worth your while to examine the Health Department statistics on 'Mothers and Babies' for your state. Data regarding intervention rates in hospitals is compiled and collated and you can see at a glance which hospitals have the lowest intervention rates. While we recognise that the high intervention rates at major teaching hospitals reflect the number of emergency or high risk deliveries which transfer from rural areas, it is easy to get caught up in the mind-set that sees so many births as complications. Chances are, if your obstetrician practises at one of the hospitals with the lowest intervention rates, you'll have a better chance of a pregnancy without all the high-tech clutter and a natural vaginal delivery. Having a look at the data can be interesting in other ways. You'll clearly see how more affluent socio-economic groups (presumably those with private health insurance) have much higher rates of medical intervention. Who said we were cynical?

ONCE YOUR DECISION IS MADE

While we definitely advocate talking to as many people as possible before you make your decision about your carer, once that decision is made, and if you have decided on low-technology midwifery care for your pregnancy and birth, it might be easier (especially if this is your first pregnancy) to keep a low profile about your choice. Unfortunately if you broadcast your choice far and wide you can stir up a real hornet's nest and the prophets of doom will be there with horror stories aplenty. They'll assure you that the technology is harmless (after all, their child is living proof). They may berate you for being selfish (just think, you could burden society with a severely disabled child). They will also question the grave risks you're taking (their baby would have died if the hospital had not been standing by to do an emergency Caesarean). There'll be more—and these doom-mongers give no thought at all to what they might be doing to your peace of mind.

Francesca finds in her clinic that even those women and couples who have stood up for their right to choose a natural approach to preconception health care or infertility treatment, often, against their own preferences, give in to social and family pressures when it comes to the pregnancy and birth. Often, those choices are later regretted. We urge you to be sure that the choices you make are those that you feel really comfortable with, whatever these may be, and not those that make everyone else comfortable at your expense!

Of course, you might be the sort of person who is prepared to stand firm and state your views loudly to one and all. You'll certainly be sure enough of your choices to withstand all the critics when you've been down the road once before. Janette was much more vocal about her decisions second time around (even though she was 42 years old by then). Of course a previous unfortunate experience with a technological pregnancy and birth can make you vociferous in your support of an alternative approach. On the other hand, numerous women (and we are among them) will be able to endorse the use of technology in emergency situations.

We hope that more women who hold strong views about a 'better' pregnancy and birth and all that follows will be heard. We hope that women who view reproduction as a normal, healthy function, which has suffered in becoming a medicalised series of events, will be heard more often. If more of those women are willing to stand up and be counted, then they will empower other women to make similarly informed choices and to regain control over their reproductive lives. We hope our book can go some way to giving women back their power.

TOWARDS THE BIRTH

Antenatal classes

Your choice of an antenatal class or a birth educator should be made as carefully as your choice of carer. Lots of classes (especially those which are run under the auspices of a maternity hospital) are little more than a preparation for a high-tech labour and delivery. Remember too that the focus of some 'preparation for childbirth' classes tends to be on breathing techniques and pain reduction, when you may wish for similar focus on some of the other factors which can contribute to a natural and fulfilling birth experience. These include thorough preconception health care (at least for the next time around), a healthy unmedicated/non-technological pregnancy, a carer who favours a supportive rather than an interventionist role during the labour and birth, and similarly supportive and nurturing family and friends.

Choosing a 'support' team

If you've made your decision to give birth at home or in a birthing centre, then you'll need to choose your support team. Just be sure that support team is really there to support you, and that they understand that this isn't a side-show or a circus. Even though you're going to be the star of the show, the rest of the cast need to be very 'supporting' indeed. When they see you in pain they need to know what they can do to give you some relief, they also need to know how to give encouragement rather than sympathy. You definitely don't need your mother saying, 'Poor little girl, I hate to see you in so much pain,' or, 'This isn't nearly as bad as when I had you.'

Children at the birth

Support people at birth also need to be truly 'there' with you, not distracting you. This applies particularly to children who are present. It is certainly true that children bond to a sibling in exactly the same way as parents do if present at the birth, and that they handle birth with great equanimity if well prepared in advance. But they must be extremely well-informed about what to expect and must also have someone present to care for them. There are some wonderful books which can be used to prepare even very young children appropriately, but the teaching needs to be done well in advance. The birth itself will take all your concentration, and if your children are upset by what they are seeing or hearing and need your attention, this will be very distracting for you.

Home or hospital?

If you have the appropriate carer and support people, the actual place of birth itself becomes largely insignificant. The focus on 'homebirth' may lead you to think that 'home' is what really matters, when in reality it is your own state of mind and the attitude of those around you which will largely determine how natural and how fulfilling that birth experience can be.

But we'd also like to emphasise that it's important not to become too attached to your preferred option. If all doesn't go to plan, you'll need to be able to 'go with the flow' and adapt to the changing circumstances. This way you can still end up with a positive experience and good memories. Make sure your support team also understands this.

For it's a fact of life that despite the most diligent care, the best laid plans can come undone. Janette's second son, who like her first, had the benefit of all that she believes in and now writes about, finished up in hospital shortly after he was born at home. This definitely wasn't an option Janette had even considered at the time, but it certainly taught her a valuable lesson. After a copybook pregnancy, an intense but short three-hour labour with a five-minute second stage and an absolutely uncomplicated delivery, Michael developed very rapid breathing about six hours into his first day of life. A 'Flying Squad' transported him to hospital, where this temporarily ailing, but otherwise robust, healthy baby was subjected to all of the high-tech stuff which Janette had wanted so much to avoid. The diagnosis—'inhaled vernix' (which could, of course, happen to any baby, no matter how healthy). However, rather than see this as a negative, Michael's short visit to the neo-natal intensive care unit only confirmed for Janette her strong belief in all that she had done both before conception and during pregnancy, the importance of the sort of birth she and her baby had still been fortunate enough to have, and the need to get those messages out to the world. She also learnt that it is important to be mentally prepared for any eventuality, and this is why we exhort you to think about all the possible outcomes.

Being able to see the positive in what you might otherwise perceive as entirely negative is very important. Francesca has treated many women for post-natal depression, where a big factor in their condition is simply unacknowledged grieving for the birth experience they wanted and expected but didn't have.

AFTER THE BIRTH

Antenatal classes which extend into the post-natal period are a very worthwhile option. Talking to other new mothers in the early weeks following your baby's birth can be a wonderful way of building your self-confidence and improving your parenting skills. Talking to some very new mothers who've just given birth while you're still pregnant yourself can also be invaluable and might clarify some things for you. Janette remembers talking to a family who spent the first week following their son's wonderful birth in the family bed. It worked well for both of us too, and our sons stayed in that bed until they chose to move out—you just need to be sure the bed is big enough to accommodate you all! We can reassure you that children will certainly be sleeping alone long before they reach puberty! Of course, you will invariably hear some birth and parenting stories from new mothers which are not so encouraging, so perhaps when you relate your positive ones you might consider sharing the reasons (and our books).

Remember too that you'll need support and help around the house after the pregnancy and birth are over, and it's wise to establish that support system now while you're still a few months away from needing it.

YOU CAN CHANGE YOUR MIND

You're only having this baby once, so you should try to get it right. Don't be afraid to change your mind about the person you want to care for you during your pregnancy. Don't be afraid to change your mind about whether you want a high-tech approach. Don't be afraid to refuse that test if it doesn't feel right. Don't be afraid to look for the antenatal teacher who fully supports all your hopes and wishes for your birth. Don't be afraid to change your mind about where you want to give birth and about whom you want to be present. To sum up: you need to remember when choosing your carer, your birth educator and your support people that this pregnancy and birth are *not* dress rehearsals.

You give yourself the very best possible chance of a 'symptom'-free pregnancy and a problem-free birth if you have attended to all aspects of your health care throughout your pregnancy. But you need to be equally thorough in finding the right people to care for you during that time.

chapter 13
Natural treatments and remedies

We'd like to think there was very little need for this chapter. We certainly believe that if you faithfully follow all of our recommendations then your use for it will be much less than it might otherwise have been. But we know even if you have done everything absolutely by the book (and even scrupulously attended to preconception health care), a minority of you will still experience some of the discomforts and complications of pregnancy.

There are many natural and effective ways to treat these common conditions and often you will not need to seek out or rely on pharmaceutical or technological solutions. A recent study comparing homoeopathic and conventional therapy in pregnancy and childbirth found little difference in effective outcome, except for fewer haemorrhages and decreased abnormal contractions in those patients who were treated homoeopathically. Herbs, of course, have a long history of use during pregnancy, labour and breastfeeding. They have been the traditional medicines of midwives for as long as we have recorded history. The midwife, whose practice was primarily concerned with pregnancy and childbirth, was often also the community healer, well versed in the 'wise woman' herbal lore of her region.

Herbs and other natural remedies work by balancing the system, by bringing it into harmony, and in that they are very different from pharmaceutical preparations which usually only mask the symptoms of a condition.

Gaining trust in your body, and knowledge of and trust in natural remedies while you are pregnant, provides very good training for family life. This knowledge and trust will allow you to follow your intuition and use naturopathic remedies, if necessary, during labour and after the birth. Once your child is born you can also avoid a lot of doctor's visits, and the various decongestants, analgesics, antibiotics and other drugs which are commonly prescribed, if you develop some understanding of natural remedies and the ways in which they act.

THERE'S ALWAYS A ROLE FOR NATURAL REMEDIES

We believe that natural remedies are able to treat effectively most, if not all, conditions of pregnancy. We also believe that where medical intervention in the form of drugs or surgery is unavoidable, there is still a role for the advice we give here, to minimise risk and aid recovery. We encourage you to seek natural treatments where possible for all health concerns during pregnancy, whether specifically related to pregnancy or not. However, treatment should be carried out with the advice of a health practitioner, trained in some form of natural therapy, who can distinguish between a complaint that is amenable to a natural approach and a condition that may justify medical intervention.

SOME NATURAL REMEDIES SHOULD BE AVOIDED IN PREGNANCY

Generally speaking, it is preferable to avoid taking any medication during pregnancy, especially in the first trimester. Although this caution also applies to natural medicines such as herbs, all the recommendations we give here are absolutely safe, and have been shown to be so through long-term and traditional usage.

Occasionally the use of a medicine (natural or otherwise), which would normally be avoided, can be justified in terms of an assessment of the risks versus the benefits. There are also many herbs, the use of which at low dosage, and where professionally supervised, may carry no risk, though self-medication may be inadvisable. We have given clear indications through the text where this is the case, and in Appendices 6, 7 and 8 you will find lists of herbs, essential oils and acupressure points to avoid in pregnancy. If you are in any doubt at all, or if you just prefer to be reassured, you can always seek professional advice from a health practitioner trained in natural medicine.

SOME NATURAL APPROACHES TO TREATMENT

Good nutrition

If you haven't yet got the message about the supreme importance of nutrition then go right back to the beginning! If you attend to your nutritional wellbeing (by following our advice in Chapters 3 and 4), then your chances of needing to treat any complaints will be substantially reduced. However, some nutrients can be used therapeutically and may be required in greater dosages for certain conditions during pregnancy. Where we have indicated single nutrients, or even a range of them, as specific treatment for a condition, this in no way changes the need for a continued balanced and comprehensive supplementation and dietary approach. It may, however, be necessary to increase the dosage of a certain nutrient temporarily. Alternatively you may find that you are already taking the required amount as part of your daily regime.

Herbal medicine

As we've already recommended, rather than visit a medical doctor you may prefer to consult with a practitioner trained in herbal medicine (of course, some medical doctors are also herbalists). In this case medicine is likely to be given as a fluid extract or tincture (liquid preparations), tablets or capsules, and the practitioner will set the appropriate dosage.

If you are self-medicating (following the advice given here) it's easier, and safer, to use herbal infusions or herbal teas, though, to be effective, herbs need to be infused (or the teabag left in the water) for at least 15 minutes. Later in this chapter we'll recommend specific herbs for specific complaints. Meanwhile, here's a generic recipe for a herbal infusion.

How to make an infusion
1. For every 30 grams (2 tablespoons) of herb, pour on 600 ml of boiling water.
2. Let it steep (infuse) for at least 15 minutes to get the full benefit of the active ingredients of the herb.
3. Strain.
4. Drink a cupful, three times daily.
5. Make a fresh brew every day, use it within 24 hours, or refrigerate.

While infusions are not as strongly active in most cases as the preparations you will receive from a herbalist, they can still be very effective, and in some cases are the preferred forms. Although you will find you can treat yourself easily in instances of mild conditions, any severe or continuing problem requires professional diagnosis and treatment.

You will also find many herbal medicines in tablet or capsule form in health food shops, and these should have clear directions (and cautions for pregnancy) on the label. The staff in these shops may also be able to help you, but we recommend strongly that you check all herbal preparations, whatever form they may take, against the list of contra-indicated herbs in Appendix 6.

Information on herbal medicine is very comprehensive and thorough these days. Not only is there a substantial and growing body of scientific research into the constituents and effects of herbs, but there is also the advantage of experience gathered over many centuries of traditional use.

Acupuncture and acupressure
The uses of acupuncture during pregnancy are many and varied, and in the hands of a skilled practitioner acupuncture can be an excellent way to treat almost any condition.

For self-help, acupressure is the easiest approach, and in this chapter we recommend specific points that can be used to treat many of the conditions of pregnancy. You will also find instructions in Chapter 10 for its use in stress control. You may wish to investigate one of the hand-held acupressure machines that are on the market which deliver an electrical impulse. Some of these even have an indicator which lights up as you hit the right spot. But whichever approach you choose, before using acupressure during pregnancy, consult Appendix 8 on which points to avoid.

How to stimulate an acupressure point
First, find the point as accurately as you can, then apply pressure in the appropriate way. Choose from the three methods below, unless specific instructions are given.

Calming: Cover the point with the palm of the hand, or gently stroke, for about 2 minutes. This method should be used where there is over-activity involved in the condition, such as for stress.

Tonifying: Apply stationary (or clockwise) pressure for 2 minutes. This pressure can be slowly increased as your tolerance to any discomfort increases (points relating to an organ or condition in need of treatment may often be tender). Pressing too hard straight away can cause you to tense. Gradually increased pressure can be better tolerated, and therefore more easily built up to effective levels. This method should be used for sluggish or depressed conditions.

Dispersing: Apply moving pressure, such as a circular anticlockwise motion, or a pumping action in and out, on the point. The pressure can be begun fairly deep, and then brought up to the surface. Take care to keep the area relaxed, and increase the pressure on successive treatments as you learn to tolerate it. This method should be used where there is congestion.

Aromatherapy
This is another very useful way to treat any malady during pregnancy. In the hands of a skilled practitioner, essential oils can be used during massage and on specific areas to relieve quite debilitating conditions. You can also apply the recommended essential oil to your skin yourself, or use it in a bath or oil burner. Although in some cultures it's common to orally ingest essential oils as therapy,

this is definitely not an option we recommend without expert supervision, and it's better avoided during pregnancy in any case. Please consult the list in Appendix 7 for contra-indicated oils before attempting any form of application.

There are four basic ways of using essential oils, and the dosages given here are appropriate for pregnancy (about half the normal dose).

Massage oil
You need a base oil (try sweet almond, grapeseed, or any good quality massage oil) to which you can add the essential oil(s) you choose, at approximately 1 drop per 2 ml of base oil.

Bath oil
You will need a dispersing base so that the oils don't collect in droplets on the top of the bath water. You can buy dispersing bath oil (without aroma) at some shops, and add your own sweet smells. You'll only need about 6 drops of essential oil in an egg-cupful of dispersing oil. If this is not available you could try vodka or full-cream milk as a base.

Compress oil
Add a few drops of your chosen oil to a bowl of very hot or ice cold water, then immerse a face cloth, wring it out and apply it over the affected area (usually the abdomen in pregnancy, especially for nausea).

Vaporisation oil
Special oil burners are widely available these days, either with a candle or electric current as a heating element. Generally, oils are added to a small amount of water in the bowl of the burner, though sometimes the oil is added directly to the heated surface. You can rig up a simple home-made version by placing a bowl of scented hot water placed over a radiator, and there are also some devices that fit over a light bulb. Other methods include placing a few drops on a hanky or the cover of a pillow. Steam inhalation is very effective, when 6 drops of the oil are added to a bowl of very hot water and a towel placed over your head, forming a tent containing your head and the bowl. This is particularly useful if you are attempting to affect the respiratory system. Alternatively, 6 drops can be added to the

top of a vaporiser (you can find these at a pharmacy) which can be left on while you sleep.

Homoeopathy

Homoeopathy works by using minute amounts of herbal or mineral substances to trigger a response in the body, and although the small amounts are not in themselves toxic, the responses they trigger can sometimes be quite powerful (as can the healing effects!).

Homoeopathic remedies are particularly appropriate during pregnancy, and we have recommended their use several times in this book. However, apart from the specific instances that we have noted, you should always consult a qualified homoeopath and not attempt to choose remedies for yourself. Where we have given alternatives, the choice of remedy can be made by consulting either a practitioner or a specific homoeopathic materia medica.

Other therapies

Osteopathy, massage, reflexology, yoga, hypnotherapy and many other therapies have a very useful role to play in treatment during pregnancy. Chiropractic, as an alternative to osteopathy, has much to offer, but we would counsel strongly that X-rays are absolutely contra-indicated in pregnancy (and in the preconception period). Since many chiropractors rely on information gleaned from an X-ray, you will need to be aware of this concern.

TREAT CONDITIONS HOLISTICALLY

Whatever approach you take to treatment, it is always more effective to treat a condition holistically. This means that all aspects of physical and mental health are examined and considered, along with the impact they may be having on the condition causing concern. We feel confident that if you fully implement the recommendations in this book you will be well on the way to a comprehensive, holistic approach to health, and to a successful and trouble free pregnancy, and that the lifestyle, nutritional and environmental changes we have already covered will form a firm basis for the specific remedies which follow.

CONDITIONS OF THE DIGESTIVE SYSTEM

Morning sickness   *Thyroid*

If you commence pregnancy suffering from food allergies, if your blood sugar levels are unstable, if your liver isn't in good health and working well, or if you are deficient in various nutrients such as vitamin B6, chromium, zinc or magnesium, you will almost certainly suffer from nausea or even vomiting.

So-called 'morning' sickness can strike at any time of the day, and if you feel constantly nauseated, you won't feel like preparing or eating nutritious meals. If you're actually vomiting then it is virtually impossible for you to ensure an adequate nutrient intake during the critical early weeks of embryonic development. Unfortunately, by the time the nausea and vomiting abate, it might not be possible for the foetus to make up the deficits, although good nutritional status before pregnancy begins will be of enormous benefit in offsetting these problems.

Quite clearly it's very important to minimise or prevent morning sickness because optimal nutrient intake in the first trimester is of supreme importance. Attending to food allergies, hypoglycaemia (low blood sugar), liver function and nutritional status before conception is one way to prevent morning sickness. But, if you're already pregnant, don't just head for the handbasin hoping the nausea and vomiting will eventually go away, although most cases do resolve by the end of the first trimester. If you adopt the attitude that morning sickness is inevitable, your baby could miss out on essential nutrients. While this may not cause severe congenital defects, it could cause subtle long-term health problems in your child.

Overall, between 50 and 90 per cent (depending on which study you look at) of pregnant women experience some form of morning sickness, and it's more common in first pregnancies, although there is also a repeating pattern from one pregnancy to the next. A small minority of women, about seven in every 2000, suffer from hyperemesis gravidarum (excessive vomiting), which is much more likely in women who are epileptic. This severe condition can lead to dehydration, and can directly threaten the health of both mother and baby. Hospitalisation may be necessary, with intravenous feeding and anti-emetic drugs, leading to a liquid diet. Most cases are, however, more easily controlled, and the nausea—which usually commences anywhere between 2 and 8 weeks of pregnancy—normally resolves naturally by 12–14 weeks, although, in the case of twins, where hormone levels are particularly high, it may last considerably longer.

Some women are definitely more susceptible than others, and there are a variety of possible causes, including:

- Poor liver function, as the liver has to process extremely high levels of hormones during pregnancy
- Poor blood sugar metabolism, as blood sugar levels fluctuate much more widely during pregnancy
- Poor nutritional status, especially of vitamin B6, magnesium or chromium (which controls blood sugar metabolism)
- Food allergies, which affect the ability to digest foods
- Stimulation of the centre for nausea control in the brain stem by HCG (the hormone produced in pregnancy)
- Relative relaxation of muscle tissue in the digestive tract
- Excess acid in stomach
- Enhanced sense of smell
- Stress or fatigue

There are other reasons, not necessarily associated with pregnancy, for nausea, which may need to be investigated. Food poisoning, tension, hepatitis, gastritis, intestinal blockage, ulcer or a variety of diseases may be responsible. There are also more serious conditions, such as ectopic pregnancy or eclampsia (the final stages of toxaemia) which can result in nausea or vomiting. We will look at these in more detail later in this chapter.

It can be difficult to differentiate between the possible causes of nausea and vomiting, but unless they become severe, they are not usually cause for concern. However, a sudden change—for example, an abrupt loss of symptoms before the end of the first trimester or an inexplicable bout of vomiting later in pregnancy, after a symptom-free period—should be checked with a medical practitioner. Also, if vomiting occurs more than two or three times daily, and doesn't respond to self-help or natural remedies, then medical help should be sought.

Usually, however, morning sickness can be naturally alleviated. Here are some ideas.

- Eat little and often. Appropriate foods for snacking include protein and complex carbohydrates, especially almonds, which are good for controlling blood sugar levels. It's important to eat before you are hungry, as when your stomach is empty, the acid it produces has nothing to digest except its own lining. Also once you are hungry, you may well start to experience fatigue and nausea, and the motivation to prepare or eat nutritious food will be undermined by the desire to lie down or vomit. Eating frequently also stops your blood sugar levels sinking so low that you reach for the nearest white flour or sugar-laden food to give you a temporary boost. This sort of food is not really helpful as, after the boost, your energy levels will fall to even lower depths. Dry biscuits or toast, which are often recommended, are only useful if they are made of whole grains.

- Eat protein last thing at night (e.g. nuts, fish, whole grains, yoghurt). Protein rich foods take longer to digest, and keep blood sugar levels stable until morning. (Levels which fall during the night have given rise to the term 'morning' sickness.) As it's not a good idea to overload your stomach just before you sleep, make this just a small snack.

- Avoid fats, sugars, acidic foods and foods to which you know you are sensitive or allergic. Also avoid the sight, smell or taste of foods that trigger nausea, and try to avoid passive smoking.

- Eat before getting up in the morning and then allow yourself time to begin your day slowly. Train your older children to come to you (rather than you to them) and see if you can organise breakfast in bed. Perhaps your husband can be persuaded to serve the breakfast and attend to the children's needs (if you achieve this, can we borrow him sometime?).

- Take plenty of fluids (especially if you are losing them through vomiting). You may also find it easier to take your food in liquid form, such as soups (avoid over-cooking and do most of the preparation in the food processor), soya milkshakes and vegetable juices.

- Try powdered or micellised (water soluble) supplements rather than tablets or capsules, and experiment with increasing the dosages of *vitamins B5* and *B6, chromium, zinc, magnesium* and *vitamin K*. We recommend 50–100 mg of vitamins B5 and B6 daily as a good general dosage level, but up to 400 mg of B6 daily can be taken in the first trimester. However, we recommend professional supervision of doses over 250 mg, since high doses of B6 can cause peripheral neuropathy (tingling in the extremities). Remember that B6 (like folic acid) should always be taken with the rest of the *B-complex* range of which it is a part. Although the higher doses, which may be necessary to alleviate nausea, are safe, prolonged use throughout pregnancy can result in withdrawal symptoms in the newborn. Chromium is particularly good when sugar cravings are strong. Magnesium and vitamin K given orally can be effective, especially if given with vitamin C. If vomiting is excessive these nutrients can be given by injection.

- Digestive remedies include the celloids (or tissue salts) *potassium chloride, sodium phosphate* (if reflux is experienced), and all *bitter herbs*, though these should not be used in excess. Herbal remedies such as *Meadowsweet* and *Chamomile* (these two herbs to be used in low dosage only), *Aniseed* and *Peppermint* will be particularly helpful if other digestive problems are experienced. *Digestive enzymes*, or papaya fruit (which contains the enzyme *papain*), are also helpful.

- Specific herbs for nausea include *Black Horehound, Meadowsweet, Wild Yam, Peppermint, Lemon Balm, Aniseed, Squaw Vine* and *Peach Leaves. Raspberry* is good for nausea which extends into the second trimester. These can be taken in fluid extract, tablet or capsule form. High doses or protracted use of Black Horehound, Raspberry and Squaw Vine are not recommended, and Meadowsweet should be avoided if you are allergic or sensitive to salicylates.

- Liver treatments can be very effective in combating morning sickness. Herbs to use here include *Fringetree, Globe Artichoke,*

Bupleurum and *Dandelion Root*. *Burdock* and *St Mary's Thistle* are very effective, but should be used with caution, under professional supervision. Dandelion Root can also be taken as a tea or coffee substitute (but make sure powdered preparations don't include sugar).

- Herbal teas, which can alleviate symptoms once nausea starts are *Ginger*, *Peppermint*, *Spearmint*, *Aniseed*, *Clove*, *Chamomile*, *Lemon Balm*, *Meadowsweet* and *Raspberry*. Don't drink excessive amounts of ginger or clove tea, as they can overly stimulate the circulation in your reproductive system. Chamomile, Meadowsweet and Raspberry should also be used in moderation.

- *Root Ginger* can be peeled and sucked, and the *juice of a lemon*, squeezed into water, can also be helpful.

- *Umeboshi plums* and *miso* soup, two Japanese foods that are used in macrobiotic diets, have a good reputation as remedies.

- Get lots of sleep to avoid fatigue, and if nausea prevents sleep, see Chapter 10 for some ideas to help beat insomnia.

- Rub some *Lavender* essential oil on your abdomen (mixed with massage oil, see page 209). Make sure this is *Lavendula officianalis*, *L. augustifolia*, *L. spika* or *L. intermedia* and not one of the contra-indicated species listed in Appendix 7. Other suitable oils include *Ginger*, *Grapefruit*, *Lime*, *Mandarin*, *Petitgrain*, *Sweet Orange*, *Chamomile* and *Tangerine*.

- The homoeopathic remedies, *Chelidonium* 6x and *Pulsatilla* 6x (in equal parts) act on the liver and have been shown to reduce nausea in 90 per cent of cases. These are very easy to take, and can be combined with *Ipecac 200c* if you are vomiting. *Sepia* and *Nux Vomica* may also help.

- Surround yourself with sweet-smelling oils to offset your heightened sensitivity to offensive odours. Try *Lavender*, *Petitgrain*, *Spearmint*, *Lemon*, *Coriander* or *Bergamot*. Use them in burners and they will create a healthy, therapeutic aroma.

- The celloid *sodium sulphate* is a good liver treatment.

- The Chinese herbal formula *Bamboo* and *Hoelen* is good for nausea in pregnancy. Chinese herbs may come as granules which can be wrapped in rice paper and chewed if you are too nauseated to swallow them directly.

- Some Australian Bush Flower essences have been found to be helpful for morning sickness. *Dog Rose* combats fear, *Crowea* and *Paw Paw* help digestion, *Dagger Hakea* helps detoxification through the liver, and *She Oak* helps to balance the hormones.

- Hypnotherapy and reflexology can also be extremely helpful. Although you will need to consult a practitioner, he or she may be able to show you how to use these treatments for self-help as well (see Contacts and Resources).

- One fairly eccentric remedy, which may seem unusual, is the tongue pull. This yoga exercise sometimes works when nothing else seems to do the trick. Grasp your tongue using a dry, clean cloth and pull it straight out, until it feels quite strained and uncomfortable, then hold it for half a minute.

Helpful acupressure points to relieve morning sickness

Instructions on how to stimulate an acupressure point are given earlier in this chapter (see page 208).

Conception Vessel 24: In the depression between the point of the chin and the lower lip, on the mid-line.

Gall Bladder 34: Bend your leg at a right angle (90 degrees). Catch your kneecap between your index finger and thumb. The middle finger is on the outside of your shin bone, and Gall Bladder 34 is at the tip of this finger, on the outside of the tibia.

Liver 2: Between the large and second toes, slightly up from the edge of the web and closer to the big toe.

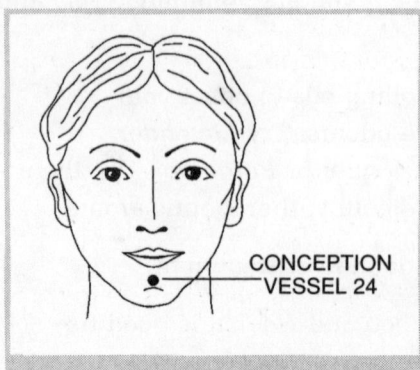
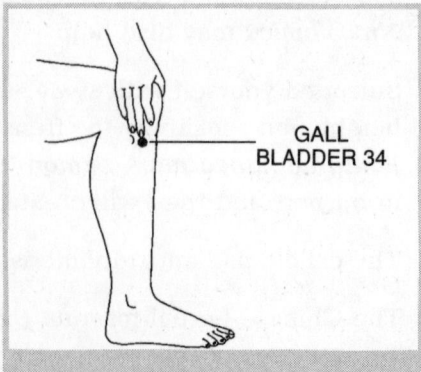

Other helpful acupressure points are Stomach 36, Stomach 45 and Pericardium 6 (see pages 163–164). You can find wrist bands, sold for travel sickness, to stimulate Pericardium 6, which is the most commonly used spot, and you can, of course, also get treatment from a trained acupuncturist.

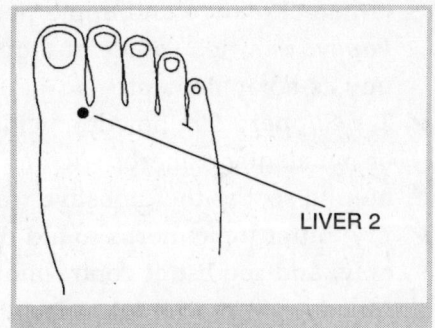

Heartburn and indigestion

It's reassuring to know that heartburn has nothing to do with your heart, though the sensation is felt close to the heart area, which is how the term arose. In pregnancy the greater incidence of both heartburn and indigestion is caused by the action of increased levels of the hormones oestrogen and progesterone. These have a softening effect on the digestive tract and one of the consequences is that the valve at the top of the stomach relaxes and allows stomach acids to rise into the oesophagus. This part of your digestive tract is not immune to acidity, and this gives rise to an uncomfortable burning sensation and sometimes results in regurgitation of sour fluid. The smooth muscle in the colon is also relaxed, leading to increased 'transit time', which in turn gives rise to bloating and indigestion. As long as constipation, which can lead to an accumulation of toxins, isn't also a problem (see next section), this increased transit time can actually benefit the baby through increased absorption of nutrients. Later in pregnancy, these symptoms can be exacerbated by the pressure exerted on your stomach and diaphragm by your growing baby.

About half of all pregnant women experience heartburn and indigestion, and it can be quite debilitating. Here's a list of do's and don'ts, in which you will find many recommendations that are similar to those in the last section on morning sickness.

- ✔ Eat little and often, snack on nuts (especially almonds), chew well and eat slowly, sit upright when eating (and afterwards while digesting).
- ✔ Use digestive aids after meals. Try *Peppermint, Spearmint, Fennel, Lemon Balm, Chamomile* or *Aniseed* teas, or chew on

(organic) orange and apple peel, dried pineapple or papaya. *Papaya* is a rich source of digestive enzymes, which you can also buy as a supplement.
- ✔ Try *Slippery Elm* powder, *acidophilus* powder, yoghurt, soya milk or mucilaginous herbs such as *Chickweed* or *Marshmallow*, which help to soothe the digestive tract.
- ✔ Try 'bitter tonic' herbs to aid digestion (but use in low dosage only, and see list of contra-indicated herbs in Appendix 6) or *Meadowsweet* (but take care if you're allergic to salicylates, which are at high levels in this herb, and use in low dosage only).
- ✔ Try increasing your intake of *B-complex vitamins*.
- ✔ Take a slow walk after meals.
- ✔ Sleep propped up on some pillows if attacks happen at night.
- ✔ Drink lots of fluids *between* meals.
- ✔ Try osteopathy, reflexology or acupuncture (for practitioner referrals, see Contacts and Resources).
- ✔ Use aromatherapy oils—*Peppermint* is a favourite, and *Sandalwood* works well too. Both of these should be used with caution, and not in excess.
- ✔ Use alkalising foods and remedies. *Cider vinegar* (1 tablespoon twice daily, before meals) can be very helpful, and so can the celloid (or tissue salt) *sodium phosphate*. Some naturally based alkalising powders can be found in health food shops, but check the 'Don't list' for other medications.
- ✔ Make sure you are taking regular *Garlic* (as a supplement as well as in your food).
- ✔ Try the homoeopathic remedies *Kali Mur, Nux Vomica, Pulsatilla, Calc Carb, Mag Carb, Mag Phos* or *Nat Phos*. Remember your homoeopath is the best person to choose the appropriate remedy.

- ✘ Don't put on too much weight or wear tight clothes.
- ✘ Don't drink with meals.
- ✘ Don't eat fatty, highly seasoned or spicy foods or drink cold fruit juices if these cause problems.
- ✘ Don't smoke or drink coffee (as if you would even think of it!).
- ✘ Don't eat lying down.
- ✘ Don't bend from the waist or lie flat on your back.
- ✘ Don't eat too late in the evening (although, if suffering from

morning sickness, you may still need a very small snack at this time).

✘ Don't use antacids if at all possible, and especially avoid those containing aluminium or high levels of sodium.

Constipation and haemorrhoids

Constipation is common during pregnancy because of the action of hormones which decrease the motility of the gut and, later on, because the expanding uterus puts pressure on the bowel. However, there is a lot you can do to alleviate constipation, and if you keep it under control, haemorrhoids will be less likely to bother you, though these can be troublesome if you let your nutrient status drop. There is a greater risk of haemorrhoids during pregnancy because of the increased volume of blood and the weakening of muscle tone. Here are some tips.

✔ Eat little and often, chew well, eat slowly.
✔ Eat as we have suggested in Chapter 3, focusing on high-fibre foods such as fresh fruit and vegetables, preferably with the skin left on (though in this case they must be organically grown), whole grains, legumes and 1–2 tablespoons of olive oil daily.
✔ Drink plenty of water; 8–12 glasses of purified water can not only prevent constipation, but can also help to keep the body free of toxins.
✔ Exercise regularly (see Chapter 9). Yoga can be especially helpful.
✔ Take *acidophilus* and *bifidus* and/or *Slippery Elm* powder, which keep the gut healthy. Bulking agents such as bran or *psyllium husks* are preferable to laxatives.
✔ Keep up a regular 1–2 grams daily dose of *vitamin C* (good for constipation) with plenty of *bioflavonoids* (especially *Rutin*), which strengthen the capillary walls. Other important nutrients are *potassium, calcium, magnesium,* and *vitamin B6* and *E.*
✔ Try the celloids (or tissue salts) *magnesium phosphate* (for constipation), *calcium fluoride* and *silica* (for haemorrhoids).
✔ Empty your bowels regularly, whenever you feel the urge, and try squatting over, rather than sitting on, the toilet.
✔ Practise your pelvic floor exercises (see Chapter 9).

✔ Use massage in a clockwise direction over the abdomen (you can add essential oils such as *Mandarin* or *Orange*), or up the stomach meridian which runs along the outside of the thigh from the hip to just below the knee, to keep the bowels regular. You can also try reflexology, massaging the foot arches in a clockwise direction, a massage of the lower back with relaxing essential oils such as *Lavender* or *Bergamot*, or osteopathy (for practitioner referrals, see Contacts and Resources).

✔ Try homoeopathic remedies. For constipation some helpful remedies are *Nux Vomica, Nat Mur, Byronia* and *Sepia*. For haemorrhoids try *Arnica, Calc Fluor, Nux Vomica, Sepia* or *Sulphur. Hamamelis* (Witch Hazel) can also be taken in homoeopathic form. As we've mentioned before, the correct choice of homoeopathic remedy is usually best left to a qualified practitioner.

✔ Sit in hot and cold sitz baths (alternating) to relieve the discomfort of haemorrhoids, and try adding salt and/or astringent herbs such as *Witch Hazel, Comfrey, Periwinkle, Oak Bark, Plantain* or *lemon juice*.

✔ Use herbal ointments on the haemorrhoids, especially if they itch or bleed. *Comfrey, Yellow Dock Root, Witch Hazel* or *Plantain* will help. You could also try *lemon juice*, a local compress of essential oils such as *Cypress, Frankincense, Lavender* or *Myrrh*, or of *grated potato* or *Slippery Elm. Baking soda* can also relieve the itching, and icepacks the pain! Fresh *garlic* and/or *ginger* can also be mashed up and used as a local compress.

✔ Keep your bowels open with herbs such as *Dandelion Root, Fennel* or *Marshmallow Root. Butternut* is a very gentle laxative but others, such as *Senna*, should only be used in small doses and if the problem has become intractable. Prunes, though rather high in sugar, are another emergency treatment.

✔ Take herbs such as *Hawthorn, Ginkgo* (both of these herbs in low dosage only) and *Bilberry*, which are high in bioflavonoids (for capillary strength) and support good circulation.

✘ Don't strain on the toilet, or let yourself go for more than one day without a bowel motion.

✘ Don't take laxatives or mineral oils.

- ✘ Don't worry about increased flatulence (common with high levels of fibre).
- ✘ Don't eat refined foods (such as white bread) or too many eggs. Red meat also takes longer to digest than fish and vegetables, and may increase constipation.
- ✘ Don't drink coffee or tea (except herbal), as they are diuretics and reduce your fluid content.
- ✘ Don't take inorganic iron supplements. In fact, don't take iron supplements at all if need is not proven (but *do* have a blood test to ascertain levels).
- ✘ Don't use haemorrhoid ointments that contain local anaesthetics or mercury (which can be absorbed and may harm the foetus).

Helpful acupressure points to relieve haemorrhoids and constipation
Instructions on how to stimulate an acupressure point are given earlier in this chapter (see page 208).

Triple Heater 6: This point is on the forearm, between the two bones, at four fingers' distance from the bend of the wrist, on the outer side. Use a clockwise motion.

The other helpful acupressure point is Gall Bladder 34 (see earlier in this chapter, page 216).

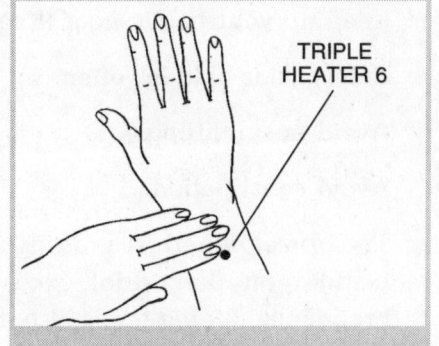

Food cravings

Food cravings indicate nutrient imbalances and are sometimes an indication of a specific requirement. Often, however, a craving can be for a food to which you have an allergy or sensitivity, so check how you feel after the food—better or worse?

If you crave chocolate, you need more *magnesium*. If you crave sugar, it may indicate a deficiency of *chromium* or *magnesium*. If you crave any strong tastes, especially sweet or salty foods, your *zinc* levels are suspect.

Bitter herbs can reduce sugar cravings though they should be treated with caution during pregnancy. *Dandelion Root* is a popular remedy, but there is a specific herb, *Gymnema*, which stops sugar cravings in their tracks. A few drops in a little water should do the trick. You can swish it around in your mouth, and then spit it out.

Some women crave quite bizarre substances in pregnancy, other than foodstuffs. This phenomenon is called 'pica', and indicates a severe nutritional lack.

CONDITIONS OF THE URINARY SYSTEM

Incontinence

About half of all pregnant women experience the problem of incontinence, which results from the pressure of the enlarging uterus on the bladder, and the loosening of the pelvic floor muscles. It then becomes difficult to stop urine leaking when extra pressure is applied—through laughing, coughing, bending over or exercising. Now you certainly can't afford to stop laughing or exercising, so try these remedies.

- Keep up your pelvic floor (Kegel) exercises (see Chapter 9).
- Empty your bladder often.
- Avoid heavy lifting.
- Avoid constipation.
- Try *Horsetail* herb tea (a rich source of silica) to strengthen your bladder, but don't drink excessive amounts of this tea in pregnancy. *Nettle* tea is also a good source of silica.
- The Ayurvedic (Indian) herb *Crataeva* is an excellent bladder tonic. Although we know of no studies or texts giving cautions about the use of this herb in pregnancy, there may be some hormonal action, so keep your dosage low.
- Take the celloids (or tissue salts) *silica, calcium fluoride* and *ferrum phosphate*.
- The homoeopathic remedies *Causticum* and *Sepia* can be helpful.

Urinary tract infections

During pregnancy you are vulnerable to urinary tract infections, which are likely to become serious and more common in the last trimester. There are two reasons for this—first, the urinary tract dilates and urine can stagnate, and second, the kidneys come under more stress during pregnancy when they have to cleanse a greatly increased volume of blood. Urinary tract infections of the bladder (cystitis), urethra and kidneys need to be promptly treated. The gentle healing approach of herbal remedies is infinitely preferable to antibiotic therapy, and extremely effective. However, there are some herbs which, although safe in low dosages and for short periods of time (for acute conditions), need to be used with care (and under professional supervision). See the lists of contra-indicated remedies in Appendix 6.

With urinary tract infections, prevention is better than cure. Here's some advice.

Prevention

- Wear loose cotton underwear and avoid tights.
- Drink plenty of fluids.
- After going to the toilet, wipe from front to back.
- Wash well before intercourse, use lubrication and adopt positions that won't irritate the urethra during intercourse, and urinate directly after intercourse.
- Avoid irritating chemicals in the bath (even some essential oils can be problematic).
- Empty your bladder well and frequently.
- Avoid all forms of sugar.
- Eat 'live' *yoghurt*, *parsley* and *garlic* (but avoid excessive amounts of parsley).
- Keep up your supplementation of *vitamin C* and *bioflavonoids*, *beta-carotene*, *zinc* and *vitamin B6* (with B-complex).
- Take *Nettle* tea as a regular drink.

If, despite your care, you experience greatly increased urination, an urge to urinate when there is no real need, burning on urination or offensive smelling urine, then look to the remedies below, which are preferable to antibiotics. However don't wait too long before seeking advice as, if these remedies don't bring relief within a day or two, it's important to stop the infection before your kidneys are involved. It's also important to start treatment as soon as you notice the warning symptoms.

Treatments

- Drink plenty of unsweetened *cranberry juice*. Take 1 glass every hour for up to 10 hours.

- *Barley water* can be very soothing, but we don't mean the sweetened cordial! Boil pearl barley in plenty of water, drain off the water and drink. Flavour with some lemon juice.

- Take 500 mg of *vitamin C* every hour (with *bioflavonoids*).

- Try reflexology, osteopathy.

- Try homoeopathic remedies (e.g. *Apis*, *Belladonna*, *Nux Vomica*).

- Try aromatherapy, with *Bergamot*, *Lavender* or *Sandalwood*.

- The celloid (or tissue salt) *ferrum phos* (iron phosphate) helps fight infection and inflammation.

- Herbal medicine is very effective. *Echinacea* and *Garlic* will help to increase the immune response. Herbs specifically recommended for the urinary tract are *Crataeva*, *Couch Grass*, *Clivers*, *Corn Silk* (use with care and for short periods only), *Buchu* (herbs teas and low doses are safe), *Uva Ursi* (not for more than 3–4 days), *Marshmallow* and *Liquorice* (small doses for short periods only and not if you're suffering from high blood pressure).

Fluid retention (oedema)

Fluid retention is a problem for many mums to be, especially in the last 10 weeks of pregnancy, when half of the extra 3–6 litres of fluid common to pregnancy is retained. It's not a serious problem, unless accompanied by elevated blood pressure or protein in the urine (for which you can test with a simple dipstick from the pharmacy). If either of these conditions exist, the fluid retention may be a forerunner to toxaemia (see 'Conditions of the cardio-vascular system' later in this chapter). Another easy self-help test is to see if the impression made by finger pressure around the ankle remains indented. If so, you should have your urine and blood pressure checked. Swelling is much less likely to be of concern if it is restricted to the evenings; if it's earlier in the day, visit your health practitioner. Fluid retention is uncomfortable, and can cause problems with vision and contact lens tolerance.

Here's what you can do.

- Drink more. Although this seems contradictory, it will flush out your kidneys and create a diuretic effect.
- Keep your weight under control, exercise to keep your circulation healthy, but stay cool.
- Wear flat, comfortable shoes; avoid standing for long periods.
- Keep your feet up when you rest (which you should try to do regularly). Put a pillow under your legs and feet when you sleep at night.
- Do some foot exercises. Bend feet up and down; rotate them clockwise and anti-clockwise.
- Raise the bottom of your bed to improve the circulation to the upper half of your body.
- Massage your legs (towards the heart) but take care if you have any varicose veins. Support hose may be helpful.
- Apply a bruised or steamed *cabbage leaf* to the afflicted area.
- Eat small but regular amounts of parsley in your food, and salt your food to taste. It's important to avoid excess salt, so you need to be sure that your need for salt is not depraved. Adequate *zinc* is essential to keep your sense of taste healthy. If you do use salt, make sure it's in modest amounts and only use *sea, rock* or *Celtic salts*. Your diet should also be high in good quality protein.
- Make sure you have adequate levels of *vitamin B6, magnesium* and *vitamin E* (for circulation).
- Try homoeopathic remedies, for example, *Nat Mur, Apis* or *Phosphorus*. Your homoeopath can help you choose.
- Try reflexology for the lymphatic system.
- Use the celloids (or tissue salts) *sodium sulphate* or *magnesium phosphate*.

⚹ Try herb teas—gentle diuretics like *Dandelion Leaf* and *Couch Grass* are appropriate at this time.

⚹ The essential oil to use now is *Geranium* (short-term use only).

Helpful acupressure points to relieve fluid retention

Use dispersing pressure on these points. This is a moving pressure, with a counter-clockwise motion, which can be begun fairly deep, and then brought to the surface. Done twice weekly, this can act as a preventative.

Gall Bladder 41: On the foot, at the peak of the angle formed by the bone of the little toe and the fourth toe.

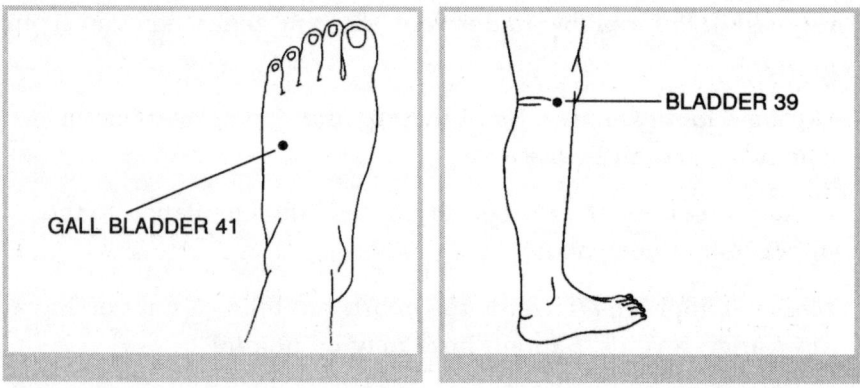

Bladder 39: On the crease behind the knee just inside the tendon on the outside of the leg.

Gall Bladder 36: One thumb width lower than halfway between the fold of the knee and the ankle, on the inner side, just in front of the fibula.

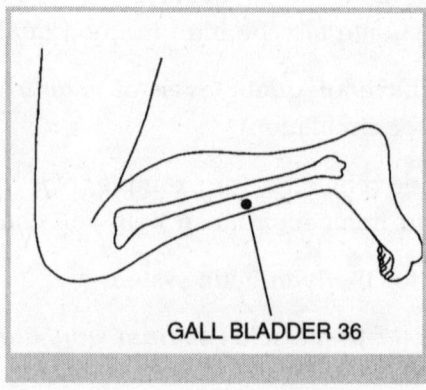

Preventative kidney support

In Chinese medicine it is traditional to treat the kidney meridian at the end of the first and second trimesters, to obtain extra energy. It is also thought that this can help to clear problems you may have inherited from your own mother. From a Western perspective, the health of the kidneys in pregnancy is of prime importance—to deal with the excess blood volume, and to avoid oedema, fatigue and toxaemia.

The spleen is working overtime during pregnancy to produce extra blood (especially if any bleeding is occurring) and, according to Chinese thought, draws energy from the kidneys. There are some preventative remedies (set out below) which can be useful to employ throughout pregnancy to avoid these problems and support the adrenals (attached to the kidneys) in order to combat stress.

- Acupuncture is a well-known Chinese preventative measure. (Once your acupuncturist has chosen the appropriate points, you may also choose to apply pressure yourself on a regular basis.) A favourite point is *Kidney 9* (see below).

- *Nettle tea* is a great tonic herb for pregnancy, and the tea can be safely drunk on a regular basis (1–2 cups daily). As well as supporting the kidneys and being high in nutrients, nettle tea helps protect against diabetes, poor digestion, fluid retention, incontinence (because it contains silica), anaemia (it's high in organic iron), hypertension, kidney stones, hair loss, leg cramps (it's high in easily absorbable calcium and magnesium), painful childbirth (because of the calcium and magnesium), hypoglycaemia and a slow metabolic rate. What more could you ask? Well, in addition to providing vitamins A, C and D, chlorophyll, copper and phosphorus, it's a superb source of vitamin K and increases available haemoglobin (thereby decreasing the chance of post-partum haemorrhage), tightens and strengthens blood vessels (helping to prevent varicose veins and haemorrhoids), helps maintain arterial elasticity and improves venous resilience. It also increases the richness and amount of breast milk and is a uterine tonic!

- The herb *Withania* is both a general and specific tonic for pregnancy, with a particular supportive action for the adrenals. This herb also has a sedative aspect and supports the immune system, as well as being an excellent tonic in tiring or stressful conditions.

⚕ Another useful herb is *Bupleurum*, which is a tonic to the kidneys and liver, an anti-inflammatory and a diuretic.

⚕ *Clivers* is a herb which is gentle to the kidneys, and helps the lymph to flow.

⚕ Reflexology can be very supportive through pregnancy (see the diagram below).

⚕ Eat plenty of cucumber (which also relieves constipation).

Helpful acupressure points and reflexology for preventative kidney support
Instructions on how to stimulate an acupressure point are given earlier in this chapter (see page 208).

Kidney 9: On the inside of the leg, at the base of the calf muscle.

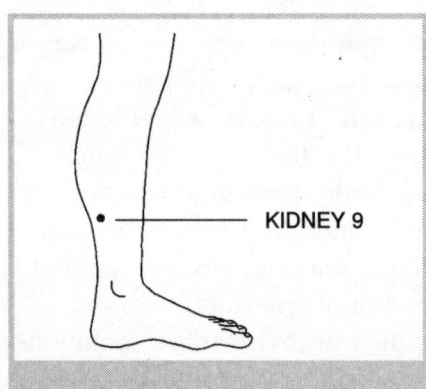
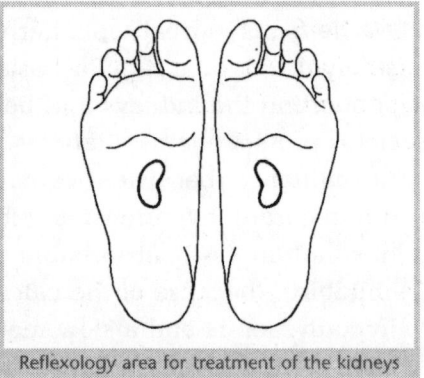
Reflexology area for treatment of the kidneys

Reflexology area for treatment of the kidneys: On the sole of the foot.

CONDITIONS OF THE CARDIO-VASCULAR SYSTEM

Palpitations

These are much more frightening than they need to be, as they are usually a symptom of stress or anxiety rather than a heart condition.

So the best way to treat them is by attending to stress (see Chapter 10). However, a few extra remedies include:

- Reflexology (see below), which can be included in an overall calming foot massage.

- *Lime Flowers* and *Zizyphus* are two useful and safe herbs to take, though Zizyphus is a warming herb and is better avoided if you feel too hot.

- Essential oils such as *Lavender*, *Lemon Balm*, *Neroli*, *Ylang Ylang*, *Peppermint* and *Rosemary* may be helpful. Peppermint and Rosemary should be used with caution (not in excessive amounts and not long-term).

- Specifically helpful herbs are *Motherwort* and *Hawthorn* but both of these need to be used with caution in pregnancy, and under professional supervision.

Reflexology for treatment of palpitations
Reflexology area for treatment of palpitations: On the soles of the feet.

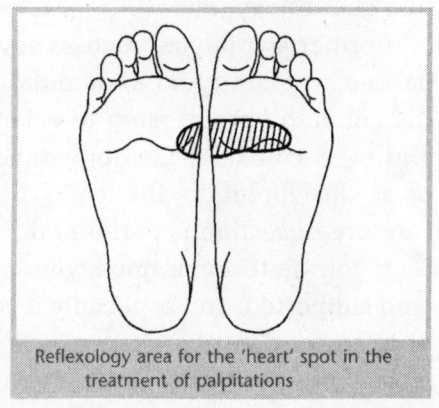
Reflexology area for the 'heart' spot in the treatment of palpitations

Hypertension, toxaemia, and pre-eclampsia

Hypertension (raised blood pressure) can take two forms during pregnancy. Chronic hypertension is a commonly experienced slight rise which occurs in pregnancy because of the extra demands on your metabolism, increased blood volume, and stress on the kidneys. This should not harm you or your baby, but needs to be watched carefully.

Gestational hypertension, or a steady rise in blood pressure after week 25, may be due to poor nutrition, especially a lack of protein (vegetarians beware, and read Chapter 3), which is commonly thought to be the main cause of toxaemia and pre-eclampsia. It can also mean that the placenta or kidneys are not functioning as well as they could. This condition has also been linked to high levels of toxic metals such as copper or lead, which of course can occur when the levels of essential minerals, especially zinc, are low. Toxaemia is more common in first pregnancies, and may not recur in subsequent pregnancies.

If your blood pressure does increase, it's important to start treating it quickly so it doesn't progress to toxaemia or pre-eclampsia. Toxaemia means literally poisoning of the blood, so it's extra important to keep your kidneys healthy, especially as they also have a role in hypertension.

Pre-eclampsia is initially diagnosed by a steep rise in blood pressure, uric acid in the blood, a low urine output, fluid retention (oedema) and sudden weight gain. Singly, these symptoms may not be a cause for serious concern, but together they indicate pre-eclampsia. They may be accompanied by a general itchiness, and progress to a situation where protein appears in the urine. At this point there is a high risk of premature labour because of placental insufficiency, and the blood flow to the foetus is severely reduced, leading to a lack of oxygen.

Further symptoms, such as severe headaches, visual disturbances, nausea, vomiting and abdominal pain, mean that there is a threat of the condition progressing to eclampsia, which is characterised by fits and even coma. At the appearance of this second level of symptoms, or if the threat to the child becomes too severe, induction or a Caesarean section is performed.

If your nutrition is good, your protein levels sufficient, your kidneys well supported, and especially if you have no personal or family history of hypertension, the chances are very good that you will not experience these problems. If you do, however, here are some remedies for the early stages. (Once it has progressed beyond these first stages more aggressive therapy and medical supervision is required.)

- First, rest. (See also Chapter 10 for more on controlling stress.)

- Avoid stimulants like cola drinks, coffee, teas and spicy foods.

- Exercise (see Chapter 9). Yoga is particularly helpful, but aerobic exercise is excellent if it has been a regular part of your routine throughout pregnancy.

- Allow yourself a healthy weight gain—certainly don't diet! But, on the other hand, make sure you aren't eating fatty and sugary foods.

- Eat calcium- and protein-rich foods, keep the ratio of protein to carbohydrate as we've suggested in the 'zone' diet in Chapter 3, and *sparingly* add salt (sea, rock or Celtic) to taste. To make sure that your salt requirements are not due to a depraved sense of taste, regularly use the zinc taste test to ascertain your zinc levels.

- Drink *Nettle*, *Dandelion*, and *Lime Flowers* teas regularly. Hops can also be helpful but only in the last trimester.

- Make sure you get adequate levels of *vitamin E* (for circulation), *Max EPA* (fish oils), *vitamin B6*, *magnesium*, *calcium*, *potassium* and *zinc*.

- If you feel that you have neglected your sources of calcium, magnesium and potassium, and need a quick boost, use the celloids (or tissue salts) *calcium phosphate*, *magnesium phosphate* and *potassium chloride*, which are the most easily assimilated forms of these minerals. Potassium-rich foods include bananas, dandelion leaves, chicory, mint and potato peel. It's important to keep your potassium–sodium ratio high, which is why you need to go easy on the salt (without restricting it altogether, if you feel a genuine need for it). Raw beetroot juice is also very helpful for this.

- Essential fatty acids (from *Evening Primrose*, *deep-sea fish* or *Flaxseed oils*), have been successfully used in the treatment of pre-eclampsia.

- Another nutrient which has been shown to be helpful is the amino acid *L-Arginine* (but don't use this if herpes is a problem).

- Herbs can help to keep your stress levels down (see Chapter 10). Try *Lemon Balm*, *Cramp Bark* and *Green Oats*.

- *Garlic* should be a regular part of your diet and supplement regimen. Onions, parsley and cucumber are excellent foods. *Cucumbers*, especially the yellow, over-ripe variety, are extremely effective in reducing blood pressure. You'll need a whole cucumber each day, or half a cup of juice, which may be easier to consume. They also relieve constipation and strengthen the kidneys.

- *Hawthorn* herb is specifically recommended for high blood pressure and is extremely effective. Its use in pregnancy should be supervised and, although there is no documented proof of problems, it should be avoided if possible in the first trimester, and used with caution in the second. *Zizyphus* is another helpful herb which is safe in pregnancy.

- Reflexology has been shown in some studies to be very effective in controlling blood pressure and treating toxaemia.

- Aromatherapy (with *Lavender*) can also help.

Varicose veins

These can be treated in a similar way to haemorrhoids, with an additional recommendation to put the legs up (against a wall when lying on your back) and not to stand up for too long. Inverted yoga poses (with guidance from a teacher) and plenty of exercise are beneficial, and you may like to use support hose.

Vitamin E, garlic, onions and *ginger* (small doses only) all help your circulation, and *bioflavonoids* (especially *Rutin*), *Oats* and *Buckwheat* are important for capillary strength. *Buckwheat* and *Elder Leaves* are good sources of Rutin, but don't take Rutin as a separate (high dose) tablet in the first trimester as it may cause miscarriage. *Nettle tea* and *Lecithin* help to keep elasticity in the veins. *Bilberry*, *Ginkgo* and *Hawthorn* are not only high in bioflavonoids, but also support healthy circulation. (Ginkgo and Hawthorn should be taken in small doses only, under supervision.) Compresses can also be helpful (see 'Constipation and haemorrhoids' earlier in this chapter).

Anaemia

If you are taking the recommended level of *folic acid* (400 mcg), and monitoring your iron levels, you should be able to sail through pregnancy with no anaemia. Foods rich in folic acid include dandelion leaves, parsley, watercress, dark green leafy vegetables and whole grains, so make sure you have plenty of these (but parsley should not be eaten in excess, so don't have a large serving of tabouli every day!). Please remember to take folic acid in balance with the rest of the B-complex vitamins.

Ferritin levels (ascertained by a simple blood test) will let you know if you need more iron. Once again, we remind you to take only organic forms of iron, and only if in proven need (though you do need to check regularly). The celloid (or tissue salt) *ferrum phosphate* is a form of iron which is easily assimilated. You may need to increase your intake of lean beef, but parsley is also a good source of iron, as is seaweed, and so are the herbs *Nettle* and *Dandelion Root*. *Vitamin C* must be present to aid absorption (remember, coffee and tea will inhibit it).

Bleeding gums

Gum disease (gingivitis) can be a sign of vitamin C and bioflavonoid deficiency, so make sure you're getting plenty of fresh fruit and vegetables. Your gums will also benefit from eating crunchy and fibrous foods, so eat raw vegetables when you can.

An effective mouthwash can be made from *Calendula*, *Echinacea*, *St John's Wort*, *Myrrh* and *Sage* in warm water, or a few drops of essential oil of *Fennel*, *Lavender* and *Myrrh*. Do not swallow the mouthwash; spit it out.

Clean your teeth extra well, and massage the gums.

CONDITIONS OF THE MUSCULO-SKELETAL SYSTEM

Backache

Lower back ache is common in pregnancy, as the increasing size of your baby changes your posture and centre of gravity, and as the ligaments and joints relax, due to hormonal output. If the kidneys are under stress, this may also contribute to backache (so pay attention to 'Preventative kidney support' earlier in this chapter). Exercise, especially yoga, and stretching exercises (see Chapter 9) can also relieve muscle spasm and contraction, and nutrition will also have an essential role to play. The following hints will do a lot to prevent or alleviate pain.

- Keep your lower back supported. Never cross your legs when sitting. Try not to stand (or sit) for long periods.

- Make sure you're getting adequate *calcium*, *magnesium* and protein.

- Get adequate exercise, and plenty of stretching. The pelvic tilt is particularly helpful—sit between your feet, or alternatively, sit on your heels. Keep your knees together. Lean back onto your hands, tightening your buttock muscles and keeping your arms straight. Tuck in your pelvis so that your pubic bone lifts up in front. Hold for a few seconds and release. Repeat several times.

- Swap massages with a friend, or treat yourself to a professional session, regularly.

- If massage isn't sufficient, try osteopathic treatment. (This is quite safe even in late pregnancy, in the hands of a professional.)

- You may like to use a herbal liniment, such as *Wintergreen* oil or *Tiger Balm*.

- Essential oils can also be used in massage—try *Lavender*, *Mandarin* or *Chamomile*.

- Sleep with pillows in strategic spots (under your knees, belly and supporting your back). Make sure your mattress is supportive and firm. If not, put a board under it.

- Don't wear high heels. Try not to reach above your head.

- Take great care, if you must lift anything at all heavy, to bend your knees, not your back. Also heed this advice when bending down for any reason.

- Your posture should be such that your lower back is as straight as possible—pull your bottom in under your tummy as much as you can. To learn more about posture consult an Alexander or Feldenkrais Technique practitioner (see Contacts and Resources).

- Try *Epsom salts* baths or heat in any form (a hot water bottle is ideal).

- If there is any nerve irritation (sciatica etc.) *St John's Wort* will help to reduce the pain in the nerve endings. The oil from St John's Wort or from *Comfrey* can be an excellent aid to massage, to relieve pain.

- Orgasm is great for any pelvic congestion—one of the more pleasurable remedies! Make sure you've discussed with your partner which positions for intercourse put least strain on your back and tummy.

- The homoeopathic remedy *Pulsatilla* may help, as may *Arnica*, *Hypericum*, *Rhus Tox* or *Bryonia*.

- Try to avoid taking pain relievers, as even over the counter drugs can have adverse side effects (see Chapter 5).

- Acupuncture can quite miraculously relieve pain, but see a professional.

Helpful acupressure point to relieve backache
Small Intestine 3: Press on the end of the fold of the little finger nearest the hand when your hand is closed like a fist. Rub clockwise.

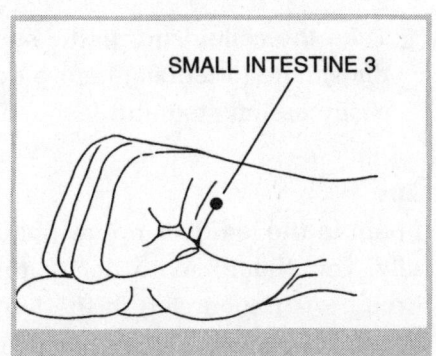

Leg cramps

There may be a combination of factors predisposing you to leg cramps in pregnancy, especially in the last trimester. The main cause is an imbalance of *calcium* and *magnesium* (too little). Your calcium and magnesium reserves take a beating in the second trimester, when your baby's bones are forming. In a few women, a lack of *sodium* (salt) can be a factor, which is why we say use salt 'to taste'. Pressure from the enlarged uterus on the nerves supporting the legs and slower circulation may also be partly to blame.

Prevention

- Keep your *calcium* and *magnesium* supplement at the recommended dosage, and eat lots of dark green vegetables, grains and seeds.

- Keep taking your *B-complex vitamins*, *potassium* and *vitamin E* for good circulation.

- Follow a regular, appropriate exercise routine, flex your calf muscles daily (see below) and do some regular foot circles (see 'Fluid retention' earlier in this chapter).

- Raise the bottom of your bed; put your feet up regularly.
- Reduce the *phosphorus* in your diet (less meat, fewer dairy products and no soft drinks).
- Be sure you're still getting plenty of protein. Fish, nuts, soy and other legumes are good phosphorus-free sources.
- Try support hose.
- Avoid heavy lifting, pointing your toes, and quick movements.
- Take the celloids (or tissue salts) *calcium* and *magnesium phosphate* (3 tablets) before going to bed. These are the most easily assimilated and fast acting forms of these minerals.

Cure

If pain in the leg does not respond to these remedies, or subside naturally, you should see a doctor to explore the possibility of a venous thrombosis (blood clot) in the leg, to which you are more susceptible during pregnancy.

- Flex your foot upwards towards the knee, and press your heel firmly into the floor, on a hard surface.
- Stand on a cold surface.
- Massage the leg (towards the heart).
- Apply hot wet towels to the calf muscle.
- Use the essential oil *Lavender* for faster recovery. After cramping you can be left with sore muscles and repeating cramps for quite a while.
- Sip tea or fluid extract (a few drops in water) of *Cramp Bark*, *Black Haw*, *Skullcap* or *Valerian*, every 10–20 minutes, until you recover.
- If leg cramps are due to a cramped nerve, try osteopathy or *St John's Wort* oil in a massage.
- For better circulation, try *Ginkgo* herb or *Ginger* tea (neither to excess).

Helpful acupressure point to relieve leg cramps

Instructions on how to stimulate an acupressure point are given earlier in this chapter (see page 208).

Bladder 57: In the centre of the back of the leg, at the base of the calf muscle.

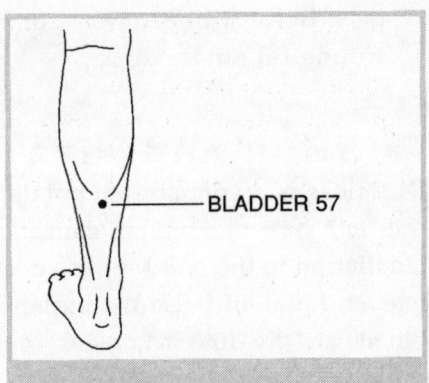

CONDITIONS OF THE NERVOUS SYSTEM

Fatigue

It's quite normal to feel a bit more tired than usual during pregnancy, and you should make every attempt to accommodate this in your daily life by resting more and cutting back on commitments where possible. Good nutrition is essential for high energy levels, and particular attention must be given to monitoring your iron stores (see Chapters 4 and 11, and 'Anaemia' earlier in this chapter). Other possible causes of fatigue include:

- Allergies (see Chapter 8).

- Low blood sugar—eat little and often, avoid foods containing sugar.

- Low thyroid function—if you suspect this (typical signs are low body temperature, excessive weight gain and fatigue, dry or thickened skin, hair loss, aching muscles, hoarse voice, pins and needles in the hands, constipation), then include *kelp*, *potassium* and *L-tyrosine* in your supplements.

- Low adrenal function, which can be the result of stress. See Chapter 10 for tips on stress control, and use *Withania* herb as a tonic. This herb, sometimes called Indian Ginseng, has the supportive and rejuvenating qualities of Ginseng, but is not overly stimulating, and has a calming action, assisting sound sleep.

- Anxiety, or nervous tension, can contribute to fatigue. As well as our suggestions on stress control in Chapter 10, try *Green Oats* (as a herb), *Oat Straw* tea or rolled oats for breakfast—a wonderful nerve 'tonic'.

Fainting and dizzy spells

Dizziness is a common complaint of pregnancy, fainting less normal, but both have a common cause in lowered blood pressure and lack of circulation to the head. These occur because blood tends to pool in the legs and feet and also the expanding uterus increases the demand for blood. In the first trimester these effects are compounded by the rapidly expanding circulatory system's demand for extra blood, and in the second and third trimesters by the pressure of the foetus on maternal blood vessels. Higher levels of progesterone also dilate the blood vessels, leading to lower blood pressure. Avoid standing up too quickly, as this can cause dizziness if blood pressure is low.

You may also feel dizzy as a result of low blood sugar levels, or if you are too hot (body heat is increased in pregnancy due to the high levels of progesterone).

Prevention

- Don't stand for too long.

- Get up slowly and gradually, especially out of a bath (which should not be too hot—high temperatures can harm your baby).

- Drink plenty of fluids.

- Eat little and often, especially almonds and other nuts, but not sugary foods.

- Keep up your intake of *vitamin E* to help circulation and decrease the need for oxygen.

- Take *Ginkgo* herb to improve cerebral circulation.

- Keep cool—seek fresh air, and wear loose clothing.

Cure

- If you feel light-headed, or that you might faint, lie down and put your feet up above your head (against a wall) or sit and place your head between your knees (if you can reach them!).

Alternatively, kneel on one knee and lean forward.

✗ If fainting occurs frequently, seek medical advice.

Insomnia
See Chapter 10 where we have dealt with this in detail.

Restless legs
This condition is often alleviated with adequate supplementation of *folic acid* and the *B-complex vitamins*. It can also be associated with allergic response (see Chapter 8). If this is particularly a night-time experience, it suggests an allergy to dust-mites, or something in your bedroom. Good results have been achieved by ensuring that all electric gadgets in the bedroom are unplugged (so there is no electro-magnetic pollution). Other people have had relief by using homoeopathic *Coffea* (caffeine), and it's very important not to indulge in coffee or other stimulants.

CONDITIONS OF THE RESPIRATORY SYSTEM

Breathlessness
You can feel short of breath as your uterus expands and places increasing pressure on your diaphragm. This can be a particular problem when lying down, and you may prefer to sleep on your side, or even propped up on some pillows. It's also important to stay calm (see Chapter 10 for stress control). Yoga can help, and osteopathy or postural techniques such as Alexander or Feldenkrais may help to alleviate the pressure.

Breathing techniques such as those taught in Yoga or antenatal classes can be useful. High levels of progesterone influence your breathing and it automatically becomes deeper—Mother Nature is really quite extraordinarily clever!

It's a good idea to practise deep breathing, which is also very calming. Place your hand on your belly (or over your belly in the later stages of pregnancy). Practise breathing by imagining your lungs as two balloons, filling and emptying. Your hand (and diaphragm area) should rise as your lungs fill and drop as they empty. It's remarkable how many people try to breathe in by contracting their diaphragm—very counterproductive!

Acupuncture can also be useful, or you can try pressure on *Pericardium* 6, the same point we recommended in Chapter 10 (but not to be used in the fourth month of pregnancy).

If breathlessness is severe, and/or accompanied by a bluish tinge around the lips or finger tips, and/or chest pain or rapid pulse, the time has come for an immediate trip to the hospital.

SKIN CONDITIONS

Stretch marks

Stretch marks may be prevented by ensuring that you supplement adequately with *zinc* and *vitamin C* with the *bioflavonoids*. Zinc is an essential nutrient in the formation of collagen which is a component of all connective tissue. If you're zinc deficient, you'll not only suffer from stretch marks as the size of your belly and breasts increases, but you'll be more likely to need an episiotomy since your perineum will be less likely to stretch adequately as your baby is born. Cracked nipples are something else you can expect if you're zinc deficient. (See Chapters 3 and 4 for more on zinc.)

Other important nutrients for skin integrity are the essential fatty acids. *Deep-sea fish*, *Evening Primrose* and *Flaxseed oils* are the richest sources, and should be taken throughout pregnancy at the recommended dosages (see Chapter 4). *Vitamin E* and *silica* are also nutrients which have a positive effect on skin condition.

Unless your skin is nourished from the inside, ointments and creams may not have much effect, but—as an adjunct to nutritional therapy—you can try rubbing your breasts and tummy with oils such as *olive*, *vitamin E*, *wheatgerm*, *jojoba*, *avocado*, *sweet almond* or *sesame*, with *lanolin*, or with *Comfrey*, *St John's Wort* and *Calendula* ointments.

Aromatherapy oils can also be used. Try *Lavender, Mandarin, Frankincense* or *Rosewood*.

Perineal and nipple preparation

To prevent perineal tearing at birth, and sore, cracked nipples afterwards, the best treatment is prevention. For helpful nutrients, and for ointments and oils that can also be used on these areas of your body, see 'Stretch marks' earlier in this section. Gentle doses of sunlight and fresh air on nipples can also help prepare them for breastfeeding. Just don't overdo the exposure to sunlight, and be aware of high ultraviolet levels at midday.

Skin pigmentation (the 'mask of pregnancy')

This condition, known as chloasma, is due to increased levels of hormones and their effect on certain nutrients such as *folic acid* and *PABA*. This is why it also affects women who take the oral contraceptive pill. Adrenal stress is also thought to be a contributing factor. Luckily (unlike the effects of the pill) the marks will disappear after pregnancy is over. The marks usually appear on the face as dark brown patches (for white skin) or white patches (for black skin). Other marks may appear, such as a dark line from the navel to the pubic area, and your nipples may darken. These changes may stay with you for ever.

Sunlight aggravates the condition, and if you have this problem, you should restrict exposure, using hats and PABA sunscreens. *St John's Wort* can protect against sensitivity to sunlight, either taken internally (in small doses and only for a limited period), or rubbed on as an ointment. Cosmetics can aggravate the condition, and should be avoided.

Homoeopathic remedies include *Calc Sulph*, *Silica* and *Sepia*, and essential oils to try are *Lavender* and *Sandalwood*.

Itchiness

Some women experience a general itchiness during pregnancy. This can be due to stretching of the skin, and the remedies given for stretch marks earlier in this section should help. Itchiness can also be a symptom of liver stress. *Yellow Dock* tea is specifically recommended for itchy conditions (use with caution, and in small amounts only), and bathing in water to which you have added *Rosemary*, *Comfrey*, *Dandelion* or *Lavender* (herbs or oils) can also help.

CONDITIONS OF THE ENDOCRINE SYSTEM

Gestational diabetes

We've already talked about the tendency to hypoglycaemia (low blood sugar) during pregnancy; now it's time to look at the other side of the coin.

Mums-to-be who already suffer from diabetes need specialised medical care, but as long as they are extremely careful about their diet there is a very high probability of a successful pregnancy.

Similar precautions can give a high level of protection against the development of gestational diabetes (that is, diabetes which develops during pregnancy), which is increasing in incidence. Women at greatest risk are older mothers, those who have a family history of diabetes, have a personal history of blood sugar disturbance, have had, or were, low weight babies, or have a history of pregnancy complications.

Prevention

- *Vitamins C, E, B5* and *B6* are preventative.

- *Chromium* stabilises blood sugar levels; *magnesium*, *manganese*, *zinc* and *potassium* are also important nutrient minerals.

- Essential fatty acids, from *Evening Primrose* and *Deep-sea fish* oils are helpful, as are digestive enzymes, such as *papain* (from papaya).

- Eliminate sugar from your diet and reduce fruit to two or three pieces daily (including those in your juice).

- Keep the liver healthy. Bitter salad vegetables and *Dandelion* tea or coffee will do the trick.

- Keep complex carbohydrate levels high in your diet, and balanced with protein as we've described in Chapter 3.

- Drink *Nettle* tea (and avoid coffee).

- Eat lots of onion and garlic.

- Eat little and often, and chew your food carefully.

- Keep your weight gain under control.
- Keep your stress levels under control.
- Get adequate exercise.

If, despite your best attempts, you are one of the 1–10 per cent of women who do develop the condition (making it the most common serious complication of pregnancy), it is still possible to use natural medicine to control the disease, though there should always be medical supervision. Take care if combining natural and orthodox medicine, as the dual approach can be over-successful, and you may develop a hypo (low) glycaemic (blood sugar) episode. Control can be achieved with the use of a glucometer. If on the meter your glucose level is 7, then you are okay; if it's greater than 9, commence natural treatment; if it's greater than 11, start medical treatment.

The first sign of diabetes is sugar in your urine, though this can also be normal in pregnancy, and is not necessarily a cause for concern. Your urine may be tested at the start of pregnancy (or before, if you practice preconception health care), though the more significant time for testing is in weeks 24–28, unless you are in a high risk category. If the test is positive, you will be sent for a glucose tolerance test to see if there is a need to treat you further. If so, you can (after consulting your natural health therapist) embark on the following treatments either as the sole therapy or as a adjunct to medical treatment, depending on the severity of your condition (but always with continued medical supervision). We don't recommend the glucose tolerance test as a routine procedure (see Chapter 11).

Other signs of gestational diabetes are unusual thirst, frequent and copious urination (unlike that of early pregnancy or urinary tract infection, when it is frequent but sparse), and fatigue (this may be difficult to distinguish from the normal tiredness of pregnancy).

Treatment

- *Vitamins B5 and B6* (with *B-complex*), *chromium, manganese* and *zinc*.
- *Vitamin E* (to avoid circulatory complications).
- Keep your stress levels under control.

- Eliminate all sugars. Avoid saturated fats (to keep the circulation healthy).

- Keep the complex carbohydrate levels and soluble fibre in your diet high by eating oats and oat bran.

- Use *psyllium husks* and *Slippery Elm* as extra soluble fibre.

- Eat bitter salad vegetables (dandelion leaves etc.).

- Consult a herbalist. He or she may use liver herbs (such as *Dandelion Root*, *Globe Artichoke* or *Fringetree*) or hypoglycaemic herbs (such as *Goat's Rue*, *Bilberry* and *Gymnema*).

In most cases, gestational diabetes resolves naturally after pregnancy, though, for those in the high risk categories, there is an increased chance of it remaining or returning in later life.

CONDITIONS OF THE IMMUNE SYSTEM

Allergies

See Chapter 8 for a detailed discussion of allergies. We'd just like to mention here that there are herbs which can be very useful to reduce their incidence, including *Hemidesmus*, an immune modulator which helps to calm the excessive immune response to allergens, and *Albizzia*, an anti-allergy herb which helps to reduce the severity of symptoms. However, the most important aspect of your health care if you have a tendency to allergies is to keep your immune system robust (see below).

Colds, flu and other infections

It's important not to get yourself into the situation where you need medication such as antibiotics. Your naturopath or herbalist should be able to help you with natural medicines, but if you keep your immune system strong, infections are less likely to affect you.

Prevention

- Keep taking your *vitamin C* every day (it's water soluble and you don't store it in your body).

- Keep your *zinc* status adequate (see Chapter 11).

- Take *Garlic* daily as a supplement as well as in your food (this helps to keep your blood pressure down too).

- Take *Withania* as a pregnancy tonic—it has immune enhancing properties, and boosts energy levels.

- Add *Shiitake* and *Reiishi* mushrooms to your salads, or use them as a supplement. These Japanese mushrooms are also very helpful in protecting you against the effects of radiation if you fly or use computers.

- *Siberian Ginseng* (Eleuthrococcus), another immuno-stimulant herb, has been shown to have beneficial effects during pregnancy. Although there are studies showing this herb to be safe, even beneficial, during pregnancy, there is also some (disputed) evidence of problems. Take it under professional supervision only. Like *Withania*, this herb is a good energy-booster, and also helps to protect against radiation effects.

- If you are in a situation where you are at risk, take *Echinacea* as a preventative. If you are susceptible to infections every winter, it won't hurt to take this wonderful herb regularly anyway.

Cure

- At the first sign of an infection, start taking *Echinacea* tablets or fluid extract.

- Increase your *vitamin C* dosage (to 2 grams, 3 times daily), and your *Garlic* intake.

- Take 2 tablets of the celloid (or tissue salt) *ferrum phosphate* every 2 hours.

- If a fever is involved, use *Elder Flowers*, *Ginger* and *Lime Flowers* as an extract or a tea. Small frequent doses are best in acute situations. Although keeping warm and inducing a sweat is a good way to reduce fever, you must take care, during pregnancy, not to let your temperature rise above 38.9°C.

CONDITIONS OF THE REPRODUCTIVE SYSTEM

Pregnancy tonics

As we're sure you are well aware by now, the accent in this book is not on how to deal with health problems as they arise, but on how to facilitate the healthiest possible environment for your baby's growth.

We've discussed how you can prepare for and support your pregnancy and your child's health through good nutrition, the avoidance and elimination of toxins, exercise and stress management, but there are also some 'tonic' remedies which support the healthy progress of your pregnancy and prepare you and your baby for a successful birth.

Nutrition comes into this category of 'tonics', but so do some traditional herbal remedies. We've discussed a few already like *Nettle* and *Withania* (see 'Preventative kidney support' earlier in this chapter), two renowned, tried and true herbs that have been used over time to enhance pregnancy and birth outcomes, and many other herbs we have mentioned have tonic actions on the systems which they affect.

Two particularly notable herbs are *Raspberry* and *Squaw Vine*. These both act specifically on the uterus, preparing it for labour. They can be safely and effectively used in the second, and particularly in the third, trimester. In our next book, on birth and bonding, we will look also at herbs and remedies to be used to encourage labour and deal with any problems associated with delivery, but these two herbs may be used by all pregnant women.

The tonic effects of Red Raspberry Leaf

This herb tones the uterus and cervix and all the pelvic muscles and acts as a 'partus preparator' (preparing the uterus for birth). It is a rich source of *calcium*, *iron*, *folic acid* and *vitamin E*. It has been used extensively to prevent miscarriage and is one of our recommended herbs for morning sickness. Taken later on in pregnancy it can facilitate safe and easy labour, during birth it can help prevent haemorrhage, and it helps the pelvic area and uterus recover postpartum. During later pregnancy, if used as a tonic, it's best taken as a tea or infusion. You should drink 1 cupful three times daily. If used as a remedy for a condition causing concern, it may be more effective as a fluid extract, or in capsule form. In this case consult a medical herbalist about dosage.

The tonic effects of Squaw Vine
This herb has many similar properties to Raspberry Leaf, being a general uterine tonic and astringent, and is helpful before, during and after birth. It's also a gentle diuretic and may help with fluid retention. It may be used safely as a partus preparator in the last trimester, and particularly in the last six weeks before birth, but also has a reputation as being useful if bleeding problems arise, and as a remedy for nausea. The method of preparation and the dosage are similar to Raspberry Leaf.

The tonic effects of reflexology
The benefits of regular reflexology treatment, especially in the latter half of pregnancy, are well established. One study performed in a London hospital showed a remarkable reduction in duration and problems of labour. The women in this study also showed a reduced level of fluid retention, backache, heartburn and hypertension and a generally increased level of overall health and wellbeing.

Candida and other genito-urinary infections

Thrush is a very common complaint during pregnancy, and we have discussed appropriate treatment in Chapter 8. Using a tea-tree cream or a local application of acidophilus yoghurt can be an effective way of keeping the vaginal problem under control, though avoidance of sugar, and regular inclusion of acidophilus yoghurt in your diet are also of importance.

Herpes

One infection that may persist into pregnancy, regardless of your preconception health care, is herpes, as the virus is impossible to eradicate. It's a particular problem if there are lesions present in the birth canal at the time of delivery. This can have severe repercussions for the health of the baby, including brain damage, blindness or death, and a Caesarean section may be necessary. If the disease is first contracted during pregnancy (rather than recurrent attacks being experienced) there is an increased risk of miscarriage. Natural remedies can be effective in keeping the virus dormant and in treating the blisters.

Dormancy
The secret is to keep your immune system strong. The following may help.

- Eat well, as we have recommended, with an emphasis on fish, though avoid nuts high in L-arginine, for example, almonds and peanuts (which are not, strictly speaking, nuts).
- Keep your stress levels under control (see Chapter 10).
- No smoking, alcohol, drugs (of course!) or chocolate.
- Keep your dosages of *zinc, manganese, magnesium, vitamins A* (or preferably *beta* or *mixed carotenes*), *B1, B6* (with *B-complex*), *E* and *C* (with *bioflavonoids*) at recommended levels as a minimum.
- Take the amino acid *L-lysine* (1200 mg daily) and avoid L-arginine. Lysine-rich foods include salmon, halibut and turkey.
- Take *Evening Primrose* and *Deep-sea fish oils* (or *Flaxseed oils*), and include raw seeds, fish and cold-pressed vegetable oils in your diet.
- Take *Echinacea, St John's Wort* (in small doses only, and under supervision), *Lemon Balm, Clivers, Reiishi* and *Shiitake* mushrooms, and *Garlic* to boost your immune response.

Warning signs
The warning signs of herpes include:
- Genital pain, itching, tingling pain with urination, vaginal discharge, tenderness in the groin
- Fever, headache, general aches and pains, depression
- Small red spots around and on the genitalia
- Lymph node swelling in groin.

Treatment
Once the warning signs are noted, and even before the blisters come out, you can apply the following remedies. Areas of severe itching and soreness are likely to be the sites of future blisters. Avoid sexual intercourse (or use a condom) to prevent infection passing back and forth.

- Take *Garlic* in high dosage as soon as warning signs are felt and repeat the dose every 3–4 hours.
- Increase dosages of immune stimulant herbs (see above).
- Apply ice to the site.
- Use *Witch Hazel, Calendula, Golden Seal* or *Solanum Nigrum* as an extract or ointment, or apply *Aloe Vera* (best taken fresh from the inside of a fleshy stem) directly to the area.
- Cotton wool balls soaked in ether can be applied to reduce the pain. (Warning: ether is highly flammable.)
- Apply *zinc sulphate* solution directly to the vaginal area.
- Essential oils which can be applied directly (though diluted or in a cream) include *Rose, Lavender, Lemon, Sandalwood* and *Bergamot*.
- *Tea tree oil* can be applied directly to blisters.
- The homoeopathic remedies *Rhus Tox* or *Nat Mur* may help.

Mastitis or sore breasts
If your breasts swell uncomfortably or become tender, try these remedies.

- Keep up your supplementation of the *B-complex vitamins* (especially *B1, B3* and *B6*). *B6* may need to be increased considerably (see Chapter 4 for more on dosage). Other important nutrients are *vitamins C* and *E, selenium, zinc, manganese, calcium* and *magnesium*.
- Keep taking and eating *Garlic, Evening Primrose* and *fish oils*.
- Useful ointments include *St John's Wort* and *Poke Root* (*not* to be taken internally).

- Steam or bruise a *cabbage leaf* and wear it inside your bra.
- Massage your breasts and under your arms.
- Drink *Clivers* tea to encourage lymphatic drainage.
- Avoid coffee, dairy food, refined carbohydrates, salt and all animal foods containing chemicals. We certainly hope you are doing this already!

Don't worry if you notice increased surface blue veins in the breast, or if your nipples become darker.

Breakthrough bleeding

This is not always a precursor to miscarriage, and although it should be heeded as a warning sign, some women bleed quite persistently throughout pregnancy without any major problems. If it is accompanied by cramping, the problem may be more serious. While it is important to seek medical advice as to the possible cause, there are several useful herbs which can staunch the flow of blood.

- *Shepherd's Purse, Beth Root, Raspberry* and *Squaw Vine* are all helpful, as are *Oak Bark, Cranesbill* and *Ladies Mantle*. They can be taken as a tea or fluid extract, every four hours. *Dong Quai* and *Peony* have also been used to great effect, though Dong Quai should not be taken in the first trimester.
- Increase *zinc* to improve collagen strength and improve connective tissue formation in the amnion (the membranous sac which encloses the foetus in the womb).
- Step up your *vitamin C* to increase the strength of the capillaries and collagen. You can increase the dosage to the level your bowel will tolerate.
- Increase your *bioflavonoids* intake to strengthen the vascular tissue of the uterus and the placenta.
- Take it easy. Bed rest is advised if the situation persists, with your legs elevated above the level of your head. If you're not in bed, try not to stand for too long, and keep your stress levels under control—try not to worry!

Premature rupture of membranes

If the amniotic fluid starts to leak, it will not necessarily lead to a miscarriage, though medical advice should be sought. *Zinc*, *vitamin C* and *bioflavonoids*, *beta* or *mixed carotenes* and *vitamin E* have all been shown to contribute to healing. It may be wise to take immune stimulant herbs (see 'Conditions of the immune system' earlier in this chapter) and *Garlic* to help prevent infection. Acupuncture and reflexology can both be very helpful.

Incompetent cervix

If the cervix has been weakened by previous terminations, or if it is inherently weak, the pressure of the baby and amniotic fluid, as the pregnancy progresses, can cause it to dilate and bring on a miscarriage. Once incompetency is diagnosed, the medical treatment is to put a stitch in the cervix during the pregnancy. Unfortunately this procedure requires anaesthesia and can itself cause miscarriage. If the pregnancy progresses through to term, the stitch is removed at around week 38 or 39 of pregnancy.

Obviously prevention is preferable to cure, and good nutrition and health care can help considerably, so if you are aware that this may be a problem, make sure that your nutritional status is good. We know of at least one case where visualisation (of a webbed hammock-type sling around the uterus) seemed to change a pattern of incompetence for the better.

Ectopic pregnancy

Again, this is a case for prevention, not cure, as, once an ectopic pregnancy has occurred, surgery is unavoidable. If the Fallopian tube is not removed, then recovery can also be assisted with natural remedies. Good nutrition, with particular attention to *zinc*, *magnesium*, *vitamin A* (or *beta-carotene*) and *vitamin E*, is essential for the health of the Fallopian tubes, and the cilia (or tiny hair-like projections) that line them. These nutrients can also assist the healing of scar tissue. Since tubal blockage or dysfunction is the principal reason for ectopic pregnancy—where the egg is prevented from reaching the uterus and implants in the tubes—preventative care, especially where there has been a previous history of the condition, is essential. Remember that high levels of copper or the heavy metals contribute to zinc deficiency.

With ectopic pregnancies there is usually severe pain, and immediate surgery is essential. One confusing factor is that the pregnancy itself may be unrecognised, as urine tests may not show positive (though blood tests will). There is certainly no place for natural treatment of the condition, but *Calendula* and *Golden Seal*, two herbs which are not advised in pregnancy, can aid recovery, helping to regenerate healthy tissue. *Silica* tissue salt (or celloid) can also be useful.

Genito-urinary infections may also be involved. See Chapter 8 for more on these.

Miscarriage

Miscarriage is most common in the first trimester, and it is estimated to affect 20 per cent of pregnancies. This rate may be even higher, as not all miscarriages are detected. The Miscarriage Association in Great Britain estimates that the rate may be as high as 35 per cent, or even 40 per cent.

Miscarriage is preventable, it is not just 'one of those things', and there is little point in giving just the advice 'to try again' unless attention is given to those factors which could cause miscarriage, and which are amenable to treatment. Miscarriage can be prevented by ensuring that the foetus is viable, the environment in which it grows is healthy, and that undue stress or trauma, of either physical or emotional origin, are avoided, especially during the first trimester.

Most miscarriages occur in the first three months of pregnancy, and are often the result of factors present at the time of conception. Because of this the best way to avoid them is to practice preconception health care for a minimum of four months before your pregnancy starts. This helps enormously to ensure that the foetus is viable and the environment in which it grows in the early weeks is healthy.

If you have been unlucky enough to lose a child during pregnancy, you can still feel very optimistic that you can prevent it happening again. Studies conducted in England by Foresight, the Association for the Promotion of Preconceptual Care, showed *no* miscarriages in a sample of 367 couples who completed the Foresight program, though the normal expectation for this sample would be 70.

If you are lucky enough to be pregnant right now, then putting into practice the advice in this book will go a long way to keeping your pregnancy and baby secure.

The first symptom of a miscarriage is bleeding, sometimes accompanied by cramping or a dull ache. Neither of these symptoms will necessarily lead to miscarriage when experienced separately, but when they come together, or if either is extreme, you should seek immediate medical advice. You can also use the remedies indicated here, though if the miscarriage is already under way, you may be too late. If these remedies are started at the first sign of spotting, or taken as a preventative if you have a history of miscarriage or have conceived under high-risk conditions (such as through IVF), there is a good chance of success.

Many women worry that they may be saving a non-viable pregnancy, and end up with a child with health problems, but this is unlikely to be the case. Natural remedies for miscarriage are unlikely, at this point in your pregnancy, to have any effect on the foetus, but can certainly affect the uterine environment to make it more hospitable and stable.

If miscarriage threatens

If you experience symptoms that concern you, if you are at risk, or if there is a sudden change in your condition, these remedies may help.

- Bed rest (with legs raised).

- Avoid intercourse.

- Ensure continued good nutrition with extra supplementation of *zinc*, 40 mg, twice daily; *vitamin C*, 2 grams, twice daily, and *bioflavonoids* (especially from cherries and citrus); *B6* (with *B-complex*) 100 mg daily (or 250 mg daily if you have a history of low progesterone); *beta-carotene* (or *mixed carotenes*), 6 mg; *vitamin E*, 1000 IU daily.

- Reflexology, acupuncture (from a professional if possible).

- Homoeopathic remedies are *Aconite*, *Arnica*, *Belladonna*, *Chamomilla*, *Ignatia*, *Pulsatilla* and *Sepia* may all be helpful—but only one remedy is required. It's best to let your homoeopath choose.

Herbs are excellent therapy. Traditionally they have been used with much success and a formula should contain remedies to deal with several possible areas of concern.

- For continued adequate progesterone levels take *Chastetree* and *Peony*. These herbs are always helpful, but are particularly indicated if there has been previous low progesterone, as shown by symptoms of pre-menstrual syndrome, an inadequate temperature rise after ovulation, or a short post-ovulatory phase of the menstrual cycle.

- For possible overactive immune response take *Reiishi*, *Shiitake*, *Hemidesmus* and *Albizzia*. These herbs are particularly recommended where there is a history of allergy or auto-immune disease, and also where conception occurred as a result of IVF or other reproductive technology.

- For uterine 'tone' and circulation take *False Unicorn Root*, *Wild Yam*, *Peony*, *Black Haw* or *Cramp Bark*.

- For cramping take *Cramp Bark* or *Black Haw*.

- For bleeding take *Shepherd's Purse* or *Beth Root* (see further recommendations in 'Breakthrough bleeding' above).

- *Raspberry* and *Squaw Vine* have been used traditionally, but are best restricted to the second (or third) trimester.

After a miscarriage, it may be necessary to proceed to a dilation and curettage (D&C). Your naturopath, herbalist, homoeopath, masseur, osteopath, acupuncturist or reflexologist can help you to recover physically, and you may need some emotional support to help you grieve and move on from what is, undoubtedly, a very traumatic experience. You should attend to your preconception health care before any future pregnancy, and refer to Appendices 11 and 12 for more information.

Preparation for labour

Well, now we've got you through your pregnancy—we're going to put you on hold while we rush off and complete our next book, on better

birthing and bonding. But we'll just mention that natural remedies can also help with the following conditions:
- Premature contractions and birth
- Delayed labour
- Breech presentation
- Premature birth
- Preparation for and facilitation of labour
- Pain control

And much more! See you there!

Sources and recommended reading

The published papers, articles and books which we have used as source material number in the hundreds. To give a complete bibliography would stretch our already large book and our publisher's patience. However, we are very happy to answer any questions (which should be addressed to the authors c/- our Australian publisher) regarding specific references. What we have included here is a list of books which can add to your knowledge and understanding, and which contain the source material for specific references.

For comprehensive catalogues of reading material on related issues you can also contact:

Australian College of Nutritional and Environmental Medicine, 13 Hilton Street, Beaumaris VIC 3193; tel. (03) 9589 6088, fax (03) 9589 5158
CAPERS Bookstore, PO Box 412, Red Hill QLD 4059; tel. (07) 3369 9200, fax (07) 3369 9299
Environment Centre Bookshop, 39 George Street, Sydney NSW 2000; tel. (02) 9247 2228

Nutrition
Bland, J. *Nutraerobics*. Harper & Row, USA, 1983.
Cheraskin, E., Ringsdorf, W.M. & Clark, J.W. *Diet and Disease*. Keats Publishing, Connecticut, USA, 1968.

Davies, S. & Stewart, A. *Nutritional Medicine*. Pan Books, London, 1987.

Davis, A. *Let's Have Healthy Children*. Allen & Unwin, London, 1968.

Foresight publications: *The Adverse Effects of Food Additives on Health; The Adverse Effects of Manganese Deficiency on Reproduction and Health; The Adverse Effects of Zinc Deficiency*. Foresight publications are available from the Foresight Association (for details, see Contacts and Resources).

Hoffer, A. & Walker, M. *Orthomolecular Nutrition*. Keats Publishing, Connecticut, USA, 1978.

Hume Hall, R. *Food for Nought*. Vintage Books, Random House, USA, 1976.

Jennings, I.W. *Vitamins in Endocrine Metabolism*. Heinemann, London, 1970.

Osiecki, Henry. *Nutrients in Profile*. Bioconcepts Publishing, Qld, 1995.

Pfeiffer, C. *Mental and Elemental Nutrients*. Keats Publishing, USA, 1975.

Pfeiffer, C. *Zinc and the Other Micronutrients*. Pivot Original Health, Keats Publishing, Connecticut, USA, 1978.

Price, W.A. *Nutrition and Physical Degeneration*. Price Pottenger Nutrition Foundation, California, USA, 1945.

Sears, Barry. *Enter The Zone*. HarperCollins, New York, 1995.

Watts, David L. *Trace Elements and Other Essential Nutrients*. Writers B-L-O-C-K, USA, 1995.

Werbach, M. *Nutritional Influences on Illness*. Third Line Press, California, USA, 1988.

Williams, R. *Nutrition Against Disease*. Bantam Books, USA, 1971.

Recipe books

There are lots of wholefood recipe books available; alternatively, you can adapt many of your favourite recipes to comply with our recommendations.

Airdre, Grant. *The Good Little Cookbook*. MacPlatypus Productions, Australia, 1998.

Alexander, Stephanie. *The Cook's Companion*. Penguin, Australia, 1997.

Brighthope, I., et al. *A Recipe for Health: Nutrient Dense Recipes*. McCullogh, Carlton, Victoria, 1989.

Buist, R. *Food Intolerance.* Angus & Robertson (HarperCollins), Sydney, 1990.
Gaté, G. *Good Food Fast.* Anne O'Donovan, Victoria, 1991.
Hay, D. & Bacon, Q. *At My Table: Fresh & Simple*, Barbara Beckett, Australia, 1995.
Katzen, M. *Moosewood Cookbook.* Simon & Schuster, Australia, 1997.
Katzen, M. *Moosewood Restaurant Cooks at Home.* Simon & Schuster, Australia, 1994.
Katzen, M. *Moosewood Restaurant Kitchen Garden.* Simon & Schuster, Australia, 1992.
Katzen, M. *New Recipes from Moosewood Restaurant.* Simon & Schuster, Australia, 1997.
Katzen, M. *Sundays at Moosewood Restaurant.* Simon & Schuster, Australia, 1991.
Kilham, Chris. *The Whole Food Bible.* Inner Traditions, UK, 1997.
Marsden, K. *The Food Combining Diet.* Thorsons, UK, 1993.
Milan, Lindley. *Plates.* New Holland, Australia, 1995.
Ombauer, Irma S. *The Joy of Cooking.* Simon & Schuster, Australia, 1998.
Sichel, G. *Relief from Candida, Allergies and Ill-Health.* Sally Milner Publishing, Sydney, 1990.
Solomon, Charmaine. *The Complete Asian Cookbook.* Lansdowne Publishing, Australia, 1992.
Solomon, Charmaine. *The Complete Vegetarian Cookbook.* HarperCollins, Sydney, 1990.
Squirrels Cookbook. Squirrels Publishing, Brisbane, 1994.

Herbal and natural medicine

Airola, P. *Hypoglycemia: A Better Approach.* Health Plus Publishers, Arizona, USA, 1977.
Alexander, P. *It Could Be Allergy and It Can Be Cured.* Ethicare, Sydney, 1988.
Bone, K. *Clinical Applications of Ayurvedic and Chinese Herbs.* Phytotherapy Press, Qld, 1996.
Bone, K. *Herbs and Pregnancy.* Mediherb, Qld, 1992.
Bone, K., Burgess, N. & McLeod, D. *How to Prescribe Herbal Medicines.* Mediherb, Qld, 1990.
Buist, R. *Food Chemical Sensitivity.* Harper & Row, Australia, 1986.

Buist, R. *Food Intolerance*. Angus & Robertson (HarperCollins), Sydney, 1990.
Chapman, E. *The 12 Tissue Salts*. Thorsons, UK, 1960.
De Ruyter, P. *Coping with Candida*. Allen & Unwin, Sydney, 1989.
Grieve, M. *A Modern Herbal*. Penguin, UK, 1977.
Gustalson, H. & O'Shea, M. *The Candida Directory and Cookbook*. Celestial Arts, Berkely, California, 1994.
Hyne Jones, T.W. *Dictionary of the Bach Flower Remedies*. C.W. Daniel Co. Ltd, England, 1976.
Ingham, E.D. *Stories the Feet Have Told Through Reflexology*. Ingham Publishing Inc., USA, 1951.
Kaminski, P. & Katz, R. *The Flower Essence Repertory*. The Flower Essence Society. California, USA, 1994.
Mills, S. *Dictionary of Modern Herbalism*. Thorsons, UK, 1985.
Mills, S. *The Essential Book of Herbal Medicine*. Arkana, UK, 1991.
Ohashi, W. *Do-It-Yourself Shiatsu*. Unwin, UK, 1979.
Segal, M. *Reflexology*. Wilshire Book Company, California, USA, 1976.
Stuart, M. *Encyclopedia of Herbs and Herbalism*. Orbis, London, 1979.
Werbach, M.R. *Botanical Influences on Illness*. Third Line Press, California, USA, 1994.

Women's health

Airola, P. *Every Woman's Book*. Health Plus Publishers, Arizona, USA, 1979.
Boston Women's Health Collective. *The New Our Bodies, Ourselves*. Penguin, UK, 1989.
Cabot, S. *Women's Health*. Pan Books, Sydney, 1987.
Curtis, S. & Fraser, R. *Natural Healing for Women*. Pandora, UK, 1991.
Federation of Feminist Women's Health Centres. *How to Stay Out of the Gynaecologist's Office*. Peace Press Inc., California, USA, 1981.
Grant, E. *The Bitter Pill*. Corgi Books, UK, 1985.
Harding, M.E. *Women's Mysteries, Ancient & Modern*. Harper & Row, New York, 1976.
Howard, J. *Bach Flower Remedies for Women*. C.W. Daniel, UK, 1992.
Llewellyn-Jones, D. *Everywoman*. Faber & Faber, London, 1971.
McQuade-Crawford, Amanda. *Herbal Remedies for Women*. Prima Publishing, USA, 1997.
Melville, A. *Natural Hormone Health*. Thorsons, UK, 1970.
The New Women's Health Handbook. Virago, UK, 1978.

Parvati, J. *Hygeia: A Woman's Herbal*. Freestone, USA, 1979.
Reuben, C. & Priestley, J. *Essential Supplements for Women*. Thorsons, UK, 1991.
Speight, P. *Homoeopathic Remedies for Women's Ailments*. Health Science Press, UK, 1985.
Tisserand, M. *Aromatherapy for Women*. Thorsons, UK, 1985.
Trickey, Ruth. *Women, Hormones and the Menstrual Cycle*. Allen & Unwin, Sydney, 1998.
Trickey, Ruth & Cooke, Kaz. *Women's Trouble*. Allen & Unwin, Australia, 1998.

Pregnancy

Barker, D.J.P. *Mothers, Babies and Disease in Later Life*. BMJ Publishing Group, London, 1994.
Eisenberg, A., Murkoff, H. & Hathaway, S. *What to Expect When You're Expecting*. Angus & Robertson, Sydney, 1987.
Enkin, M., Keirse, M. & Chalmers, I. *A Guide to Effective Care in Pregnancy and Childbirth*. Oxford University Press, Oxford, 1989.
Gardner, Joy. *Healing Yourself During Pregnancy*. The Crossing Press, California, USA, 1987.
Griffey, H. *The Really Useful A–Z of Pregnancy & Birth*. Thorsons, UK, 1996.
Kitzinger, S. & Bailey, V. *Pregnancy Day by Day*. Doubleday, Sydney, 1990.
Plater, Diana. *Taking Control*. Doubleday, Sydney, 1997.
Reid, E. & Elzer, S. *Maternity Reflexology: A Guide for Reflexologists*. Born to be Free & Soul to Sole Reflexology, Sydney, 1997.
Rodwell, L. & Kon, A. *Natural Pregnancy*. Salamander Books, London, 1997.
Stoppard, M. *The New Pregnancy & Birth Book*. Viking (Penguin), Melbourne, 1996.
Weed, Susan. *Wise Woman Herbal Childbearing Year*. Ash Tree Publishing, New York, 1986.
Wesson, Nicky. *Alternative Maternity*. Vermilion (Random House) London, 1989.
Wesson, N. *Morning Sickness*. Vermilion-Random House, London, 1997.

Sources and recommended reading 261

Preconception health care

Bradley, S.G. & Bennett, Nicholas. *Preparation for Pregnancy*. Argyll Publishing, Scotland, 1995.

Barnes, B. & Bradley S.G. *Planning for a Healthy Baby*. Ebury Press, London, 1994.

Brewer, Sarah. *Planning a Baby? A Complete Guide to Preconceptual Care*. Optima, UK, 1995.

Doyle, Wendy. *Healthy Mum: Healthy Baby*. Hodder & Stoughton, London, 1995.

Ford, Judy. *It Takes Two*. Environmental & Genetic Solutions, South Australia, 1997.

Naish, Francesca & Roberts, Janette. *The Natural Way to Better Babies*. Random House, Sydney, 1996.

Stewart, Maryon. *Healthy Parents, Healthy Baby*, Headline, UK, 1995.

Natural fertility awareness

Billings, E. & Westmore, A. *The Billings Method*. Anne O'Donovan Melbourne, 1980.

Naish, F. *The Lunar Cycle*. Nature & Health Books Australia and New Zealand; Prism Press, UK, 1989.

Naish, F. *Natural Fertility*. Sally Milner Publishing, Sydney, 1991.

Ostrander, S. & Schroeder, L. *Astrological Birth Control*. Prentice-Hall, New Jersey, USA, 1972.

Lifestyle and environmental factors

Books marked with an asterisk* contain safe alternatives to use in the kitchen, bathroom, laundry and garden.

Archer, John. *The Water You Drink: How Safe Is It?* Purewater Press, Australia, 1996.

Ashton, J. & Laura, R. *The Perils of Progress: The Health and Environment Hazards of Modern Technology and What You Can Do About Them*. University of New South Wales Press, Sydney, 1998.

Colborn, Theo, Myers, John Peterson & Dumanoski, Dianne. *Our Stolen Future*. Dutton, USA, & Little Brown & Co., UK, 1996.

Elkington, J. & Hailes, J. *The Green Consumer Guide*. Penguin Books, Australia, 1989.*

Hodges, J. *Harvesting the Suburbs*. Nature & Health Books, Australia, 1985.*

Ott, J. *Health and Light*. Pocket Books, Simon & Schuster, New York, USA, 1976.

Powerwatch. *Living with Electricity*. Powerwatch, 2 Tower Road, Sutton, Ely, CB62QA Cambridgeshire, UK.

Salminen, S. et al. *Safeguards (Home Chemicals Guide)*. McPhee Gribble (Penguin), Melbourne, 1991.

Smith, R. & Total Environment Centre. *Chemical Risks and the Unborn: A Parents Guide*. Total Environment Centre, Sydney, 1991.

Foresight publications: *The Adverse Effects of Alcohol on Reproduction*; *The Adverse Effects of Tobacco Smoking on Reproduction*; *The Adverse Effects of Lead*; *The Adverse Effects of Agrochemicals on Reproduction and Health*; *The Adverse Effects of Genito-urinary Infections*. Foresight publications are available from the Foresight Association (for details, see Contacts and Resources).

Medical technology and drugs

Chitty, Hunt & Moore, cited in Adams, C. & Parsons, M. 'Prenatal Testing', *Birthings Newsletter*, no. 57, pp. 12-17.

Foreman, R., Gilmour-White, S. & Forman, N. *Drug Induced Infertility and Sexual Dysfunction*. Cambridge University Press.

Landymore-Lim, Lisa. *Poisons Prescriptions*. PODD, Subiaco, WA, 1994.

McTaggart, Lynne. *What Doctors Don't Tell You*. Thorsons, London, 1996.

What Doctors Don't Tell You is also a monthly newsletter and is available by subscription only. For further details contact: Wallace Press, 4 Wallace Rd., London N1 2PG, England; tel. 0011 44 171 354 4592. For the full report on travel vaccines send 7.80 pounds Sterling.

Meditation and exercise

Anderson, B. *Stretching*. Shelter Publications, California, USA, 1980.

Shakti, Gawain. *Creative Visualisation*. Bantam New Age Books, USA, 1979.

Shandler, N. & M. *Yoga for Pregnancy and Birth*. Schocken Books, NY, 1979.

Health issues from a holistic perspective

The following is a list of journals and newsletters which report on studies and research findings regarding health issues from a holistic perspective. Many of the studies we have mentioned have been reported in these journals.

Alternative & Complementary Therapies, available from Mary Ann Leibert Inc, 2 Madison Avenue, Larchmart NY 10538, USA; tel. (914) 834 3100, fax (914) 834 3582

Alternative Medicine Digest, available from Future Medicine Publishing Inc. Editorial Office, 21½ Main Street, Tiburon CA 94920, USA; tel. (415) 789 8700

Australasian Society of Oral Medicine and Toxicology, available from ASOMAT, PO Box A860, Sydney South NSW 2000; tel. (02) 9867 1111, fax (02) 9665 5043

Australian Health & Healing, available from Australian Health Newsletters, PO Box 427, Paddington NSW 2021

Australian Journal of Medical Herbalism, available from Anne Cowper, PO Box 403, Morisset NSW 2264; tel. (02) 4973 4107, fax (02) 4973 4857

Birth Issues, available from CAPERS, PO Box 412, Red Hill QLD 4059; tel. (07) 3369 9200, fax (07) 3369 9299

Birthings, available from Homebirth Access Sydney, PO Box 66, Broadway NSW 2007

Environment & Health News, available from The Environment Health Trust, PO Box 1954, Glastonbury, Somerset BA6 9FE; tel. (0176) 762 7038

Health & Wellness Report, available from Tapestry Communications, Spectrum Marketing Services, PO Box 264, Toorak VIC 3142; tel. (03) 8247 7938

Herbalgram, available from American Botanical Council & Herb Research Foundation, PO Box 201660, Austin TX 78720, USA; tel. (512) 331 8868

International Clinical Nutrition Review, available from Integrated Therapies, PO Box 370, Manly NSW 2095

International Journal of Alternative & Complementary Medicine, available from Green Library, 9 Rickett Street, Fulham, London; tel. (0171) 385 0012, fax 0171 385 4566

Journal of Health Sciences, available from PO Box 6200, South Penrith NSW 2750

Journal of Nutritional & Environmental Medicine, available from Carfax Publishing Ltd, PO Box 25, Abingdon, Oxfordshire OX143UE, UK

Journal of the Australasian College of Nutritional & Environmental Medicine, available from ACNEM, 13 Hilton Street, Beaumaris VIC 3193; tel. (03) 9589 6088, fax (03) 9589 5158

Life Spirit, available from Tracey Harris, PO Box 312, Fortitude Valley QLD 4006; tel. (07) 3854 1286

Metagenics Phenolic Desensitisation and Homoeopathic Detoxification Therapy, available from Metagenics, 8/633 Kingsford Smith Drive, Eagle Farm QLD 4009; PO Box 830, Hamilton QLD 4007; tel. (07) 3868 1119, fax (07) 3868 1808.

Natural Parent; *Proof!*; and *What Doctors Don't Tell You*, available from WDDTY, 4 Wallace Road, London N1 2PG; tel. (0171) 354 4592, fax (0171) 354 8907, e-mail: wddty@zoo.co.uk

Soma Newsletter, available from PO Box 7180, Bondi Beach NSW 2026; tel. (02) 9789 4805, fax (02) 9922 5747

Contacts and resources

We have given national contacts wherever possible. NSW contacts, when given, can usually supply you with appropriate addresses in your own state or territory. Natural health journals also contain service directories and advertisements which will give many more names and addresses than we have been able to list here. All addresses and phone numbers are up to date at time of publication.

Francesca and Janette also offer the following services which can augment and update the information in this book.

For information on the following you can contact our website: www.fertility.com.au

The Natural Way to Better Babies

The Natural Way to Better Babies: Preconception Health Care for Prospective Parents, by Francesca Naish & Janette Roberts, is available in all good book stores or by mail order. Cost is $24.95 plus postage (add $6.00 NSW; $8.50 VIC, QLD, SA; $9.50 WA, NT, TAS). Send cheque/money order or credit card details (VISA, Mastercard or Bankcard) to: Better Babies, Mail Box 16, 133 Rowntree Street, Birchgrove NSW 2041; fax (02) 9818 3734

'Better Babies' nutritional supplements

Formulated in conjunction with Efamol, *Efanatal*, an essential fatty supplement, is now available. This is specifically designed for use before conception, during pregnancy and while breastfeeding. We expect that 'Better Babies' multivitamin and mineral supplements will be available in the future. For information contact: Better Babies, Mail Box 16, 133 Rowntree Street, Birchgrove NSW 2041; fax (02) 9818 3734.

Natural Fertility Management

Francesca is the director of Natural Fertility Management (NFM), which offers programs for contraception, conscious conception and overcoming fertility problems, as well as holistic health care for all reproductive concerns, including pregnancy and threatened miscarriage. A comprehensive range of medical and holistic therapies is provided by highly qualified practitioners, using natural and non-invasive therapies.

For enquiries and bookings, please contact: The Jocelyn Centre, 1/46 Grosvenor Street, Woollahra NSW 2025; tel. (02) 9369 2047, fax (02) 9369 5179

For those unable to attend the Jocelyn Centre, Natural Fertility Management provides a referral service to NFM-accredited counsellors throughout Australia, New Zealand, USA and the UK. Contraception and conception kits are also available by mail order. Send stamped, self-addressed envelope for enquiries and referrals to: Jane Bennett, National Co-ordinator, NFM, 70 Bowden Street, Castlemaine VIC 3450; tel. (03) 5472 4922, fax (03) 5470 5766

Natural Fertility Management counsellor training

Seminars are conducted by Francesca Naish and Jane Bennett to train health professionals in NFM techniques. All accredited counsellors have access to NFM kits for their clients. Please send for details and dates of training sessions in Australia, New Zealand, USA and the UK to: Jane Bennett, National Co-ordinator, NFM (address, above).

Further reading

The Lunar Cycle, Francesca Naish. Available by mail order from the Jocelyn Centre (address, above). $14.00 includes postage and packing within Australia. $A20.00 includes postage and packing outside Australia.

Natural Fertility, Francesca Naish. Available in all good bookshops or by mail order from the Jocelyn Centre. $32.00 includes postage and packing within Australia. $A35.00 includes postage and packing outside Australia.

Send cheque/money order (in Australian dollars) or credit card details (VISA, Mastercard or Bankcard) to Natural Fertility Management (address, above). International orders—send international money order/bank draft/credit card details.

Balmain Wellness Centre

Janette is co-founder and director of one of the first wellness and longevity centres in Australia. The centre offers comprehensive naturopathic programs for: vitality and longevity, weight management, preconception care, pre and post-natal care, breastfeeding care, allergy treatment and corporate health care. The centre offers its clients a comprehensive 'wellness program' which is in direct contrast to traditional 'crisis care' treatments for illness and chronic conditions. All programs incorporate the use of sophisticated bio-impedance analysis (BIA) techniques developed in Canada. Each program is individually tailored and includes initial BIA testing with regular re-assessment, comprehensive health appraisal, naturopathic consultations with full nutritional support, spinal health care and fitness appraisal with individualised exercise program. Regular workshops on topics including nutrition, lifestyle, environment, stress and exercise are designed to enhance client compliance and ensure program maintenance. Postal consultations are also available.

For further details, contact: Balmain Wellness Centre, Mail Box 16, 133 Rowntree Street, Birchgrove NSW 2041; tel. (02) 9555 9967, fax (02) 9818 6073.

'Better Babies' preconception health care: lectures and workshops

Janette also presents lectures to prospective parents and workshops for health professionals such as midwives, birth educators and lactation consultants who are involved in counselling couples planning a pregnancy. Length and type of presentation, time, date and place can be tailored to suit the audience. For further details, contact: Better Babies, Mail Box 16, 133 Rowntree Street, Birchgrove NSW 2041; tel./fax (02) 9818 3734

The Foresight Association

Janette is the Australian representative of Foresight, The Association for the Promotion of Preconceptual Health Care.

Foresight membership costs $A35.00 per annum. Members receive regular newsletters with updated research results from the UK.

Foresight brochures are available on request for distribution by health practitioners. Fully referenced booklets are available, detailing the adverse effects on reproduction of the following: alcohol, tobacco, zinc deficiency, manganese deficiency, food additives, genito-urinary infections, lead, agrochemicals. Cost is $A5.00 per booklet (includes postage).

The Foresight video 'Preparing for the Healthier Baby' (running time 85 minutes) is suitable for viewing by preconception couples. Cost is $A50.00 (includes post and packing within Australia).

For any/all of the above, send cheque/money order/credit card details (VISA, Mastercard or Bankcard) to: Foresight Association, Mail Box 16, 133 Rowntree Street, Birchgrove NSW 2041; fax (02) 9818 3734

Other contacts and resources

To find a doctor trained in nutritional and environmental medicine, contact:

Australian College of Nutritional and Environmental Medicine (ACNEM), 13 Hilton Street, Beaumaris VIC 3193; tel. (03) 9589 6088, fax (03) 9589 5158

For names of appropriate natural health practitioners, contact:

Acupuncture Ethics and Standards Organisation (AESO) and Australian Acupuncture Association (AACA), PO Box 5142, West End QLD 4101; tel. (07) 3846 5866

Aromatherapists, International Federation of, PO Box 107, Burwood NSW 2134; PO Box 400, Balwyn VIC 3103; IFA National Information Line, tel. 190 224 0125

Association of Massage Therapists (NSW), PO Box 1248, Bondi Junction NSW 2022; tel. (02) 9300 9405

Association of Remedial Masseurs, 1/120 Blaxland Road, Ryde NSW 2112; tel. (02) 9807 4769

Australian Association of Reflexology, 2 Stewart Avenue, Matraville NSW 2036; tel. (02) 9311 2322

Australian Council for Experiential Therapies and the College of Experiential Psychotherapy, 141 Beattie Street, Balmain NSW 2041; tel. (02) 9818 4188

Australian Feldenkrais Guild Inc., 276b Johnston Street, Annandale NSW 2038; tel. (02) 9555 1374

Australian Hypnotherapists Association, tel. 1800 067 557 (free call)

Australian Natural Therapists Association, PO Box A964, Sydney NSW 2000; tel. (02) 9283 2234; country and interstate tel. 1800 817 577

Australian Osteopathic Association, PO Box 699, Turramurra NSW 2074; tel. (02) 9449 4799

Australian Psychological Society, 30 Atchison Street, St Leonards NSW 2065; tel. (02) 9906 6504

Australian School of Reflexology, 15 Kedumba Crescent, Turramurra NSW 2074; tel. (02) 9988 3881

Australian Society of Teachers of the Alexander Technique (AUSTAT), PO Box 716, Darlinghurst NSW 2010; tel. 1800 339 571 or (03) 9853 1356

Australian Society of Clinical Hypnotherapists, 30 Denistone Road, Eastwood NSW 2122; tel. (02) 9874 2776

Australian Society of Hypnosis (members are doctors, dentists, psychiatrists, psychologists) and Academy of Applied Hypnosis, 300 George Street, Sydney NSW 2000; tel. (02) 9231 4877

Australian Traditional Medicine Society, PO Box 1027, Meadowbank NSW 2114; tel. (02) 9809 6800

BKS Iyengar (Yoga) Association of Australia Inc., PO Box 159, Mosman NSW 2088; tel. (02) 9948 2366

Chiropractors Association of Australia, tel. 1800 803 665 (free call)

Homoeopathic Association of NSW, 90 Pitt Street, Sydney NSW 2000; tel. (02) 9231 3322

International Yoga Teachers Association Inc., PO Box 207, St Ives NSW 2075; tel. (02) 9484 2256

Natural Health Society, Suite 28/541 High Street, Penrith NSW 2750; tel. (02) 4721 5068

Natural Herbalists Association of Australia, PO Box 61, Broadway NSW 2007; tel. (02) 9211 6437

Reflexology Association of Australia, 22 Lagoon Street, Narrabeen NSW 2101; tel. (02) 9970 6155

Reiki Network, 187a Avenue Road, Mosman NSW 2088; tel. (02) 9969 1623; 1800 804 529 (free call)

Shiatsu Therapy Association of Australia, 332 Carlisle Street, Balaclava VIC 3183; tel. (03) 9530 0067; PO Box 47, Waverley NSW 2024; tel. (02) 9314 5248

Tai Chi Australian Academy, PO Box 1020, Burwood North NSW 2134; tel. (02) 9797 9355

To receive an organic products directory, contact:
Royal Easter Show Exhibit and Directory, Organic Promotions, Consultation & Education, tel./fax (02) 9365 7668

To find a supplier of organically grown produce near you, contact:
The National Association for Sustainable Agriculture, Australia (NASAA)
Head Office: PO Box 768, Stirling SA 5152; tel. (08) 8370 8455, fax (08) 8370 8381
New South Wales and ACT: c/- PO Box 770, North Sydney NSW 2060
Queensland: PO Box 733, Emerald QLD 4720
South Australia: c/- PO Box 207, Stirling SA 5152
Western Australia: PO Box 8387, Stirling Street WA 6849
Tasmania: Post Office, Lower Longley TAS 7109
Victoria: c/- RMB 1299, Blampied VIC 3363

To find out if drugs you need to take are safe during pregnancy, contact:
Australian Drug Evaluation Committee, PO Box 100, Woden ACT 2606

If you have trouble stopping smoking, contact:
Smokers' Clinic, St Vincent's Hospital, 73 Boundary Street, Darlinghurst NSW 2010; tel. (02) 9361 2625

If you need help overcoming an addiction to drugs or alcohol, contact:
Alcohol, Drug and Nicotine Treatment Centre, Nobbs Street (cnr South Dowling Street), Surry Hills NSW 2010; tel. (02) 9331 2196
Alcohol and Drugs Education and Information Centre, Balmain Road, Rozelle NSW 2039; tel. (02) 9818 0444
Alcoholics Anonymous National Office, Joynton Avenue, Zetland NSW 2017; tel. (02) 9663 1206

For information on hazards at work, contact:
Total Environment Centre, 1/88 Cumberland Street, Sydney NSW 2000; tel. (02) 9247 4714
Toxic Chemicals Committee, 1/88 Cumberland Street, Sydney NSW 2000; tel. (02) 9247 8476
Worksafe Australia, National Occupational Health and Safety Commission, 92 Parramatta Road, Camperdown NSW 2050; tel. (02) 9565 9555

To find out about occupational health and safety entitlements during pregnancy, contact:
Worksafe Australia, 92 Parramatta Road, Camperdown NSW 2050; tel. (02) 9577 9555 or 1800 252 226 (free call), fax (02) 9577 9202

For advice on procedures to remove lead safely, contact:
Environmental Protection Authority, 66–72 Rickard Road, Bankstown NSW 2200; tel. (02) 9793 0000 or (02) 9793 0250
The LEAD Group, PO Box 161, Summer Hill NSW 2130; tel. (02) 9716 0014, fax (02) 9716 9005

For advice on safe removal of dental amalgam, contact:
Australian Society of Oral Medicine and Toxicology (ASOMAT), PO Box A860, Sydney South NSW 2000; Dr Roman Lohyn, President, tel. (03) 9650 1660; Dr Robert Gammal, Secretary, tel. (02) 9264 5195

For alternative pest extermination, contact:
Academic Pest Control, 282 Oxford Street, Bondi Junction NSW 2022; tel. (02) 9389 7844
Systems Pest Management, 4 Jarrett Street, Leichhardt NSW 2040; tel. (02) 9564 1614

For information about antiradiation and anti-electro-magnetic devices, contact:
Electra Medica, PO Box 705, Sunbury VIC 3429; tel. (03) 9740 9917
ELF Cocoon Australia, Health and Environment Services, PO Box 405, Merimbula NSW 2548
Harmonic Products, Teslar Tech, 31 Jasper Terrace, Frankston VIC 3199; tel. (0418) 990 539
Harmonology, 57/59 Brown Street, West Wallsend NSW 2286; tel. (02) 4953 2726

To order non-toxic household cleaners and personal products, contact:
Trinature, Box 304, Hunter Region Mail Centre NSW 2310; tel. (02) 4928 2199, fax (02) 4928 2405

To order EM Power modulator for use with your computer, contact:
EMR Cleares, PO Box 686, Alstonville NSW 2477; tel. 1800 804 714 (free call), fax (02) 6628 3202

For information about water filters and water deliveries, contact:
All Clear Water Aust (08) 9257 2241
Aqua One Water Filters (07) 3890 2900
Crystal Clear Purification Systems (08) 8331 3376
Crystal Flow (03) 9866 8222
Culligan (02) 9316 4142
Neverfail Spring Water Co (02) 9712 1022
Raindance Water Purifiers(07) 3849 1577
The Freshly Squeezed Water Co (02) 9712 1022; (07) 3856 0988
The Pure Water Shop (08) 8373 2096
The Water People (03) 9885 0222
The Water Shop (02) 9956 5677
Unicorn—The Water Filter Advisory Centre (08) 9242 1066
Water One (02) 9181 2983

If you're painting your house, contact:
Bio-paint, Bio-products Australia Pty Ltd, tel. (08) 8339 1923
Planet Ark (also mail order), tel. (02) 9516 4681, (08) 9430 5054

For information about full spectrum lighting, contact:
Interlight Australia, 20 Nulgarra Street, Northbridge NSW 2063; tel. (02) 9958 6378

For (practitioner) information about heavy metal test systems and homoeopathic chelation, contact:
Hemperton Management, 37 Blaxland Street, Hunters Hill NSW 2110; tel./fax (02) 9817 0239

For Bach Flower remedies and Australian Bush Flower essences, contact:
Australian Bush Flower Essences, 45 Booralie Road, Terrey Hills NSW 2084; tel. (02) 9450 1388, fax (02) 9450 2866
Martin and Pleasance, 135 Swan Street, Richmond VIC 3121; tel. (03) 427 7422
'Rose of Raphael' Flower Essences, PO Box 410, Bellingen NSW 2454; tel. (02) 6656 1447

For meditation and yoga classes, contact:
Siddha Yoga Foundation, 50 Garnet Street, Dulwich Hill NSW 2203; tel. (02) 9559 5666

For ambient music and relaxation tapes, contact:
Natural Symphonies, PO Box 252, Camden NSW 2570; tel. (02) 4655 1800, fax (02) 4655 9434
Phoenix Music, PO Box 98, Bondi NSW 2026; tel. (02) 9211 5891

For DIY acupressure machines, contact:
ELF Cocoon Australia, Health and Environment Services, PO Box 405, Merimbula NSW 2548
SHP International P/L, 5/212 Glen Osmond Road, Fullarton SA 5068; tel. (08) 8379 0700

For information about chelation therapy, contact:
Dr Ian Brighthope, Australian Detox Centre, 199 North Road, Elsternwick VIC 3185; tel. (03) 9598 5699
Omnicare, 2 Brady Street, Mosman NSW 2088; tel. (02) 9960 4133
Whole Health Medical Clinic, 31 Dunstan Street, Clayton VIC 3168; tel. (03) 9562 7558

The Sydney Natural Medical Centre, 15 South Steyne, Manly NSW 2095; tel. (02) 9977 7888

For information about hair trace mineral analysis, contact:
Clinical Assays, PO Box 394, Hornsby NSW 2077; tel. (02) 9482 2933, fax (02) 9987 4144
Interclinical Laboratories Pty Ltd, PO Box 630, Gladesville NSW 2111; tel. (02) 9214 2525, fax (02) 9635 1352

Alternative diagnostic tests including allergy testing available from:
Australian Biologics Testing Services, Suite 401, 4th Floor BMA House, 135 Macquarie Street, Sydney NSW 2000; tel. (02) 9247 5322, fax (02) 9247 5453
Clinical Assays, PO Box 394, Hornsby NSW 2077; tel. (02) 9482 2933, fax (02) 9987 4144

If you have, or suspect, an allergy and need help or support, contact:
Allergy Information Network, 370 Victoria Road, Chatswood NSW 2067; tel. (02) 9419 7731

For information about toxoplasmosis, contact:
The Toxoplasmosis Trust, 61–71 Collier Street, London N1 9BE; tel. (071) 713 0663, fax (071) 713 0611, helpline (071) 713 0599

If you have experienced pregnancy loss or the death of a child, contact:
Bonnie Babies Foundation, PO Box 222, Knoxfield VIC 3180; tel. (03) 9563 4004 fax (03) 9563 4002
Pen-Parents of Australia, PO Box 574, Belconnen ACT 2616; tel. (06) 261 6459 or (06) 292 4292
SANDS (Stillbirth and Neonatal Death Support) in your state
Sudden Infant Death Association, tel. 1800 651 186 (free call)

For antenatal support, contact:
Birth Awareness, tel. (02) 9797 6808
Birthing Rites Australia, tel. (02) 9387 3615 or (03) 9899 3311
Associates in Childbirth Education, 148 Hereford Street, Forest Lodge NSW 2037; tel. (02) 9660 5177

For parenting preparation courses, contact:
B. J. Larson Seminars (Parenting Preparation Courses), PO Box 587, Woollahra NSW 2025; tel. (02) 9319 0847, (015) 432 288

For information on homebirth options, contact:
Homebirth Access Sydney Inc., PO Box 66, Broadway NSW 2007; tel. (02) 9792 8345, (02) 9888 7829 or (02) 9314 5738

For comfortable, attractive maternity underwear, swimwear and nightwear, contact:
Full Bloom Pty Ltd, tel. 1800 068 870

For information on levels of toxins in breast milk, contact:
Reply Paid AAA51, Greenpeace Australia, PO Box 139, Surry Hills NSW 2010; tel. 1800 815 151

For full reports on travel vaccines and alternatives, contact:
What Doctors Don't Tell You, Wallace Press, 4 Wallace Road, London N1 2PG (cost of report is 7.80 pounds Sterling); tel. 0011 44 171 354 4592

APPENDIX 1

Reproductive health diet summary

All foods should be fresh and organically grown/fed whenever possible (such food is higher in nutritional value and lower in toxins). To help make positive choices, try an affirmation such as: 'I am making a positive choice for my health and wellbeing and that of my child.'

Protein

You need an appropriate-sized serving of protein-providing food at least 3 times a day during pregnancy (see page 45 to estimate this size). This should be food giving you either:

1. A primary protein, which comes from an animal source, and is a complete protein (i.e. one which contains all the amino acids) *or*

2. A combination of secondary proteins, which come from a plant source, and are incomplete proteins (i.e they do not contain the full range of amino acids). By combining two of the following food groups, you will have a complete protein source, as each group has a different range:

   - Nuts
   - Grains and seeds
   - Legumes and pulses

Protein-providing foods

Fish
Eat 2–3 times weekly. Fish is low in saturated fats and high in essential fatty acids, especially deep-sea, ocean and cold-water fish, which are also less polluted (e.g. mackerel, mullet, salmon, taylor, trevally and sardines). Avoid large fish, which are too high in mercury (e.g. tuna, shark and swordfish). Fresh fish are definitely preferable to tinned or frozen fish.

Chicken
Trim the skin to avoid fats. Use only free-range/organically fed poultry (which is not necessarily the same thing, as some free-range poultry are still fed hormones and antibiotics).

Eggs
Eat 2–3 weekly, maximum. However, if you are confident you are not allergic or sensitive to eggs, you can increase consumption, as eggs are a good protein source. Make sure they are free-range/organically fed (see above).

Dairy foods
Avoid cow's milk and cheese. They create mucus in tubes and malabsorption. Natural acidophilus non-flavoured yoghurt is good. Eat goat's or soy milk and cheese where possible.

Red meat
Eat in moderation and avoid the meat from non-organically fed animals, especially organ meats (such as liver), sausage and mince (or get the butcher to mince non-organ meat for you). Organ meats contain high levels of pesticides and hormones. Avoid delicatessen meats (which are high in fats, offal content and toxic preservatives). Trim all fat.

Legumes and pulses
Lentils, beans, soya, tofu and tempeh are good vegetable protein and good sources of detoxifiers. Avoid high-aluminium soya brands.

Whole grains
These are also a good source of plant protein. Eat only whole grains (organically grown whenever possible), such as brown bread, rice, pasta, pastry. (Green pasta might be white with dye added.) Avoid refined flour products; they leach nutrients. Read bread packets carefully and avoid those containing preservatives/additives.

Nuts and seeds
These should be raw, unsalted and fresh. Store in fridge, away from light, and eat within 2 weeks (nuts should not taste bitter). Use in stir-fries, salads, pasta dishes, as a snack.

Vegetables
Eat lots every day. They should make up a minimum of 40 per cent of your total food intake. Use organic produce whenever possible. Consume a wide variety, especially dark green leafy vegies and red and orange ones, as well as avocado. Eat both raw and cooked vegetables on a regular basis.

Juices
Try juices as a great way of ensuring adequate vegetable intake. Carrot, celery and beetroot taste good, but any vegetable you have can be added.

Salads
Use a wide variety of vegetables in your salads. Pale lettuce is not highly nutritious. Add chopped fresh herbs (e.g. parsley and watercress).

Cooked vegies
You can steam, stir-fry or dry-bake. Do not cook or defrost with microwaves. Discard green potatoes (they are toxic).

Fruit
Eat 2–3 pieces daily, maximum (because of high sugar content). This includes fruit that is juiced, which should be diluted 50/50 with purified water. Avoid dried fruit. Eat organic fruit whenever possible.

Fats
Use lots of cold-pressed oils on salads (extra virgin olive or flaxseed, safflower, sunflower, pumpkin or walnut). These oils are high in essential fatty acids if never heated. They should be kept out of the light (in dark containers) and in the fridge (except olive). You can add lemon, pepper, garlic and herbs to dressing.

Avoid saturated fats. This means heated and animal fats. These will upset your prostaglandin / hormone / mineral balance.

Avoid eating fried food, except stir-fries. Cook with olive oil, which is a mono-unsaturated fat and will not saturate on heating. Canola and sesame oils are possible alternatives.

Avoid butter and margarine. They are both saturated fats. Margarine is even worse than butter—it saturates during processing and is also full of chemicals. Try avocado, banana, hummus, tahini or nut spreads (if fresh and refrigerated and kept away from light).

Avoid non-organic produce whenever possible. As most toxins are stored in fat, this is a major source of chemicals, hormones etc.

Purified water
Drink 8–12 glasses of purified water daily. Spring (still) water is a reasonable substitute. Mineral (sparkling) water is okay occasionally, but may be high in salt. Unpurified tap water is high in many toxins and heavy metals which are concentrated, not destroyed, by boiling.

Tea
You can drink a maximum of 2 cups of weak, naturally low caffeine (not decaffeinated) tea daily. Green and herb teas preferred.

Coffee
Avoid coffee—it is related to problems in pregnancy and foetal health, including miscarriage. We don't recommend decaffeinated. Cereal-based substitutes and dandelion root are okay (but check for added sugar).

Alcohol
Avoid alcohol—it is both toxic to the foetus and leaches nutrients.

Sugar

Avoid sugar and all sweet things, including honey, artificial sweeteners such as Nutrasweet, undiluted fruit juices, cakes, biscuits, soft drinks. Sugar leaches nutrients from your body.

Salt

Only add salt 'to taste', not routinely in cooking or on food. Use rock, sea or Celtic salt rather than ordinary table salt. Avoid highly salted pre-prepared food.

Junk foods

Avoid fats, sugars, salt and chemical additives. Read labels carefully.

Acid/alkali balance

This should be okay if you eat lots of vegetables and moderate amounts of animal products.

N.B. Individuals may have additional or different dietary needs—your naturopath can advise you.

This diet summary may be photocopied by the book's purchaser provided that it is for personal use only. (*The Natural Way to a Better Pregnancy*, by Francesca Naish and Janette Roberts, published by Doubleday (Transworld Publishers (Aust) Pty Limited), Sydney, 1999. Copyright © Francesca Naish and Janette Roberts, 1999.)

APPENDIX 2

Nutritional content of organic versus non-organic foods

Nutritional content of organically grown foods in comparison to inorganic (conventionally grown) foods

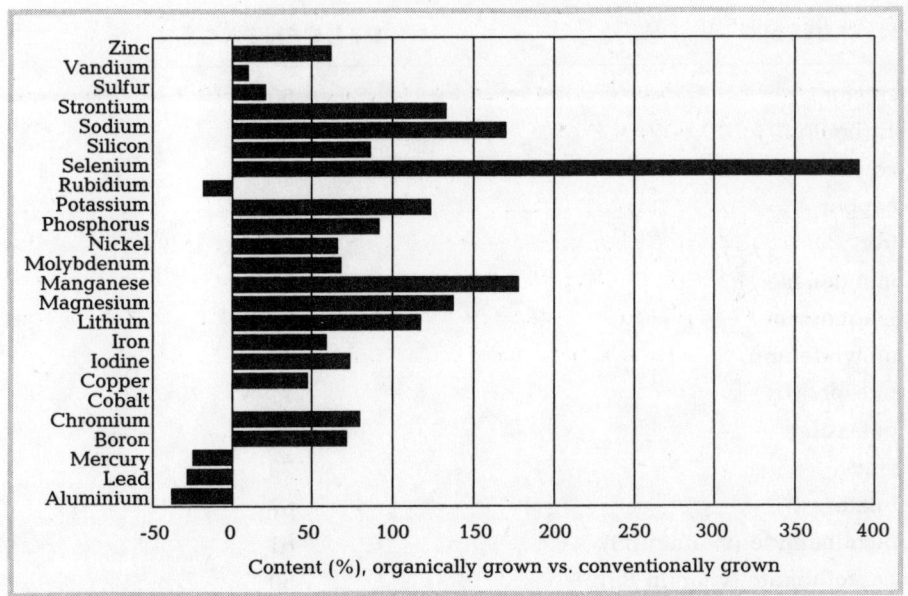

Adapted by John Bolk, *Cancer and Natural Medicine*, Oregon Medical Press, 1995, from data in B.L. Smith, 'Organic Foods vs Supermarket Foods', *Journal of Applied Nutrition*, 1993, vol. 45, no. 1, pp. 35–9.

APPENDIX 3

Nutrients lost when wheat is refined

When white flour is produced from whole wheat, the following amounts of nutrients are removed.

NUTRIENT	PERCENTAGE
calcium	60
chromium	40
cobalt	89
copper	68
iron	76
manganese	86
magnesium	85
molybdenum	48
phosphorus	71
potassium	77
zinc	78
folate	67
nicotinamide (vitamin B3)	81
pantothenate (vitamin B5)	50
pyridoxine (vitamin B6)	71
riboflavin (vitamin B2)	80
thiamine (vitamin B1)	77
vitamin E	86

From Foresight (UK) Newsletter Autumn 1997

APPENDIX 4

Nutritional deficiencies and symptoms

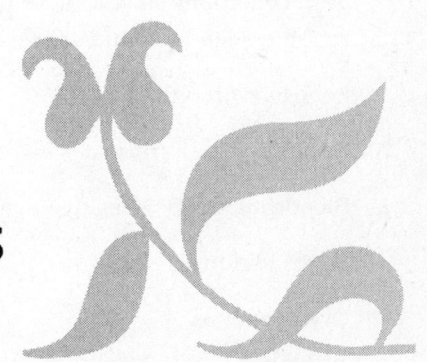

Below we have listed some common signs and symptoms and their corresponding nutritional deficiencies. We certainly hope you're not suffering from too many (or any) of these symptoms; but if you are, seek advice from someone who has experience in nutritional and environmental medicine. All these signs and symptoms can be caused by other medical conditions, and self-help is best not attempted.

SIGN OR SYMPTOM	DEFICIENCY
Cracking at the corners of the mouth	iron, vitamins B2, B6, folic acid
Recurrent mouth ulcers	iron, folic acid, vitamin B12
Dry, cracked lips	vitamin B2
Smooth, sore tongue	iron, vitamins B2, B12, folic acid
Fissured tongue	vitamin B3
Enlargement (prominence) of taste buds at the tip of the tongue (red, sore)	vitamins B2 or B6
Bruising or enlargement of veins under the tongue	vitamin C
Red, greasy skin on face, especially sides of nose	vitamins B2, B6, zinc or essential fatty acids

Rough, sometimes red, pimply skin on upper arms and thighs	vitamin B complex, vitamin E or essential fatty acids
Scrotal and vulval dermatitis	vitamin B2, zinc
Skin conditions such as eczema, dry rough cracked peeling skin	zinc, essential fatty acids
Poor hair growth	iron or zinc
Dandruff	vitamin C, B6, zinc, essential fatty acids
Bloodshot, gritty, sensitive eyes	vitamin A or B2
Night blindness	vitamin A or zinc
Dry eyes	vitamin A, essential fatty acids
Brittle or split nails	iron, zinc or essential fatty acids
White spots on nails	zinc
Pale appearance due to anaemia	iron, vitamin B12, folic acid (it's essential to consult a doctor if you are anaemic)
Poor dream recall	vitamin B6

APPENDIX 5

Diet and lifestyle questionnaire

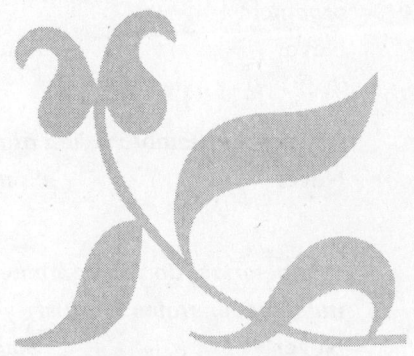

Circle your answer to each question and score 1 point for each answer in the left-hand column, score 2 points for each answer in the middle column, and score 3 points for each answer in the right-hand column.

What sort of bread do you eat most frequently?
White   Wholegrain/brown   Organically grown/
                                          stoneground

Which type of rice and pasta do you eat predominantly?
Don't eat rice, pasta   White rice, white pasta   Brown rice/wholemeal
                                                    pasta

How many portions of fruit and vegetables do you eat daily?
Two servings or fewer   Four servings   More than four servings

Are your vegetables . . . ?
Don't eat vegies   Canned/frozen   Fresh

Are your fresh vegetables . . . ?
Don't eat vegies   Non-organically grown   Organically grown

Do you eat large amounts of natural sugars (e.g. fresh or juiced fruits)
10+ pieces daily   4–10 pieces daily   2–3 pieces daily

Do you trim the fat off your meat and the skin off your chicken?
Never   Sometimes   Always

Do you avoid eating organ meats, sausages and deli meats (except if organic)?
Never   Sometimes   Always

Is your beef/lamb/chicken organically raised and fed?
Never   Sometimes   Always

If vegetarian, do you combine legumes (beans, split peas, lentils, chickpeas), nuts, seeds, grains to satisfy your protein requirements?
Never   Sometimes   Often

How many times per week do you eat deep-sea fish?
Never   Once or twice   Three times at least

Do you eat fried food?
Every day   Two or three times a week   Rarely

What spread do you use on your bread?
Margarine   Butter   Neither

What oils do you use on your salads?
Pre-packaged dressings   Olive/flaxseed/safflower/sunflower/pumpkin/walnut   Cold pressed, organically grown olive/flaxseed/safflower/sunflower/pumpkin/walnut

What oils do you use for cooking?
Polyunsaturated   Olive/canola/sesame   Cold pressed, organically grown olive/canola/sesame

Do you salt your food?

| Heavily | Lightly | Sometimes (to taste) |

Do you cook, heat or defrost your food in a microwave?

| Always | Quite often | Rarely/never |

How often do you eat out or get take-away?

| Usually | Once or twice a week | Occasionally |

Do you purify your water?

| No | Only drinking water | Drinking water and water for cooking |

How much purified water do you drink daily?

| Fewer than 3 glasses | 3–8 glasses daily | 8–12 glasses daily |

Do you cook/brew tea in aluminium pots and pans?

| Yes | Sometimes | Never |

Do you eat desserts/sugar snacks (biscuits, candy bars etc.)?

| After every meal and in between | Most days | Very occasionally/never |

Do you drink tea/coffee/cola, soft drinks (which contain caffeine)?

| More than 3 cups daily | Fewer than 3 cups daily | Very occasionally/never |

Do you use sugar/sweetener in your tea/coffee?

| Lots | A little | Never |

Do you smoke?

| More than 10 cigs per day | Fewer than 10 cigs per day | No |

Do you drink alcohol?

| More than 1 drink per day | Fewer than 7 drinks per week | Non/occasional drinker |

Do you take (or have you taken) drugs for a chronic condition (e.g. asthma, high blood pressure, birth control–oral contraceptives)?

| Yes | In the past | Never |

Do you use drugs (e.g. aspirin, paracetamol, antacids, laxatives etc.) for minor conditions?

| Yes | In the past | Never |

Do you use recreational drugs?

| No—but my best friend has a big habit! | No—but I might if it was legal. Anyway, I don't inhale! | Never |

Are you exposed to chemicals, heavy metals, or copper or iron in the workplace?

| Regularly | Occasionally | Never |

Do you use chemical cleaning products in the home?

| Regularly | Occasionally | Use non-toxic alternatives |

Are you exposed to chemicals/solvents during leisure pursuits or hobbies?

| Regularly | Occasionally | Use non-toxic alternatives |

Have you had your house fumigated recently?

| In last 3 months | In last 3 years | Never |

Have you recently renovated or painted your house?

| Ongoing painting/renovation | In last 3 years | Never |

If renovating or painting are you using any of the following?

| Products which contain toxins (such as solvents) | Some non-toxic products | All non-toxic products |

Do you travel in rush hour traffic (without air conditioning)?

| Often | Occasionally | Never |

Do you live/work near a major road/flight path?

| Very close | Not too close | Far away |

Do you live/work near the source of any industrial pollution?

| Very close | Not too close | Far away |

How many hours per day do you spend in front of your computer monitor?
2–8 hours   No more than 2 hours   0 hours

If you use a computer monitor, do you . . . ?
Use all the protective   Use some protective   Use no protective
measures suggested in   measures   measures
Chapter 6

How often do you use a mobile phone?
Several times daily   Once or twice a week   Never

Do you carry an activated phone near your body?
On my hip   Away from my body   No

Do you have active electrical gadgets in your bedroom (clock-radio, electric blanket, waterbed etc.)?
Several   1–2   None

Do you have a fuse box near your bed (or on the other side of the wall)?
Very close   Quite close   Far away

Have you been exposed to X-rays in the last five years?
Regularly   Occasionally   Never

Do you fly often?
Frequently   Once a year   Never

Do you exercise?
Not if I can help it!   Occasionally   Regularly

Do you consider that you lead a stressful lifestyle?
Always   From time to time   No

Do you practise any forms of stress reduction (meditation, regular exercise, yoga, tai-chi etc.)?
No   Occasionally   Regularly

How would you rate your overall general physical health?

| Always/frequently below par | OK I guess | Feel on top of the world! |

Do you consider yourself to be overweight?

| Considerably | A little | No |

Do you consider yourself to be underweight?

| Considerably | A little | No |

How would you rate your overall general mental health?

| Depression/insomnia | Irritable, nervous | Stable |

Do you get 6–8 hours of unbroken sleep at night?

| Almost never | Some nights | Almost every night |

Do you take a comprehensive multivitamin/mineral nutritional supplement?

| Never | From time to time | Every day without fail |

Do you take single supplements (e.g. iron, calcium, zinc, folic acid) on their own?

| Every day | Occasionally | Never/only with a multivit/mineral |

Your total score?

The closer your score to 168, the better your pregnancy is likely to be. Aim to improve your score as quickly as you can!

APPENDIX 6

Herbs to avoid during pregnancy

All medication, even natural medicine such as herbs, is to be treated with caution during pregnancy, especially in the first three months. There are, however, occasions when those herbs which have a long tradition of safe use can be very helpful. This is a comprehensive list of herbs which could be problematic in pregnancy, and has been taken from many different sources. Some of these herbs are avoided traditionally, some are contra-indicated because of scientific findings. We have divided them into three categories.

In *Category 1* we have listed those herbs which are known teratogens (that is, which can cause foetal abnormalities) and those herbs which are highly toxic. Sometimes these toxic herbs can be used medicinally in small doses in the adult (by a qualified herbalist) but not during pregnancy, as the foetus is much more vulnerable than you are. These herbs must definitely be avoided.

In *Category 2* we have listed those herbs where there is documented evidence of some adverse effects in pregnancy. In many cases this is only true of large doses, and a herbalist might possibly use some of these herbs under certain conditions, where the problematic actions of the herb were clearly understood. These herbs should be avoided except when professionally prescribed and supervised.

In *Category 3* we have listed those herbs for which there is little concrete evidence of problems, though some anecdotal evidence or concern. In many cases the actions of these herbs (usually beneficial) are perceived to pose a possible threat even though there is a considerable history of safe traditional use.

You will find we have included some of these herbs in our advice on remedies for various ailments, though always with a reminder to use with caution (in low doses, not for extended periods, and sometimes only under certain conditions).

Remember that, although caution is necessary, many of these herbs have been used for centuries to alleviate problems in pregnancy, and be assured that, taken as we suggest, there is no threat to your pregnancy or your child.

Category 1: Herbs to avoid

KNOWN TERATOGENIC PLANTS	HIGHLY TOXIC HERBS
Datura (Johnson Weed)	Aconitum
Ferula	Belladonna
Gelsemium	Bryonia
Nicotiana (Tobacco)	Conium
Prunus species	Convallaria (Lily of the Valley)
Senecia	Digitalis
Sorghum	Ephedra (Ma Huang)
Trachymene	Germander
	Lupinus
	Oleander
	Phytolacca (Poke Root)
	Poison Ivy
	Pteridium (Bracken Fern)
	Sanguinaria
	Solanum (Bittersweet)
	Veratrum (American Hellebore)

Category 2: Herbs contra-indicated, with documented risk

Adhatoda vasica—contra-indicated in pregnancy except at birth (an abortifacient, especially as a douche)

Alfalfa (Lucerne)—seeds have haemolytic activity

Aloes—anthraquinone content, cathartic, reputed abortifacient (avoid high doses)

American Mandrake (Podophyllum)—teratogenic especially from weeks 23–29

Ammi Visnaga

Andrographis paniculata

Angelica archangelica—avoid high doses

Arnica montana—vasodilator

Baical Skullcap (Scutellaria baicalensis)—very high doses found to have teratogenic effects, avoid in early pregnancy

Barberry (Berberis species)—berberine content; avoid high doses

Blue Cohosh (Caulophyllum thalictroides)—except during labour to assist birth, oxytocic

Boerhaesca diffusa—teratogenic in rats

Boldo (Peumus boldo)

Broom (Sarothamnus scopamus)—oxytocic

Buckthorn (Rhamnus frangula)—laxative, avoid high doses or non-standard preparations

Bugleweed, Gypsywort (Lycopus species)

Cascara (Rhamnus purshiana)—laxative, avoid high doses; also avoid during lactation

Celery (Apium graveolens)—Apiol, volatile oil content

Corydalis ambigua

Dan Shen (Salvia miltiorrhiza)

Dong Quai (Angelica sinensis)—contra-indicated in first trimester, tendency to spontaneous abortion, vasodilator

Embelia Ribes

Feverfew (Tanacetum parthenium)—volatile oil, avoid doses greater than 500 mg per day

Fumitory (Fumaria officianalis)—also avoid during lactation

Ginseng (Eleutherococcus)—has hormonally active constituents, though some studies show high degree of safety, even benefit, and adverse studies may have been in error

Ginseng (Panax)—has hormonally active constituents, affects hypothalamus/pituitary

Golden Seal (Hydrastis canadensis)—berberine content; mucosa and uterine stimulant, may age placenta, possibly increase blood pressure, oxytocic (in high doses)

Greater Celandine (Chelidonium majus)—avoid high doses (greater than 1000 mg per day)
Horsechestnut (Aesculus hippocastanum)—vasodilatory effects (in high doses)
Ipecac (Cephaelis ipecacuanha)—homoeopathic use in vomiting permitted
Juniper (Juniperus communis)—volatile oil, vasodilator (in high doses)
Kava (Piper Methysticum)
Lobelia (Lobelia inflata)—toxic at high doses
Lomatium (Lomatium dissectum)
Mistletoe (Viscum album)—except in last 6 weeks to assist birth, vasoconstricting
Mugwort (Artemesia species)—abortifacient, avoid high doses
Nutmeg (Myristica fragrans)—avoid high doses (greater than 1000 mg per day)
Parsley (Petroselinum crispum)—Apiol/volatile oil, culinary use safe
Pau D'arco—teratogenic/anthraquinone glycoside
Pennyroyal (Mentha pulegium)—abortifacient, volatile oil
Periwinkle (Vinca species)—vasoconstrictor (in high doses)
Poppy (Papaver somniferum)
Pulsatilla, Pasque Flower (Anemone pulsatilla)—affects menstrual cycle, irritant, uterine activity in vitro and in vivo, anti-dopaminergic; also avoid during lactation
Purslane (Portulacca)
Rauwolfia
Red Sage (Salvia officinalis vox Purpureum)
Rhubarb (Rheum palmatum)—laxative, avoid high doses, culinary use safe; also avoid during lactation
Rue (Ruta graveolens)—abortifacient, volatile oil
Sage (Salvia officinalis)—thujone containing varieties
Schisandra Chinensis—except in last 6 weeks to assist birth
Senna (Cassia species)—laxative, to be used in pregnancy and lactation only after medical advice
Snake Root, Birthwort (Aristolochia species)
Squill (Urginea species)
Sweet Flag (Acorus calamus)—may interfere with prostaglandins
Tansy (Tanacetum vulgare)—volatile oils, vasodilating, abortifacient
Thuja (Thuja occidentalis and species)—volatile oils

Wormwood (Artemesia absinthium and species)—vermifuge, vasodilator, abortifacient in doses greater than 500 mg per day or equivalent

Yarrow (Achillea millefolium)—thujone containing varieties; reputed abortifacient (avoid high doses)

Category 3: Herbs to use with caution

Agave—has hormonally active constituents
Apricot—cyanide toxicity
Asafotehda—reputed abortifacient and affects menstrual cycle
Astragalus—possibly teratogenic, though probably not the root commonly used in herbal medicine
Autumn Crocus—uterine vasodilator
Avens—reputed to affect menstrual cycle
Black Cohosh—oestrogen receptor binding in vitro, uterine vasodilator; not long-term use, only in last 6 weeks; also avoid during lactation
Bladderwrack, Kelp (Fucus)—thyroid activity, possible heavy metal contamination; also avoid during lactation
Blood Root—vasodilator
Blue Flag—irritant, cathartic
Bogbean—irritant, purgative
Boneset—cytotoxic constituents
Borage—pyrrolizidine alkaloids
Buchu—volatile oils (avoid greater than 3 g per day)
Burdock—uterine stimulant
Calendula—uterine action in vitro
Cat's Claw
Cayenne (Capsicum)
Chamomile (German)—reputed to affect menstrual cycle, uterine stimulant with excessive use
Chamomile (Roman)—reputed abortifacient and to affect menstrual cycle with excessive use
Chaparral—uterine activity, possibly hepatotoxic, haemolytic potential
Chastetree—hormonal action, with safe traditional use to promote progesterone
Chinchona
Cinnamon—culinary use safe

Citrus Seed
Cocoa—caffeine
Cola—caffeine
Coltsfoot—pyrrolizidine alkaloids
Comfrey—pyrrolizidine alkaloids, external use only
Cornsilk—uterine stimulant in vitro, questionable
Cotton Root
Culvers Root (Leptandra)—cathartic, laxative; also avoid during lactation
Damiana—cyanogenic glycosides, risk of cyanide toxicity in high doses, vasodilatory
Devils Claw—oxytocic
Elecampane—questionable; also avoid during lactation
Eucalyptus—oil to be avoided internally
Euphorbia—smooth muscle activity in vitro
False Hellebore
False Unicorn Root—uterine vasodilator, traditional use to prevent miscarriage
Fenugreek—oxytocic, uterine stimulant in vitro
Feverfew—volatile oils, reputed abortifacient (avoid high doses)
Gentian—highly bitter, possibly oxytocic
Ginger—blood-thinner; avoid doses more than 2000 mg, excellent for morning sickness, culinary and tea use safe
Ginkgo biloba—unpredictable effect on vasculature, but traditionally very safe
Gotu Kola (Hydrocotyl)—abortifacient, reputed to affect menstrual cycle
Ground Ivy—irritant oil
Guaicum—unpredictable vasodilation
Hawthorn—uterine activity in vivo and in vitro
Holy Thistle
Hops—uterine activity in vitro, oestrogenic activity, not in first trimester or for regular use
Horehound (Black)—reputed to affect menstrual cycle, however used traditionally for nausea in first trimester
Horehound (White)—reputed abortifacient, mildly hypertensive, reported to affect menstrual cycle
Horseradish—irritant oil; avoid high doses
Horsetail

Hyssop
Jamaican Dogwood—uterine activity in vivo and in vitro
Lad's Hore (Artemesia ubrotanum)
Life Root (Senecio species)—pyrrolizidine alkaloids
Liquorice—oestrogenic activity, mineralocorticoid activity, reputed abortifacient, can contribute to raised blood pressure
Male Fern
Mate—caffeine
Meadowsweet—possible uterine activity in vitro, salicylate content
Motherwort—uterine activity in vitro, oxytocic, affects menstrual cycle
Myrrh—affects menstrual cycle
Nettle—reputed to discourage implantation (in high doses only); affects menstrual cycle; very safe in lower doses (e.g. as a tea), with long-term traditional use as a pregnancy tonic
Papaya—in large doses
Passionflower—alkaloids (harmaline, harmine) uterine stimulant
Peach Tree—cyanogenic constituents (amygdalin)
Peruvian Bark
Plantain—uterine activity in vitro, laxative
Pleurisy Root—uterine vasodilator
Poplar—conflicting reports, salicylate content
Prickly Ash—coumarin content, alkaloids
Quassia
Queens Delight—irritant
Queens Root (Stillingia)—vasodilator
Raspberry—possible uterine activity, caution in first trimester; recommended in second and third trimesters
Red Clover—oestrogenic activity
Rosemary—volatile oil
Sassafras—oil is abortifacient, 'safrole' is hepatotoxic
Shepherds Purse—reputed abortifacient, oxytocin synergist, but traditionally used to prevent bleeding/miscarriage
Skullcap—to eliminate afterbirth and promote menstruation, potential hepatotoxicity
Skunk Cabbage—reputed to affect menstrual cycle
Southernwood
Squaw Vine—possible uterine activity, caution in first trimester; recommended in second and third trimesters
St John's Wort—slight uterine activity

St Mary's Thistle—may cause problems in pregnancy

Thyme—volatile oils, culinary use safe

Uva Ursi—large doses oxytocic, uterine vasoconstrictor if used for more than 3–4 days

Vervain—abortifacient, oxytocic

Wahoo—vasodilator

Wild Carrot—oestrogenic, irritant, vasodilator

Wild Cherry—cyanogenic

Wild Indigo—theoretically teratogenic

Willow—conflicting reports, salicylates

Withania—conflicting reports, long history of safe traditional use as pregnancy tonic

Yellow dock—anthraquinones, non-standardised preparations to be avoided, glycetract preferable

APPENDIX 7

Essential oils to avoid during pregnancy

To be avoided

Ajowan
Angelica Root
Aniseed
Basil
Birch
Bitter Almond
Boldo
Buchu
Bulgar Rose
Camphor
Cedarwood species (Virginian and Atlas)
Cinnamon
Clary Sage
Clove
Cornmint
Fennel
Horseradish
Hyssop
Jasmine
Lavender Cotton*
*Lavendula stoechas**

Mugwort
Mustard
Myrrh
Oregano
Parsley seed
Pennyroyal
Pimenta racemosa
Plecanthrus
Rose (in first trimester)
Sage
Savin
Savory
Star Aniseed
Sweet Marjoram
Tansy
Tarragon
Thuja
Thyme
Wintergreen
Wormseed
Wormwood

To be used with caution
Chamomile—only use small amounts in first and second trimester
Cypress
Geranium—only use small amounts
Juniper
Peppermint
Rose—only use in last two trimesters; safe to use in last three weeks
Rosemary
Sandalwood—very slight risk

---

* *Lavendula spika* (Spike Lavender) and *L. officinalis*, *L. augustifolia* and *L. intermedia* are safe, but use in small amount only in the first trimester.

APPENDIX 8

Acupressure points to avoid during pregnancy

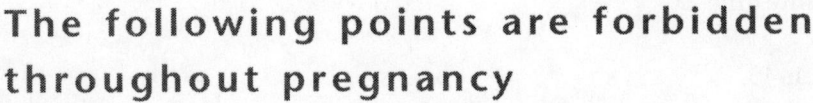

The following points are forbidden throughout pregnancy

Colon 4
Stomach 12
Spleen 1, 6, 9 and 15 (but Spleen 6 may be used during childbirth)
Bladder 60 and 67 (but Bladder 67 is used as labour approaches to reposition a foetus that is transverse or breech)
Governing Vessel 1
Liver 3
It is also preferable to avoid any points on the abdomen

The following points are forbidden in pregnancy during the indicated months

1st month
Conception Vessel 2
Gall Bladder 2
Colon 4
Small Intestine 1

2nd month
Gall Bladder 3

3rd month
Pericardium 8
Triple Heater 4

4th month
Triple Heater 10
Pericardium 6*
Gall Bladder 9

5th month
Stomach 4
Spleen 4, 8 and 9

6th month
Small Intestine 10
Lung 7
Stomach 45
All Triple Heater points to be used with caution

7th month
Lung 2

8th month
Colon 2 and 10

9th month
Kidney 1, 2, and 7
Stomach 36*

---

* Pericardium 6 and Stomach 36 are used in the first trimester for nausea.

APPENDIX 9

Tips for travellers

The following is summarised from an article in the monthly medical newsletter *What Doctors Don't Tell You* (see Contacts and Resources).

Where the real risks are

The risk of *malaria* is high if you're travelling to Africa, though in South America and Asia the only significant risk is if you're in a rural area after dark. You are at little risk of *typhoid* in industrialised countries, though at quite high risk in countries with primitive sanitation, especially developing countries in Africa, Asia and South America. *Yellow fever* is a risk in tropical areas of South America and Africa. The risk of *cholera* infection is high in countries with poor sanitation, especially in Africa and the Middle East, Asia and South America. However, the vaccine is only recommended if you're travelling to these areas across remote (overland) borders. You may be at risk of *polio* in developing countries in Africa, Asia, the Middle East and Eastern Europe. You could risk *rabies* in South and Central America, the Indian subcontinent, Asia and Africa, though the pre-trip vaccination is usually only recommended for those who are putting themselves at high risk through their chosen activity (such as bush treks). *Meningitis* is common in Asia and Africa, though there are different strains, not all covered by the vaccine. Immunisation is required by Saudi Arabia for Muslims on the annual holy pilgrimage. *Hepatitis A and B* are only slight risks in industrialised countries (except if you indulge in unsafe sex or sharing of needles). Developing countries, or those where sanitation is poor, may pose more of a risk.

Homoeopathic and natural remedies

Homoeopathic nosodes are like a homoeopathic vaccine. Their advantage over regular vaccines is that they give only the smallest nudge to your immune system, prompting it to produce its own protection. Unlike regular vaccines, which kick start your immunity by introducing to your system a mild dose of the disease you wish to avoid, nosodes introduce only the tiniest trace of the disease, or in some cases avoid the disease altogether, relying instead on creating an energy pattern. Nosodes work very well, and studies show their use is associated with greatly reduced incidences of disease, with no side effects.

The following information dealing with the use of homoeopathic nosodes to ward off disease is also extracted from the monthly medical newsletter *What Doctors Don't Tell You* and was acquired by the newsletter from Helios Pharmacy in the UK.

DISEASE	NOSODE 'VACCINE'
Cholera	1 dose of *Camphor 30* at bedtime, and another on rising, two weeks before departure
Hepatitis	1 dose of *Chelidonium 30*, eight days before departure and another dose every week of your stay
Polio	1 dose of *Lathyns Satirus 30*, seven days before departure
Yellow Fever	1 dose of *Arsenicum Album 30*, five days before departure
Typhoid	1 dose of *Manganum 30*, three days before departure
Malaria	1 dose of *Natrum Mur 30*, six days before departure and another dose every week of your stay
Meningitis	1 dose of *Belladonna 30* weekly, if this becomes epidemic during your stay
Cuts or puncture wounds	1 dose of *Ledum 30*

APPENDIX 10

Drinking water

What are the alternatives to tap water?

Distilled water
Distilling removes bacteria, viruses, chemicals, minerals and pollutants. It is not effective for chemicals whose boiling point is higher than water and volatile substances such as chlorine by-products. Note, however, that *all* minerals, not just the toxic variety, have been removed and that trace mineral supplementation may be necessary.

Boiled water
Boiling will destroy a broad range of bacteria and micro-organisms. If water is boiled for 10 minutes approximately 95 per cent of the organic compounds will be removed, however this method does not remove heavy metals or toxic chemicals and will concentrate the remaining substances. It is therefore important to purify water even if you boil it.

Mineral water
The mineral content depends on where the source is. Avoid mineral waters high in sodium and keep sulphates, chlorides, nitrates and fluorides low. If you are drinking a lot of mineral water containing minerals (especially sodium) that you do not lack, there is a danger of ingesting excessive levels.

Spring water

Spring waters are naturally occurring and their composition depends on the geography of the source. They undergo general sediment filtration, and must pass general ion analysis and testing for bacterial and other contamination. These are the waters found in offices and clinic waiting rooms and can be supplied to your home at a significant cost.

Purified water

The price of purified water depends on the filter efficiency and the volume of water required.

Activated carbon Provides very effective removal of organic and inorganic contaminants, asbestos and chlorine. Improves taste, colour and odour. Does not remove bacteria or viruses unless specifically stated. Ensure that you know the capacity of the filter and the approximate amount of water you put through each week. It is essential that the cartridge be replaced regularly before it has expired, *not* after, as it can then begin to dump the removed contaminants back into the water and become a breeding ground for bacteria. Keep filter jugs in the fridge to prevent bacterial overgrowth and discard first jugful if left for more than 48 hours without use. Recent developments in carbon filtration technology have greatly increased efficiency (see comparison table below).

Ion exchange This effectively removes nitrates, fluoride, sulfates, calcium, magnesium, cadmium, barium, lead and some forms of radium. It does not remove dirt, rust, sediment, pesticides, microorganisms or chlorine by-products. Ideally a carbon filter should be used in conjunction with this to make it an efficient broad spectrum filter. However, the ion-exchange component may become ineffective faster than the carbon, deeming it essential that the whole filter be replaced regularly to prevent dumping of removed heavy metals back into the water.

Reverse osmosis The most effective but often slow way of filtering impurities from the water. It results in some water wastage and the removal of beneficial as well as unwanted minerals. Except for distillation, reverse osmosis is the only process which is effective in removing sediment and dissolved solids, toxic metals, radioactive elements, pesticides and herbicides. Sediment and carbon filter needs replacing every 4 to 12 months, depending on the manufacturer, and membranes every 2 years.

Ceramic filters Usually contain a carbon shield. They are moderately effective filters, but being open to air makes them highly susceptible to algal growth. They must be scrubbed thoroughly inside and out regularly and not kept in dark positions. Glazed ceramic filters have similar performances and are much less prone to algal growth.

(The major reviews in *Choice* of water purifiers (May 1989) and filter jugs (Feb and Sept 1993) found that most units lived up to the claims.)

Comparative effectiveness of filters in removing a spectrum of contaminants

	Jug #	Activated carbon 1	Activated carbon 2	Reverse osmosis
Volatile organic chemicals	†	86–99%	98%+	†
Phenols	†	85–98%	98%+	†
Chlorine	85%	100%	100%	†
Chlorine by-products	†	96%	99%	†
Herbicides & pesticides	70%	99%	98%+	†
Lead	80%	81–96%	91%+	98.2%
Iron	†	81%	†	†
Cadmium	†	99%	†	99.4%
Arsenic	†	96%	†	99.0%
Copper	95%	98%	99%+	99.9%
Mercury	†	99%	90%+	96.0%
Aluminium	67%	96%*	50–99%*	†
Nitrates	†	98%	>85%	95.5%
Fluoride	†	†	44%	95.5%
Bacteria, Giardia, Cryptosporidium	No	No	Yes	Yes

\# Results for jug at 27 litres only. These figures are assumed to be maximal and do not include 'drop-off' due to ageing cartridge. There seems to be no data available regarding effectiveness of removal of more complex chemicals such as organic chemicals. Considering the minimal long-term price difference between this and the more effective filters, the latter are recommended. Some water filter jugs now use a more efficient carbon system with fractal polymers, which they

state removes three times more contaminants across the board than their competitors.
☦ Percentages not available.
* Aluminium tests—50% removal at water flow of 3.5 litres per minute. Rates vary according to flow and aluminium level. American results of 96% and 99% refer to removal of spiked aluminium.

N.B. For parasites to be removed the filter must be a 'block', not a 'loose' packed cylinder, and be 1 micron or less.

This appendix is extracted from an analysis that was prepared by Melanie Koeman for Natural Fertility Management.

APPENDIX 11

Preconception health care

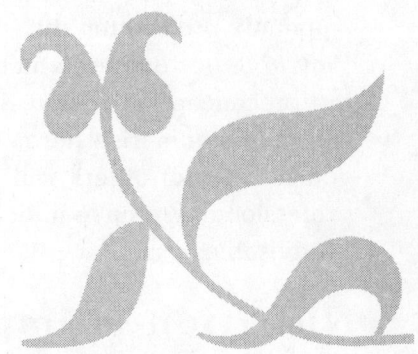

Your better pregnancy can start before you fall pregnant!

If your pregnancy isn't a reality yet, then you've got the perfect opportunity to practice preconception health care which is the very best foundation for a better pregnancy and a better baby. It's often much simpler to implement the appropriate changes, which include an improved diet, a healthier lifestyle and a cleaner environment, in those months before you actually conceive. These measures can also be more effective if implemented fully then, because they can involve both of you equally. You can be in this quest for a better pregnancy and a better baby together. To do that you and your partner should give yourselves a minimum period of four months before you make any attempt to conceive. But you must use that time productively. Really use those months to 'clean up your act'. A healthy egg and healthy sperm will improve your chances of having a really healthy pregnancy and healthy baby, and those healthy cells don't just appear overnight!

The four months immediately preceding conception are when the greatest benefits can be obtained because ova are susceptible to damage for about 100 days before ovulation, and sperm formation can take up to 116 days. If both you and your partner are non-toxic, free from infection and allergy, eating a highly nutritious diet and living a healthy lifestyle in a pollution-free environment during the whole of that critical four-month period, then the health of your pregnancy and baby will benefit enormously.

All of our recommendations for a better pregnancy apply equally before conception, so please read the whole book carefully. However, there are some specific recommendations which apply only to the preconception period, or conditions which can be treated a little differently during that time, and we'll talk about those issues in this Appendix. But better still, you can buy our earlier book, *The Natural Way to Better Babies*, which is a comprehensive step-by-step guide to the preconception period. It covers in detail all the issues which we can only summarise here. You can address many of those issues by yourselves, but others will be more effectively managed by a health professional. We have indicated when the help of a health practitioner is advisable.

Nutrition is important

What you eat (and digest and absorb) is of primary importance. Every aspect of reproduction, from the formation of sperm and the maturation of the egg, right through to the production of adequate amounts of high quality breast milk, is dependent on a sufficient supply of all the nutrients, which include vitamins, minerals and essential amino and fatty acids.

All the eggs a woman will need during her lifetime are present when she is born. Once she reaches sexual maturity, an egg ripens every month in anticipation of fertilisation. But even though that egg developed long ago, it is actually susceptible to harmful effects for about three months before ovulation takes place. As well, the development of a mature egg depends on hormonal stimulation, and the formation of these hormones depends on an adequate supply of numerous nutritional factors.

Unlike the ova, sperm are not present at the time of a man's birth. After the man reaches puberty they are manufactured in his testes. The formation of sperm can take up to four months and adequate numbers of really healthy sperm can only be achieved when all the essential nutrients are present in plentiful supply and when there is a complete absence of toxic substances.

A really nutritious diet is one of the most important factors in your preconception health care program and is essentially the same as the diet we recommend during pregnancy. You should pay particular attention to the balance of carbohydrate, protein and oil and acid/alkali balance (as acidity kills sperm). See Chapter 3 for more on all aspects of diet. Comprehensive nutritional supplementation for both of you is just as important before conception as it is during pregnancy, although some of the dosages may be a little different, and we have included guidelines for appropriate supplementation in the preconception period in the table below. See Chapter 4 for more on all aspects of supplementation.

Supplementation for both prospective parents

VITAMIN	DAILY DOSAGE
Vitamin A	10,000 IU, or beta-carotene 6 mg (or mixed carotenes if available)
Vitamin E	500 IU
Vitamin D	200 IU
Vitamin B complex	B1, B2, B3, B5—up to 50 mg each B12—400 mcg B6—up to 250 mg Biotin—200 mcg Choline, inositol, PABA—25 mg
Folic acid	500–1000 mcg (0.5–1.0 mg) (1 mg daily if you have had a previous miscarriage, if there is a history of neural tube defects in your family, or if you are over 40 years of age)
Vitamin C & Bioflavonoids	Vitamin C—2000–3000 mg (2–3 g) (upper levels if you are suffering from infection or toxicity) Bioflavonoids—300 mg
Calcium	800 mg daily (twice the amount of magnesium)
Magnesium	400 mg daily (half the amount of calcium)
Potassium	15 mg daily or as potassium chloride cell salt
Iron	15 mg daily with ferrum phos. cell salt (supplement should be organic and chelated, but should only be taken if need is proven)
Manganese	10 mg
Zinc	20–60 mg (depending on result of Zinc Taste Test. Take separately on an empty stomach, last thing at night)

Chromium	100–200 mcg daily (upper levels for those with sugar cravings)
Selenium	100–200 mcg (upper levels for those exposed to heavy pollution—you will need a prescription in Australia)
Iodine	75 mcg daily (or as kelp—150 mg daily)
Evening primrose oil	500–1000 mg three times daily
Max EPA (deep-sea fish oil)	500–1000 mg three times daily, especially if your diet contains little deep-sea fish
Acidophilus & Bifidus	½–1 teaspoonful of each, once or twice daily (upper level for those with candida problems)
Garlic	2000–5000 mg (upper levels for those exposed to toxins)
Silica	20 mg
Copper	1–2 mg (only if zinc status is adequate)
Hydrochloric acid & digestive enzymes	for those with digestive problems (take as directed on packaging labels)

Appropriate weight before you conceive

Before conception it is important that both of you have a weight which falls within the normal range, because excess weight is a significant contributing factor to infertility, particularly for the female. Studies have shown that even quite modest weight losses can reverse infertility without resort to stricter measures.

If all aspects of your preconception health care are attended to faithfully, then appropriate weight loss (or gain in some instances) will inevitably occur. But it's important to know what is your 'normal' weight range.

You can calculate whether your weight is within the normal range very simply.

$$\text{Quetelet (Q) index} = \frac{\text{Weight in kilograms}}{(\text{Height in metres})^2}$$

For example, if someone weighs 65 kilograms and is 167 cm tall (you guessed it—that's Janette), the calculation looks like this:

$$\frac{\text{Q index} = 65}{1.67 \times 1.67} = \frac{65}{2.8} = 23.2$$

Janette's weight is within the normal range (20 to 25). If your Q index is less than 20, you need to gain weight; if it's greater than 25, you need to lose weight.

Lifestyle factors

Avoid cigarettes, alcohol, caffeine, other drugs
The recommendations for a better pregnancy apply equally to the time before conception, and both of you should completely avoid cigarettes, alcohol, caffeine and other drugs in that important four-month period. All of these factors can adversely affect the health of egg and sperm, and can also seriously compromise your nutritional status, which you're working hard to optimise.

Some drugs affect cervical mucus
Many commonly used pharmaceutical preparations may have possible adverse effects on cervical mucus as well, which is an important factor to be aware of if you haven't yet conceived. The cervical mucus must be fertile (thin and watery) at the time of ovulation, and of a general consistency which will allow the sperm to penetrate it easily. Any drying or thickening of the mucus, which can be caused by anti-histamines or compounds such as pseudoephedrine, could prevent conception from occurring. These substances are found in many common cold and cough remedies which dry up nasal congestion. On the other hand, expectorant cough mixtures which contain potassium iodide or guaphenesin could increase or thin mucus.

Environmental factors

Test for heavy metal burden
Toxic or heavy metals should be avoided before conception, and you'll find a comprehensive list of sources of contamination in Chapter 6. Fortunately, the preconception period presents an ideal opportunity to

rid your body thoroughly of any burden of these substances.

A hair trace mineral analysis is recommended for both of you. This is a simple test which involves sending a tablespoonful of the most recent growth of your hair (preferably untreated with colour or bleach) to a laboratory for analysis (see Contacts and Resources for further information). This test will also give valuable information about levels of essential trace minerals and may indicate malabsorption, thyroid and adrenal stress. If the test reveals that either of you has a heavy burden of any of the toxic metals, dietary measures and non-toxic medicines can be used to reduce this load, and the source of the this contamination needs to be traced and removed if possible.

The foods which can help reduce toxic levels include garlic, onions, legumes (lentils, chickpeas and all the dried beans), and apples stewed with their pips. Supplementation with antagonistic minerals can expedite the detoxification process. This means that you take extra calcium and zinc to reduce high levels of lead; zinc to remove cadmium; selenium to remove mercury; and magnesium and silica to get rid of aluminium. The anti-oxidants vitamin C, selenium and zinc can help to remove all toxic metals and need to be taken at our maximum recommended dosage. Oral or intravenous chelation might be necessary to reduce a very high toxic load (see Contacts and Resources for further information). Both of you must have levels within the normal range for a minimum period of four months before you make any attempt to conceive.

Avoid chemicals and radiation

Chemicals in the home, the garden and the workplace should be avoided as far as possible by both of you in the preconception period. Radiation (both ionising and non-ionising) should also be avoided. It is well recognised that ionising radiation (X-rays) must be avoided during pregnancy, but few doctors think to ask you if you might be contemplating getting pregnant in the near future.

Dr Judy Ford, head of the Genetics Department at Flinders University in Adelaide, has clearly shown that there is an increased risk of miscarriage if either partner has undergone an X-ray to abdominal or pelvic region in the five years preceding the conception. There will be some instances in which diagnostic X-rays are absolutely necessary, but many more instances in which they are not. If an X-ray becomes necessary during that critical four-month period, then your full preconception health care program and four-month lead-up time should be begun all over again.

Electro-magnetic radiation should also be avoided as far as possible by both prospective parents. In Chapter 6 we outlined the importance of limiting your exposure to radiation from computer monitors and other devices during pregnancy, so read that chapter and put those same protective measures in place before conception.

Detoxification

Unfortunately, avoiding harmful lifestyle and environmental factors isn't enough. Detoxification for both partners is a very important part of preconception health care. If detox is carried out before conception, you will be able to employ a more rigorous approach than is possible during your pregnancy. Depending on the levels of toxicity and past exposure, you may need the help of a practitioner, but all the self-help methods discussed in Chapter 7 will be helpful.

During any rigorous detoxification program, there will be a release of toxins into the body, which may increase symptoms temporarily. Therefore, *the best possible approach is to undertake and complete the bulk of the detox process a minimum period of four months before a conception is attempted*, to avoid the sperm and egg being contaminated.

There are many herbs which can be used to stimulate detoxification through the liver, kidneys, bowel, blood, lymph, lungs, skin and immune system. Although these are very safe when administered by a medical herbalist, *it is better not to self-prescribe*. Some of the most effective herbs may not be appropriate, or even safe, during pregnancy, so you need to be sure you haven't conceived yet, or stick to those herbs which are gentle enough not to harm your baby.

As well, the following detox measures should only be used before conception, so if you are in any doubt at all about whether you have conceived, stick to the gentle measures we recommend during pregnancy.

Colonic irrigation is a particular form of enema, where water under pressure penetrates deeply into the colon, cleansing from rectum to caecum. Toxins and putrefactive matter are loosened and eliminated, and acidophilus and other lactobacilli are then administered to re-colonise the gut. Colonics and conventional enemas must be carried out by trained practitioners, and can be helpful in eliminating parasites, which can also be treated with herbal medicine.

Fasting is also best supervised by a health professional—although, before conception, a fast for one day per week, where only freshly purified water and/or vegetable juices are taken, is quite safe. Prolonged fasting can affect hormone levels, and is definitely not recommended. Colonics or enemas, used in conjunction with a fast, can ensure that old food is eliminated when the gut is inactive.

Chelation therapy is a process whereby agents are introduced into the body via intravenous drip or oral administration, and bind to heavy metals and remove them. Chemical agents are often combined with vitamin C and other helpful nutrients, and there are homoeopathic versions of these remedies which can be effective for the less severe levels of contamination. See Contacts and Resources for further information.

Treating allergies, candida and genito-urinary infections

Allergic conditions should be detected and treated (in both of you) before conception occurs. Untreated allergies or sensitivities can adversely affect your health and nutritional status because they impair your body's ability to absorb nutrients. What's more, if you are both allergic, then you have about a 60 per cent chance of having an allergic child.

The simple methods of detecting allergenic compounds, such as the pulse test, muscle testing and the food diary (which we've outlined in Chapter 8) are applicable in the preconception period. These tests may allow you to detect the offenders quite easily yourself, and should be carried out before you or your health practitioner embark on more sophisticated detective work.

Provocation tests (which involve introducing a sample of the suspected substance and observing your reaction) can detect airborne or contact allergens, although this type of testing is not recommended during pregnancy.

An elimination diet (which involves complete avoidance of all but low-reactive foods), when followed faithfully, should bring about an improvement in allergic symptoms. To identify offending foods, the likely suspects are re-introduced, one at a time, and your reaction is observed each time. However, this type of diet should not be considered as treatment, nor should it be followed once you are pregnant.

Candida—a condition which we describe in Chapter 8—is best treated before conception, when it will be much easier to get it under control. It's also possible, at this time, to use more aggressive treatments, which will speed up the process.

For a local (vaginal) infestation, douching can be most effective, but this can only be carried out if there is no chance of pregnancy. You can both douche and dunk with the same (well, not actually the very 'same') tea tree and vinegar mixture we describe in Chapter 8. A useful herbal mixture which can also be used before conception is equal parts of: *Golden Seal* (anti-bacterial), *Calendula* (anti-bacterial and anti-fungal), *Uva Ursi* (disinfectant) and *Witch Hazel* (astringent and anti-viral). This can be used instead of, or with, the tea tree/vinegar douche.

Aloe Vera gel can be very effective, especially if a few herbs or essential oil of *marjoram* (an anti-fungal) are added. A clove of *garlic* (unchipped and wrapped in gauze) can be inserted into the vagina. Leave a 'tail' on the gauze so you can pull it out. Don't use vinegar if you have any cuts or abrasions.

If the infection is external rather than internal, you can sit in a basin or shallow bath and 'swish' the mixture up into the vagina, or soak a tampon in the mixture and insert it, instead of using a douche. *Never* leave a tampon in place for longer than eight hours, as it could lead to toxic shock syndrome, and *never* use these treatments inside the vagina if you are, or could be, pregnant.

Useful herbs for internal treatment (before conception) only are *Golden Seal*, *Pau D'Arco* and *Calendula* (to kill the yeast), *Vervain* and *Yarrow* (to stabilise blood sugar levels) and *Siberian Ginseng* and *Cat's Claw* (to boost the immune system).

Genito-urinary infections (GUIs) are a common cause of infertility, miscarriage and other reproductive problems, including ill-health in the new-born. They are frequently undiagnosed because they may cause few (if any) symptoms. Thorough screening for a comprehensive range of bacterial infections, ureaplasma and mycoplasma, should be carried out through a urine test (for chlamydia), a colposcopy or high cervical swab for women (vaginal swabs are not as informative), and a urethral smear for men. A blood test can determine the presence of HIV, Hepatitis B and C or syphilis if the personal history suggests there is a risk. Treatment of GUIs will need help from a professional and is most easily carried out before conception, as the treatments that can be used at that time will be most effective. Antibiotic therapy is often the only option since some of these infections are very stubborn and this should be completed well before conception. It is important that acidophilus and bifidus lactobacilli are given concurrently and afterwards, and that naturopathic immune support is also implemented. Herbs can be used to great effect for this purpose. Try *Echinacea*, *Astragalus*, *Picrorrhiza*, *Siberian Ginseng*, *Cat's Claw* with specific anti-viral herbs *St John's Wort* and *Thuja*. Other guidelines for treatment can be found in Chapter 8.

Toxoplasmosis and cytomegalovirus (CMV) are also more easily and more effectively treated before conception. As well as the treatments outlined in Chapter 8, additional treatments can be used in the preconception period. The herbs we have found useful in eradicating toxoplasmosis before conception act to eliminate parasites and stimulate the immune system. Any of the following may be used: *Echinacea*, *Pau D'Arco*, *Astragalus*, *Golden Seal*, *Siberian Ginseng*, *Euphorbia*, *Picrorrhiza*, *Cat's Claw*, *Wormwood* or *Citrus Seed Extract*. You may also choose to use the homoeopathic nosode to help give protection if no immunity exists.

To treat CMV, anti-viral herbs such as *St John's Wort*, *Phylanthus*, *Picrorrhiza* and *Liquorice* can be added to the treatments outlined for use during pregnancy. The homoeopathic nosode could also form part of preconception treatment, though it is *not* recommended during pregnancy, as with viral diseases there can be a 'trigger' effect from such a remedy. It can be used to treat an existing infection, or as a preventative measure to help give immunity.

If you have no immunity to *rubella*, alternatives to vaccination, if you prefer not to follow this path, are covered in Chapter 8. However, if you're not already pregnant, you can also use the homoeopathic nosode and the herbs we've mentioned for the treatment of CMV.

Avoid oral contraceptives and IUDs

Most women who have been taking the Pill just decide to stop taking it and get pregnant. We recommend that you stop taking oral contraceptives for at least six months before you want to conceive, and ideally for longer. This is because the Pill has an adverse effect on a very wide range of nutrients, including vitamins A, B1, B2, B6, folic acid, biotin, B12, C (and the bioflavonoids), E and K, and the minerals iron, calcium, magnesium, potassium, selenium, copper and zinc. The prostaglandins and blood lipids are also affected. These adverse effects may contribute to the greater incidence of birth defects and problem pregnancies experienced by mothers who conceive soon after taking the Pill.

IUDs are not considered a suitable alternative to the Pill since they irritate and inflame the uterus and incline it to infection. Spermicides are not recommended either—they may contain mercury and other toxic chemicals.

Natural Fertility Management

We recommend that you use Natural Fertility Management during the six (or more) months that precede conception. The observation and charting of cyclical cervical mucus changes and the basal or body-at-rest temperature, known as the sympto-thermal method, coupled with calculation of a woman's bio-rhythmic lunar cycle, are together known as Natural Fertility Management. This method can be used extremely effectively to pinpoint potentially fertile days. On these days if you are trying to avoid conception, you can use barrier methods of contraception or you may choose to abstain from sexual intercourse. Of course, this same method of charting and observation can also be used when you actually want to conceive. You can then time intercourse to avoid conceiving when eggs or sperm may be old and potentially defective, or too late in your cycle, which can predispose to miscarriage. You can also conceive consciously and thus welcome your child from the very earliest days of its life.

In carrying out the necessary charting and observations which form the basis of Natural Fertility Management it is also possible to obtain a very clear picture of your reproductive health. Essentially, you should be ovulating in all (or most) of your cycles, your cycles should be regular with a pre-ovulatory phase which is not more than 17 days long and a post-ovulatory phase which is not less than 12 days in length.

You should also be free from conditions like PMS, dysmenorrhoea, menorrhagia, endometriosis, fibroids or pelvic inflammatory disease. If your cycles are irregular, or if you are suffering from these or other conditions, it is not only possible, but highly desirable, with the use of natural medicine and other therapies, to correct imbalances and disease states which can lead to a less than successful pregnancy outcome. Our previous book, *The Natural Way to Better Babies*, enlarges on these aspects of preconception health care in detail.

Most women find it simple to observe and record the changes in their cervical mucus, basal temperature and other symptoms. They find it empowering and of great interest to know what is happening in their bodies and to be able to make decisions based on these observations. Another advantage for a woman who knows exactly when she is or is not fertile is that she can have prompt confirmation of her pregnancy. Once the basal temperature, which responds to progesterone levels, has been significantly elevated above its pre-ovulatory level for 18 days, and shows no sign of dropping, or indeed is still rising, a pregnancy is probable. Once the temperature has been elevated for 20 days, you can be fairly certain that you are pregnant.

An even more important advantage is that once you are familiar with the signs of fertility in your cycle, and know when it is necessary to avoid conception, this information can be used with great confidence to predict returning fertility after childbirth.

What's involved in NFM?

There are three observations that give you most of the important information about your fertility: cervical mucus, basal temperature and the lunar bio-rhythmic cycle.

In response to changing levels of oestrogen, the cervix produces different types of *cervical mucus* at different points in the menstrual cycle. This mucus has a role in preventing or achieving conception, and gives clear warning of the approach to ovulation. This indicator is critical for effective contraception and also for a successful conception, and it will also inform you when ovulation is over. This is the symptom which will also warn of returning fertility during breastfeeding.

The *basal temperature* (or body-at-rest temperature) will rise in response to progesterone. This is why you always feel so hot during pregnancy. Its use in fertility management is to confirm that ovulation has occurred (and that it is over, so you are infertile again). This is the symptom which will confirm whether a mucus change has actually resulted in an egg being released, and as such is very useful during breastfeeding when there can be several 'false alarms'.

The *lunar bio-rhythmic cycle*, which peaks at the same point in the lunar month that occurred at the time of your birth, seems to have an underlying effect on your fertility. Not only does it frequently synchronise with your menstrual cycle, which is also a lunar monthly rhythm, but it seems to boost fertility when this is the case. There is also much evidence that when the peak in this cycle falls separately from the mid-cycle ovulation, a spontaneous (or extra) ovulation is likely to be triggered by sexual stimulation. This may explain (and in our experience often does) the phenomenon of non-identical twins, especially where one twin appears to be much further developed than the other. These lunar peaks can be easily calculated from your birth data (date, place and preferably, exact time).

For more comprehensive information on Natural Fertility Management you should read *Natural Fertility* by Francesca Naish (Sally Milner Publishing) and *The Natural Way to Better Babies* by Francesca Naish and Janette Roberts (Random House). The latter also gives you complete details of all the preconception health care measures which we have only briefly outlined here.

Exercise, stress reduction and thinking positively

Establishing a regular program of aerobic and strengthening exercise before conception makes it much more likely that you will be able to continue to exercise throughout your pregnancy, and in doing so, reap all the benefits. If you also put in place some sort of stress reduction program and if you're already thinking positively about the implementation of the full preconception health care program and consequently about the eventual outcome of your pregnancy, you're well on the way to having a better pregnancy and a better baby too!

Some tests before you conceive

Also refer to Chapter 11, where many of these tests are discussed fully.

Tests which you can do for yourselves (both prospective parents):
- Zinc taste test (Chapters 4 and 11)
- Urine screen for heavy metals (Chapters 6 and 11)
- Hair trace mineral analysis (Contacts and Resources)
- Dental check-up

For the prospective mother only:
- Basal (body-at-rest) temperature
- Cervical mucus observations

Tests which your doctor or midwife can perform (both prospective parents):
- Blood pressure
- Urine-protein, sugar
- Full blood count (ESR, Rh factor, blood group) (Chapter 11)
- Toxoplasmosis (Chapters 8 and 11)
- Cytomegalovirus (CMV) (Chapters 8 and 11)
- Iron stores (serum ferritin) (Chapters 4 and 11)
- Thyroid/liver function
- Genito-urinary infections (Chapters 8 and 11)
- Sperm antibodies

For prospective mothers:
- Pap smear
- Ovulation status
- Rubella (Chapters 8 and 11)

For prospective fathers:
- Semen analysis

APPENDIX 12

How to prevent miscarriage

Many of the causes of birth defects and premature births (and indeed, infertility) are also reasons for miscarriage, and preconception health care (for *both* parents) can make a profound difference. In a recent study conducted by Foresight, the Association for the Promotion of Preconceptual Care, in England, of the 367 couples involved, 327 (i.e. 89 per cent) gave birth, and there were *no* miscarriages. At our clinic in Sydney (The Jocelyn Centre) we also have a great deal of success treating this problem, even with those women or couples who have had a history of repeated loss in pregnancy.

As the Foresight study shows, *most* cases of miscarriage are preventable, by ensuring that the foetus is viable, the environment in which it grows is healthy and that undue stress or trauma, of either physical or emotional origin, are avoided, especially during the first trimester. So—preconception health care, in place for a minimum of four months before conception, for both parents, is the best way to avoid miscarriage.

Here is a table to help you see what might have caused your miscarriage, and how to deal with it.

CAUSE	REMEDY
Incompetent cervix	See 'Incompetent cervix' in Chapter 13.
Rupture of membranes	See 'Premature rupture of membranes' in Chapter 13.

Placenta praevia	See 'Breakthrough Bleeding' in Chapter 13.
Abruptio placenta	See 'Breakthrough Bleeding' in Chapter 13.
Nutrient deficiency—leading to poor quality eggs and sperm, poor uterine tone, poor hormonal output etc.).	See Chapters 3 and 4. Remember the preconception period is even more important, and this applies to *both* parents (see Appendix 11).
Toxicity—through exposure to drugs (social and medical), radiation and electro-magnetic pollution, heavy metals and dust, chemicals (including solvents, glues, paints, fertilisers, industrial pollution, renovating materials, pesticides).	Preconception and pregnancy health care with respect to lifestyle, protection and detoxification. See Chapters 5, 6 and 7. Preconception health care applies to *both* parents (see Appendix 11).
Hormonal insufficiency—especially where there's been a history of PMS, short post-ovulatory phase, inadequate temperature rise (all of which indicate low levels of progesterone).	Preconception health care to balance hormones. Particular attention to *vitamin B6*, *Chastetree* and *Peony* herbs, both before and during pregnancy. A phenolic (homoeopathic) preparation of progesterone may help, as may a progesterone cream (as an emergency measure).
Uterine dysfunction—possibly due to poor tone or health, to anatomical abnormalities, or to fibroids if they are placed so as to interfere with implantation and growth.	Preconception health care to tonify uterus and treat fibroids. Particular attention to all nutrients, *True* and *False Unicorn Root*, *Peony*, *Blue Cohosh*, *Dong Quai*. The last two herbs only to be used with caution (and under professional supervision) in pregnancy.

Chromosomal abnormalities	These can respond to nutritional and detoxification remedies in the preconception period for *both* parents (see Appendix 11).
Infections—candida, genito-urinary infections, toxoplasmosis, cytomegalovirus, rubella.	See Chapter 8 for discussion and therapy during pregnancy, and Appendix 11 for the preconception period.
Auto-immune factors—particularly anti-cardiolipin and lupus anti-coagulant antibodies (not necessarily indicating auto-immune disease as such), and a lack of maternal blocking antibodies to stop rejection of the foetus. This is particularly likely to be a problem where there is a history of auto-immune disease or allergy, or persistent infection.	Treatment of the immune system, preferably *before* conception to reduce susceptibility. Before conception—herbs such as *Astragalus, Siberian Ginseng, Reiishi, Hemidesmus, Rehmannia, Withania, Feverfew, Baical Skullcap* and *Albizzia*, combined with *zinc, vitamin C* and the complete range of nutrients. During pregnancy—see herbs in Chapter 13. Some doctors give an injection of the father's white blood cells to stimulate blocking antibodies. Aspirin can be given when lupus anti-coagulant or anti-cardiolipin antibodies are present. Possible natural alternatives to aspirin include *Garlic, Ginkgo* or *White Willow Bark*, as these have a similar effect, though we know of no direct evidence of benefit. For Lupus anti-coagulent antibodies, steroid treatment can be successful. Herbs which have a similar effect include *Turmeric* and *Liquorice*, though, again, there is as yet no study showing how effective these may be. Phenolic desensitisers help to treat allergy, as do acupuncture, reflexology and homoeopathy.

Excessive heat	Avoid hot tubs, saunas, hot baths. Treat fevers promptly with diaphoretic and immune stimulant herbs such as *Echinacea*, *Ginger*, *Elder Flowers* or *Lime Flowers*.
Diabetes	See section in Chapter 13 for remedies.
Hypothyroidism—this may be a problem if the temperature recorded in monthly charts is below 36°C in the first half of the cycle.	Treat *before* conception with *Sarsaparilla*, *Blue Flag*, *Poke Root* (neither of the last two herbs are safe for use in pregnancy, and *Poke Root* to be used always with extreme caution in small doses). Also use *L-tyrosine*, phenolic remedies, *potassium iodide*, *Bladderwrack* (kelp), reflexology, acupuncture.
Age	Good preconception health care has been shown to prevent age-related congenital malformation and miscarriage.
Poor quality eggs and sperm—due to poor nutrition, toxicity, poor timing (see below).	For discussion and therapy during pregnancy, see Chapters 3–7; for the preconception period, see Appendix 11.
Poor conception timing—old eggs and sperm, or eggs released later than day 17 in the cycle, are more likely to lead to problems and miscarriage.	Natural Fertility Management—charting of cyclical symptoms such as mucus and temperature—to identify problems of hormonal balance and to give guidance for timing of conception. See Appendix 11.
Amniocentesis and chorionic villus sampling	Preconception health care to give confidence of low risk. See Appendix 11.

Defective sperm—indicated by low levels of motility and morphology (percentage of normally shaped sperm). Studies show clear link with male health, the proportion of abnormally shaped sperm and miscarriage rates.	Good preconception health care, nutrition, detoxification and lifestyle adaptation. Herbal and other natural remedies. Screening of toxins and their origin.

Glossary

abruptio placenta placenta which has detached or broken away from the uterine wall
acidophilus lactobacilli type of bacteria present in natural yoghurt; used to re-establish normal bowel flora
acupressure pressure applied to specific points to bring relief for specific complaints; also called 'shiatsu'
acupuncture needles, rather than pressure (as in acupressure), are applied to specific points to bring relief for specific complaints
albumin the most abundant of the proteins dissolved in blood
alpha fetoprotein (AFP) blood test performed at approx. 16 weeks to test for neural tube defects and Down syndrome; see page 179
amniocentesis see page 184
amniotic bag/sac membranous bag containing amniotic fluid
amniotic fluid watery liquid in which a baby floats in the uterus until birth
amygdalin toxic compound found in bitter almond and the kernels of aprocots, peaches and plums
anaemia shortage of haemoglobin, the oxygen carrying pigment of red blood cells
antenatal before birth
anti-dopaminergic having an inhibitory effect on dopamine, a neuro-transmitter
anti-oxidant protects against the damaging effects of oxidative reactions; important as a detoxifier

antibody substance formed by the body in the presence of an antigen or allergen
antio-cardiolipin an antibody which affects blood-clotting mechanisms, and can cause miscarriage
Apgar score the measure of your baby's health at birth
auto-immune disease abnormal, injurious reaction by the body to its own tissues
beta-carotene/mixed carotenes precursors of vitamin A
bifidus lactobacilli type of bacteria present in natural yoghurt; used to re-establish normal bowel flora
bioflavonoids compounds occurring with and working with vitamin C
birthing centre centre with home-like atmosphere attached to maternity unit and staffed by midwives
blood sugar level of glucose in blood
Braxton-Hicks contractions trial (practice) contractions of the uterus
breakthrough bleeding vaginal bleeding occurring at an inappropriate time (e.g. during pregnancy)
celloid/tissue salts minerals in the biochemical form found in the body tissues or cells
cervix neck of the uterus which projects into the upper part of the vagina
chelate form of trace mineral which is well absorbed by the body
chorionic villi initial tissue of the placenta
chorionic villus sampling (CVS) *see* page 183
conjugated oestriol oestrogenic substance that has been metabolised through the liver
cyanogenic constituents toxic constituents (cyanide) found in some herbs, bitter almond and the kernels of aprocots, peaches and plums (e.g. amygdalin)
cytomegalovirus a viral infection
cytotoxic toxic to cells
detoxification removal of accumulated toxins from the body
eclampsia convulsions occurring at end of pregnancy as result of toxaemia
endocrine system glands which release hormones directly into bloodstream
endometrium the lining of the uterus which builds each month after menstruation

essential amino acids proteins are composed of amino acids and 'essential' ones must be obtained from the diet

essential fatty acids fatty acids are part of the wall of every cell in the body and 'essential' ones must be obtained from the diet

ferritin levels iron stores

folic acid/folate part of B-complex group of vitamins

free radical highly reactive, damaging compound; damage can be quenched by anti-oxidants

fundus the top of the uterus

gestational diabetes diabetes which develops during pregnancy

glucagon hormone that tells the body to burn fat

glucose tolerance factor chromium (GTF chromium) the most effective way to supplement with chromium

glycaemic of glucose; *see* hypoglycaemic (low glucose) *and* hyperglycaemic (high glucose)

glycetract a liquid herbal remedy made with glycerine instead of alcohol as a preservative

glycoside an active constituent in herbal medicine

haemolytic activity action which breaks down red blood cells

hair trace mineral analysis (HTMA) method for determining body burden of heavy metals, such as lead, by analysing the mineral content of recent growth of scalp hair

hepatoxic toxic to the liver

homebirth birth which takes place at home and usually in presence of midwife only

homoeopathic nosodes a form of homoeopathic remedy made from the actual disease tissue

homoeopathic phenolic desensitising remedies homoeopathic doses of phenolics, which are commonly occurring natural compounds found to be responsible for 90 per cent of allergies; *see also* page 113

homoeopathic remedies remedies which use a minute, dilute concentration of a substance (usually of herbal or mineral origin) to trigger a healing reaction in the body

homoeopathy *see* page 210

homoeostatic mechanisms mechanisms by which constant conditions in the body are maintained

human chorionic gonadotrophin (HCG) hormone which maintains the pregnancy

hydrochloric acid with pancreatic enzymes acid, secreted by stomach, together with enzymes produced by pancreas; used as aid to digestion
hyperglycaemia high blood glucose
hypertension of pregnancy high blood pressure (of pregnancy)
hypoglycaemia low blood glucose
hypothyroidism underactivity of thyroid gland
in vitro in a test tube
in vivo in the living body
insulin hormone secreted by pancreas to remove glucose from bloodstream
listeriosis a flu-like disease which can cause miscarriage and stillbirth
lupus anticoagulant antibodies an antibody which affects blood-clotting mechanisms, and can cause miscarriage
micelles water soluble forms of vitamins and minerals
micellised made into micelles
midwife nurse specifically trained to assist women at birth
midwifery centre *see* birthing centre
mineralocorticoid activity activity that increases excretion of minerals such as potassium through the adrenals
mutagenic agent agent which affects chromosomes in eggs and sperm
neural tube tube which encloses central nervous system
neuro-transmitter a substance which transmits effects through the nervous system
oedema excess fluid in tissues
oestriol one of the family of oestrogen hormones occurring in the placenta and in pregnancy urine
osteopathy correction of structural defects by manipulation
oxidative stress damage caused by oxidative reactions or free radicals
oxytoxic having action which stimulates contractions of the uterus
oxytoxin synergist agent which enhances action of oxytoxin
perinatal period shortly before, during, or shortly after birth
placenta praevia placenta lies across the opening of the uterus instead of high up; may mean birth by Caesarean section
placenta organ by which the unborn infant receives nourishment from its mother

post partum after birth
pre-eclampsia condition preceding full-blown eclampsia
prematurity born significantly before full term
progesterone the hormone secreted after ovulation, necessary for pregnancy
prostaglandin group of substances derived from fatty acids, having effects on inflammation and hormonal activity
Quetelet (Q) index number which can be calculated to indicate whether individual's weight is within the appropriate range
reflexology similar to acupressure, but using pressure points on the feet
Rh factor see page 175
shiatsu see acupressure
sitz bath a hip bath
sub-clinical not yet presenting definite symptoms
synergistic combined effects which are greater than sum of individual parts
teratogen agent capable of producing birth defects (also teratogenic/teratogenicity)
tonify increase 'tone' of an organ or system (i.e. bring back to healthy functioning) or one of the ways to apply acupressure
toxaemia symptoms include high blood pressure, protein in urine and swelling of ankles; can lead to eclampsia
toxoplasmosis see page 121
trans fatty acids chemical configuration of fatty acids which is foreign to the body
trimester a 12-week period during pregnancy (first, second and third trimesters)
ultrasound scan see page 181
vasoconstricting having a constricting effect on the vascular system
vasodilating having a dilating effect on the vascular system
vermifuge a remedy for expelling parasites from the gut
visualisation a similar technique to meditation, in which a positive or calming picture is created in the mind

Index

A
abdominal muscle 131
abdominal palpation 177
abnormalities, chromosomal 3, 183
abruptio placenta 328
acid/alkali balance 280
acidophilus lactobacilli
   anti-oxidant 100
   candida treatment 117
   definition 328
   dosage 60
activated carbon filters 306
active birth 135–38
acupressure
   to avoid in pregnancy 301–2
   backache 235
   definition 328
   fluid retention 226
   haemorrhoids and constipation 221

acupressure (contd)
   kidney support 228
   leg cramps 237
   morning sickness 216
   stress reduction 163–64
   use during pregnancy 207–8
acupressure machines 208, 273
acupuncture
   definition 328
   stress reduction 163–64
   use during pregnancy 207–8
addictions, breaking 76, 271
additives 43–44
aerobic exercise 124–30, 321
affirmation 169–71
AFP (alpha fetoprotein) test 179, 328
age 3–4, 189
albumin
   definition 328
   test 177

alcohol
    before conception 313
    giving up 76–77, 271
    risks 70–72, 279
allergens, identifying 109–10
allergies 107–15, 244, 274, 316–18
alpha fetoprotein (AFP) test 179, 328
aluminium 82, 83
ambient music 273
amino acids, essential *see* essential amino acids
amniocentesis 7, 184, 184–85
amniotic bag/sac 328
amniotic fluid
    definition 328
    leaking 251
amygdalin 328
anaemia 232–33
    definition 328
    sickle-cell 183
animal fats 42
animal protein 38
ant repellents 89
antenatal classes 200
antenatal, definition 328
antenatal support 274
antenatal tests 172–91
    adverse effects 186–89
    alternatives 274
    anxiety about 150
    before conception 321–22
    diagnostic procedures 181–86
    non-invasive 172–76
    routine tests 176–78
    screening procedures 178–81
antibiotics
    adverse effects 75
    colds and flu 244
    effect on nutritional status 73
    genito-urinary infections 318
    replenishing gut flora 120
    Strep B 180

antibodies 329
anticonvulsants 73
anti-dopaminergic, definition 328
antihypertensive drugs 75
anti-inflammatory drugs 74–75
antio-cardiolipin 329
anti-oxidants 100, 328
anxiety 151, 228
Apgar score 329
appetite 54
areola 14
aromatherapy 164, 208–10
aspirin 73, 74
astrology 94
attitude, positive 2–3, 11, 321
Australian Bush Flower essences 165–66, 273
auto-immune disease 329

B

Bach Flower essences 165, 273
backache 233–35
Baddha Konasana pose (yoga) 139
baking 48
Balmain Wellness Centre 267
Barker, Professor 28–29
basal temperature
    natural fertility management 319, 320
    sign of conception 13
    sign of fertility 6
bath oil 209
bathroom chemicals, alternatives to 87–88
beetle repellents 89
benzodiazepine 75
beta-carotene 37, 329
b-hCG (beta-human chorionic gonadotrophin) test 179
bifidus lactobacilli 60, 100, 329
bioflavanoids 37, 59, 329
bio-impedance analysis (BIA) 267

biophysical profile (BPP) test 180
birth
    approach of 24–25
    preparing for 154–56
    stretching exercises for 135–38
birthing centres 196, 200, 329
bladder
    during exercise 142
    infections 223
    pressure on 15
bleeding 250
blood count test 174
blood pressure
    benefits of aerobic exercise 125
    check-up 177
    high 28, 229–32, 331
blood sugar
    avoiding stress 159
    definition 329
    stability 44
body-at-rest temperature *see* basal temperature
body image 149–50
boiled water 305
bonding 187–88
bones
    benefits of exercise 125
    osteoporosis 38
bottled food 43–44
bowel function
    benefits of aerobic exercise 125
    detoxification 101–4
BPP (biophysical profile) test 180
Braxton-Hicks contractions 17, 329
breads 38, 44
breakthrough bleeding 250, 329
breastfeeding
    preparation for 14–15
    toxins in milk 275
breasts
    changes 14–15
    sore 249–50

breathing techniques
    for detoxification 105–6
    overcoming breathlessness 239–40
    stress reduction 161–62
breathlessness 239–40
Busnel, Dr Marie-Claire 23
butter 42, 279

C

cadmium 82, 83
caffeine 47, 72–73, 76–77, 313
calcium
    benefits of aerobic exercise 125–26
    cow's milk 112
    dosage 59
    effect of sugar 36
    non-cow's milk sources 112
    overcoming stress 158
    supplements 63
calming (acupressure) 208
calories 35
candida 115–19, 247, 316–18
canned food 43–44
capsules 66
carbohydrates
    balance 44, 45
    complex 31, 44
    refined 34
carbon filter 306
cardio-vascular system 228–33
cardiotocograph (CTG) 177
cardiovascular disease 28
carer
    choosing 192–203
    types 196
    what to look for 196–98
cell division 19, 21
celloid salts 329
ceramic filters 307
cervical mucus 6, 313, 319, 320
cervical swab 317

cervix
   definition 329
   incompetent 251
Chamberlain, Dr David 24
chelate 329
chelation therapy 273–74, 316
chemicals
   before conception 314–15
   food additives 43–44
   in the home 87–90, 261–62, 272
   pollutants 85–90
chicken 39, 277
children
   present at the birth 157, 200–201
   reactions to pregnancy 157
chiropractic 210
chlamydia 317
chloasma 241
chocolate 72, 221
cholera 303
chorionic villi 184, 329
chorionic villus sampling (CVS) 7, 183–84, 329
chromium 31, 60
chromosomal abnormalities 3, 183
cigarettes *see* smoking
cilia 19
circulation, benefits of exercise 125, 142
classes
   aerobics 129
   antenatal 200
   meditation and yoga 273
   parenting preparation 275
cleaning products 88, 261–62, 272
clothes 149, 275
cockroach repellents 89
co-enzyme Q10 60
co-factors 32
coffee 47, 72, 279
colds 244–46
colonic irrigation 315–16

colostrum 14
colposcopy 317
complex carbohydrates 31, 44
compress oil 209
computers, protection from radiation 90, 91–92, 272
conception
   importance of zinc 32
   natural fertility management 319–21
   planned 6–8
   sign of success 13
   sources 266
confidence 2–3
congenital defects 3, 28, 69, 183
conjugated oestriol 179, 329
constipation
   benefits of exercise 125
   detoxification 102–3
   natural remedies 219–21
contacts 265–75
contaminants
   see also pollution
   in drinking water 305–8
   in fat 49
contemplation 168
contraceptive pill 73, 318–19
contraceptives 266, 318–19
contractions, Braxton-Hicks 17
cooking methods 48, 278
coping mechanisms 145
copper 24, 60
cosmic radiation 94–95
counselling 150–51, 168
cow's milk 39, 40, 111–12, 114, 277
cracked nipples 14
cramps, leg 235–37
cravings 50–51, 109, 221–22
CTG (cardiotocograph) 177
CVS (chorionic villus sampling) 7, 183–84, 329
cyanogenic constituents 329

cystitis 223
cytomegalovirus 121–22, 174, 318, 329
cytotoxic, definition 329

D

dairy foods 39, 40, 111–12, 114, 277
daylight 105–6, 162
death of a child 274
deficiencies, nutritional
    see also supplementation, nutritional
    effects of 27–28
    refined foods 35
    sub-clinical 56
    symptoms 283–84
    zinc 61
degenerative disease 28
dental amalgam 83, 271
dental check-up 176
depression 151, 167
detoxification 97–106
    before conception 315–16
    bowel health 101–4
    definition 329
    liver health 104
    need for 97–98
    nutrients for 99–102
    skin 104–5
    water for 98–99
diabetes 28, 242–44, 330
diagnostic tests *see* antenatal tests
dietary fibre 101–2
diets
    see also food; nutrition
    anti-candida 117
    elimination 316–17
digestive enzymes 60, 66
digestive system 211–22
dilation and curettage (D&C) 254
discomfort 149
dispersing (acupressure) 208

distilled water 305
distress 146
diuretics 73, 75
dizzy spells 238–39
DNA 19
doctors trained in nutritional and environmental medicine 268
Doppler ultrasound 177
Down syndrome 3, 179, 189
dowsing 110
dreams 152
dried fruits 37
drugs 68–77
    giving up 76–77
    pharmaceutical *see* pharmaceutical drugs
    recreational *see* street drugs
    social 69–73
due date 13
duration of pregnancy 12–13

E

eating disorders 150
eating out 51–52
eclampsia 329
ectopic pregnancy 251–52
Efnatal 266
egg health (ova) 309, 310, 313, 315
eggs (food) 277
electro-magnetic radiation 92–93, 272, 315
elimination diet 316–17
embryo 13, 19–21
emotions
    flower essences for 165
    herbal remedies 166–67
    swings 151–52
endocrine system 242–44, 329
endometrium 20, 329
endorphins 127
endurance 126
enemas 315–16

energy
   benefits of aerobic exercise 126
   early weeks 13–14
   whole foods 31
environment
   before conception 313–16
   pollution *see* pollution
   reading material 261–62
enzymes, digestive 60, 66
erythrocytes 183
essential amino acids
   animal protein 38
   definition 330
   plant protein 40
essential fatty acids 42, 65, 240, 330
essential oils 208–10, 299–300
eustress 146
evening primrose oil 60
exercise 124–43
   aerobic 124–30
   before conception 321
   benefits 7
   for detoxification 105–6
   effect on appetite 54
   fathers 134–35
   improving bowel function 104
   late pregnancy 142–43
   muscle strengthening 131–32
   pelvic floor muscles 133–35
   reading material 262–63
   stress reduction 161
   stretching 135–42

F
fainting 238–39
Fallopian tube 19–20
family reactions 156–57
fasting 316
fat
   balance 44, 46
   contaminants 49
fathers *see* partners

fatigue 6–7, 126, 148–49, 237–38
fats 41–43, 279
fatty acids 42, 65, 240, 330
fears 150–51
ferritin levels 330
fertilisers 33
fertility *see* conception; natural fertility
fibre 101–2, 103
filtered water 99, 306–8
fish 40, 277
flea repellents 89
flexibility 135–42
float tank therapy 161
flour, white 35, 282
flower essences 165–66, 273
flu 244–46
fluid retention (oedema) 43, 224–26, 331
fluorescent lighting 162
fly repellents 89
flying 78, 94–95
Foetal Alcohol Effect 71–72
Foetal Alcohol Syndrome 71–72
foetus
   assessing size 182
   awareness 23–24
   development 18–24, 21–23
   effect of ultrasound scan 181–82
   embryo 13, 19–21
   screening tests 178–81
   sex 187
   size and position check 177
folic acid
   cell division 21
   definition 330
   effect of sugar 35
   requirements 57
   supplements 63
food
   see also diets; nutrition
   additives 43–44

food *(contd)*
   allergens 109–10
   changing habits 48–54
   chemicals in 85–86
   cravings 50–51, 109, 221–22
   diary 109
   and exercise 142
   preparing 48, 53
   refined 34–36
   whole 30–32
Ford, Dr Judy 87, 314
Foresight Association 252, 268, 323
fortified foods 34–35
free radicals 330
fried foods 42, 48, 279
fruit 36–38
   amounts 278
   non-organic 33–34
full spectrum lighting 162, 273
fundus 142, 177, 330

G

Gardner, Robert W. 113–14
garlic 60
genes, influenced by nutrition 28
genetically engineered food 41
genito-urinary infections
   diagnosis and treatment 119–20, 316–18
   natural remedies 222–24, 247
   tests 174
gestational diabetes 180, 242–44, 330
gestational hypertension 229–30
gingivitis 233
Glover, Dr Vivette 24
glucagon 44–45, 330
glucometer 243
glucose 31
   urine test 177
glucose tolerance factor (GTF)
   chromium 330
glucose tolerance test (GTT) 179–80

glycaemic, definition 330
glycetract 330
glycoside 330
GPs 196
grains 38, 40–41, 278
grandparents 156
green leafy vegetables 37, 278
green tea 47
group B haemolytic streptococcus test 180
GTT (glucose tolerance test) 179–80
gum disease 233
gut flora 119, 120
gynaecologists 196

H

haemolytic activity 330
haemorrhoids 125, 219–21
hair trace mineral analysis 274, 314, 330
hearing, foetus's 23
heart 228–33
heatburn 217–19
heavy metals 82–85
   before conception 313–14
   detoxification 100–102
   tests for 174, 273
hepatitis 303–4, 317
hepatoxic, definition 330
herb teas 47, 166–67
herbal medicine
   to avoid in pregnancy 291–98
   emotional states 166–67
   reading material 258–59
   using 206–7
herpes 247–49
HIV 317
holistic treatment
   benefits 210
   reading material 263–64
   sources 266
home birth 200, 201–2, 275, 330

homoeopathic chelation 273
homoeopathic nosodes 304, 330
homoeopathic phenolic desensitising remedies 330
homoeopathic remedies
　allergies 113–15
　definition 210, 330
　stress 166
　for travellers 304
　use 210
homoeostatic mechanisms 330
hormones 151
hospital birth 198, 201–2
house renovations 84, 88
household chemicals 87–90, 261–62, 272
human chorionic gonadotraphin (HCG) 179, 183, 330
hydrochloric acid 60, 66, 331
hyperemesis gravidarum 211–12
hyperglycaemia 331
hypertension 28, 229–32, 331. *see also* toxaemia
hypnotherapy 77, 168, 210
hypnotics 75
hypoglycaemia 243, 331
hypothyroidism 331

I

immune system 244–46
implantation of the embryo 20
in vitro, definition 331
in vivo, definition 331
incompetent cervix 251
incontinence 133, 222
indigestion 217–19
infections
　consequences during pregnancy 122–23
　genito-urinary tract *see* genito-urinary infections
　immune system 244–46

infections *(contd)*
　vaginal 175–76
infusions 207
inhalation, steam 209
inorganic iron supplements 63
inorganic produce
　nutritional content 281
　source of nutrients 33–34
insect repellents 89
insomnia 16, 149, 163–64
insulin 44–45, 331
intervention rates 198
intestinal candida 116, 118
intuition 5
iodine 60
ion exchange filters 306
ionisers 105–6
ionising radiation 94–95, 314–15
iron
　dosage 59
　supplements 63
　test 175
itchiness 241
IUDs 318–19

J

Jocelyn Centre 266
Jonas, Dr Eugen 94
juices 37, 278
junk foods 280

K

kick charts 177
kidney function
　benefits of aerobic exercise 125
　infections 223
　preventative support 227–28
kinesiology 110
kitchen chemicals, alternatives to 87–88

L

labels on packaged food 51
labour, preparation for 254–55
lanugo 22
laundry chemicals, alternatives to 87–88
laxatives 73, 101–2
lead 82, 83, 271
legs
   cramps 235–37
   restless 239
legumes 40–41, 277
lethargy 14
lifestyle
   before conception 313
   effect on nutrient levels 58
   importance 4
   questionnaire 285–90
   reading material 261–62
ligaments 143
light therapy 161–62
lighting 161–62, 273
listeriosis 40, 331
liver health 104
lunar bio-rhythmic cycle 321
lupus anticoagulent antibodies 331
lying down 143
lymphatic massage 106

M

McTaggart, Lynne 181
magnesium
   overcoming stress 158
   supplementation 59
   whole foods 31
malaria 303
manganese 59
margarine 42, 279
'mask of pregnancy' 241
massage
   for detoxification 105–6
   improving bowel function 104

massage *(contd)*
   lymphatic 106
   oil 209
   role 210
   stress reduction 162
mastitis 249–50
maternity wear 149, 275
MaxEPA 60
meat 34, 38–39, 277
medical technology
   evaluating 150
   inappropriate use 5
medication *see* pharmaceutical drugs
meditation
   classes 273
   reading material 262–63
   for stress 168
mega-doses 62–63
membranes, rupture of 25, 251
Mendelsohn, Dr Robert 189
meningitis 303
mercury 82, 83
metals, heavy 82–85
mice 89
micelles 66, 331
microwaving 48
midwifery (birthing) centres 196, 200, 329
midwives 7, 196, 331
migraine preparations 74
milk, cows' 39, 40, 111–12, 114, 277
mineral water 47, 305
mineralocorticoid activity 331
minerals
   refined foods 34, 35
   whole foods 30–31
miscarriage
   effect of stress 145
   prevention 252–54, 323–27
mobile phone safety 93
mono-unsaturated oils 42
Montgomery's tubercles 14

mood swings 151
morning sickness 6, 15–16, 211–17
mosquito repellents 89
moth repellents 89
mothers' groups 157
muscle strengthening exercise 131–32
muscle testing 110
musculo-skeletal system 233–37
music therapy 161–62, 273
mutagenic agents 73, 331
mycoplasma 317

N
nappies 155
native peoples' diet 27
natural fertility 319–21
   contacts 266–67
   reading material 261
natural remedies 204–55
   to avoid in pregnancy 205–6, 291–302
   practitioners 268–70
   reading material 258–59
   for travellers 304
   use 4–5
Natural Way to Better Babies 265
nausea 15–16, 211–17
neonatal sepsis 180
nervous system 237–39
nesting instinct 18, 152
neural tube
   defects 179
   definition 331
   development 21
neurotransmitter 331
nipples
   changes 14–15
   preparation 240–41
non-ionising radiation 90–93
non-stress test 177
nosodes 304, 330

nutrition 276–80
   see also diets; food
   balance 44–46
   before conception 310–12
   benefits of aerobic exercise 125
   for cell division 21
   deficiencies *see* deficiencies, nutritional
   for detoxification 99–102
   effect of pollution 57–58
   effect of stress 145
   embryonic development 19
   essential 36–47
   fighting allergies 108–9
   importance 26–54
   increased needs 27, 56–57
   insufficient 27–29
   nutrient content of food 57
   organic versus non-organic foods 281
   partner's 29
   questionnaire 285–90
   reading material 256–57
   refined wheat 282
   sources of nutrients 29–36
   stress reduction 150, 158–59
   supplementation *see* supplementation, nutritional
   therapeutic use 206
nuts 40–41, 278

O
obstetricians 196, 198
occupational health and safety entitlements 271
oedema (fluid retention) 43, 224–26, 331
oestriol
   conjugated 179, 329
   definition 331
oils (aromatherapy) 208–10, 299–300
oils (food) 41–43, 279

older mothers 3
olive oil 42
oral contraceptives 73, 318–19
organ meats 40, 277
organic produce
   benefits 29–30
   nutritional content 281
   shopping for 49
   sources 270
organophosphates 33
orgasm 158
osteopathy 210, 331
osteoporosis 38
Ott, Wayne 87
overheating 128
ovum health 309, 310, 313, 315
oxidative stress 331
oxygen 125
oxytoxic, definition 331
oxytoxin synergist 331

P

packet food 43–44
painting 84, 272
palpitations 228–29
pancreatic enzymes acid 331
PAPP-A test 179
parenting
   discussion with partner 153
   preparation courses 275
parents-in-law 156
parents, mother's 156–57
partitioned foods 34–36
partners
   deciding on type of care 193–94
   exercise 134–35
   involvement 10
   nutrition 29
   sexual relationship 157–58
   stress 153–54
partus preparator 246
passive smoking 70

pelvic floor muscles 133–35
pendulum 110
perinatal, definition 331
perineal preparation 240–41
peristalsis 125
pest eradication 88–90, 271
pesticides 33
pharmaceutical drugs
   before conception 313
   dangers 73–75
   reading material 262
   reducing need 77
   safety 270
phenolic desensitisation 113–15
pica 222
pigmentation 241
placenta 20, 331
placenta praevia 182, 331
plant protein 40–41
polio 303
pollution 81–96
   see also detoxification
   chemicals 85–90
   effect on nutrients 57–58
   heavy metals 82–85
positive thinking 2–3, 321
post partum, definition 332
potassium 59
Pottenger, Francis 27
power walking 129
prayer 168
preconception health care 309–22
   contacts 267–68
   preventing miscarriage 252
   reading material 261
pre-eclampsia 229–32, 332
pregnancy associated plasma protein
   see PAPP-A
pregnancy loss 274
pregnancy tonics 246–47
prematurity 332
preparing for motherhood 154–56

Price, Dr Weston 27–28, 65
processed food 72
progesterone 20, 332
prostaglandin 332
protein 38–40, 276–80
    balance 44, 45
provocation testing 110, 316
pulse test 109
pulses (vegetables) 40–41, 277
purified water 47, 98–99, 279, 306–8

Q
questioning health care workers 197–98
Quetelet (Q) index 332

R
rabies 303
radiation
    before conception 314–15
    ionising 94–95
    non-ionising 90–93
    resources 272
raspberry leaf 246–47
reading material 256–64
rebirthing 161
rebounding 130
recipe books 257–58
recreational drugs *see* street drugs
rectus muscle 131
recycling 155
red meat 38, 277
red raspberry leaf 246–47
refined foods 27, 31, 34–35
reflexology
    definition 332
    kidney support 228
    palpitation 229
    role 210
    stress reduction 163–64
    tonic effect 247

relaxation
    aromatherapy 164
    overcoming fatigue 148
    tapes for 273
relaxin 143
renovations 84, 88
reproductive system 246–47
resources
    organisations and products 265–75
    reading material 256–64
respiratory system 125, 239–40
responsibility 10
rest 13–14, 148
restless legs 239
reverse osmosis filters 99, 306
Rhesus factor 175
roasting 48
roughage 103
rubella 122, 174, 318
rupture of the membranes 251

S
salads 37, 278
salt 43, 280
saturated fats 42, 279
screening tests 178–81
seeds 40–41, 278
selenium 60
serotonin 36
serum ferritin test 175
sex of child, determining 187
sexual fantasies 152
sexual relationship 157–58
sexually transmitted diseases *see* genito-urinary infections
shiatsu *see* acupressure
shopping for food 51
sickle-cell anaemia 183
signs of pregnancy 13
silica 60
sitz bath 332
skeletal system 233–37

skin 104–5, 240–41
sleep
   benefits of aerobic exercise 126
   insomnia 16, 149, 163–64
   stress 145, 159–61
slug repellents 89
smoking
   before conception 313
   giving up 76–77, 270
   risks 69–70
snacks 46, 52
soft drinks 47, 50, 72
soil 29–30, 33, 57
sperm health 309, 310, 313, 315
spermicides 319
spina bifida 21, 179
spleen 227
sporting activities 132
spring water 98–99, 306
squat exercise 140
squaw vine 247
stamina 126
steam inhalation 209
steaming food 37, 48
stir-frying 37, 42, 48
stretching exercise 135–42
street drugs
   before conception 313
   giving up 76–77, 271
   risks 75–76
Streissguth, Dr Ann 71
strengthening exercise 131–32, 321
Strep B organism 180
stress 144–71
   acupuncture 163
   before conception 321
   benefits of exercise 126
   causes 146–48
   effects of 144–45
   foetus's 23–24
   herbs for 167
   natural remedies 158–71

stress *(contd)*
   palpitations 228
   resolving 148
   symptoms 145–46
stretch marks 240
sub-clinical deficiencies 56, 332
sugar
   cravings 50, 221
   fruit 37
   threats 35–36, 280
sunlight 105–6, 162
supermarket shopping 51
supplementation, nutritional 55–67
   avoiding allergens 111
   beginning a program 66–67
   doses 58–60, 62–66
   preconception 311–12
   reasons for 56–58
   sources 266
   stress reduction 150
'support' team 200
surgery 251–52
swimming 129–30
sympto-thermal method 319
synergistic, definition 332
syphilis 317

T

T-test 179
tablets 66
talking through your problems 168
tapes, music 273
tea 47, 72, 279
teas, herbal 47, 166–67
technology, medical *see* medical technology
teenage mothers 3–4
temperature
   body *see* basal temperature
   external 128
teratogens
   alcohol 71

teratogens *(contd)*
    definition 332
    herbs 291, 292
    pharmaceutical drugs 74
tests, antenatal *see* antenatal tests
tetracycline 75, 176
thalidomide 74
thrush 116
tiredness 6–7, 126, 148–49, 237–38
tonics 246–47
tonifying
    acupressure 208
    definition 332
toxaemia 125, 229–32, 332
toxins
    breast milk 275
    eliminating *see* detoxification
toxoplasmosis 121, 174, 274, 318
trace elements
    hair trace mineral analysis 274, 314, 330
    inorganic produce 33
    organic produce 30
traditional communities 27
trampoline 130
tranquillisers 75
trans fatty acids 42, 332
travelling 77–80, 94–95, 275, 303–4
'treating' pregnancy 192–93
trimester, definition 332
typhoid 303

U

ulcer treatments 73
ultrasound scan (USS) 181–83
    adverse effects 181–82
    alternatives to 182
    avoiding 93
    definition 181
    Doppler 177
    false readings 182–83
unrefined foods 30–32

Upavista Konasana pose (yoga) 141
ureaplasma 317
urethra infections 223
urinary system 222–28
urinary tract infections *see* genito-urinary infections
urination, frequent 15
urine tests 177, 243
USS *see* ultrasound scan (USS)
uterus tonics 246–47

V

vaccinations
    homoeopathic 304
    travellers 78–80, 275
vaginal discharges 175–76
vaginal infections 116, 175–76, 317
vaporisation oil 209–10
varicose veins 125, 232
vasoconstricting, definition 332
vasodilating, definition 332
vegetables 36–38
    amounts 278
    non-organic 33–34
    organically grown 29–30
    preparation 48
vegetarian diet 40–41
vermifuge 332
vernix 22
Virabhadrasana pose (yoga) 140
Virasana pose (yoga) 141
visualisation 148, 169–71, 332
vitamins
    refined foods 34
    whole foods 30–31
vitamin A
    dosage 58
    in oils 41
    supplements 64–65
vitamin B group
    dosage 58–59
    overcoming stress 158–59

vitamin B group *(contd)*
    refined foods 34, 35
    whole foods 30–31
vitamin B6 35
vitamin C
    dosage 59
    overcoming stress 159
    supplements 64
vitamin D 41, 59
vitamin E 41, 59
vomiting 16, 211–12

W
walking 129
water
    alternatives to tap water 305–8
    detox measure 98–99
    filters and deliveries 272
    nutritional value 46–47
    purified 98–99, 279, 306–9
    staying cool 128
water birth 196
water purifiers 99, 306–8
water therapy 161–62
weight
    before conception 312–13
    gain 54

wellness centres 267
wheat, refined 35, 282
white flour 35, 282
White, Ian 165
whole foods 27, 30–32
whole grains 278
workplace
    chemicals in 85–87
    hazards 271

X
X-rays 185, 210, 314–15

Y
yeast infection 117
yellow fever 303
yoga 138–41, 161, 210, 273
yoghurt 40

Z
zinc
    dosage 60
    supplements 61–62
    taste test 172–74
    whole foods 31, 32
zinc taste test 61
'zone diet' 46